| AUTHOR | CLASS |
|---|---|
| HONIGSBAUM, M. | 616.9362HON |

**TITLE**  The fever trail

MARK HONIGSBAUM

# THE FEVER TRAIL

*The Hunt for the Cure for Malaria*

MACMILLAN

First published 2001 by Macmillan
an imprint of Pan Macmillan Ltd
Pan Macmillan, 20 New Wharf Road, London N1 9RR
Basingstoke and Oxford
Associated companies throughout the world
www.panmacmillan.com

ISBN 0 333 90185 1

1 3 5 7 9 8 6 4 2

A CIP catalogue record for this book is available from
the British Library.

Typeset by SetSystems Ltd, Saffron Walden, Essex
Printed and bound in Great Britain by
Mackays of Chatham plc, Chatham, Kent

FOR JEANETTE

# Acknowledgements

Researching this book gave me a licence to travel widely in South America and spend many contented hours browsing libraries and archives I would never otherwise have entered. But without the advice and support of a number of key people I would not have got very far and the browsing would have lacked a certain direction.

First, the logistics. For helping me navigate Venezuelan bureaucracy, the Orinoco and the Casiquiare canal my thanks to Alejandro Reig, Hugo Perdomo and Sixto, and for the loan of her jungle-strength mosquito net to Yasmin Rubio Palis. For guiding me over Chimborazo and nursing me through the dreaded 'soroche', I am indebted to the best expedition planners in Ecuador, Robert and Daisy Kunstaetter, and for their hospitality in Vilcabamba to Orlando and Alicia Falco of the Ruimi Huilco nature reserve.

For chauffeuring me safely along some of the worst roads in Bolivia, and for their unfailing good humour, my thanks to Isaac and Eulogio and their Toyota 'that could'. In Colombia, I am indebted to Alberto Gomez Mejia and Jesus Idrobo of the Bogotá Botanical Garden for showing me the finest cinchona tree 'in captivity', and to Dr Manuel Patarroyo for taking time out of his busy schedule to fly with me to Leticia.

Now the facts. The research for this book was carried out principally at the Wellcome Trust Library in Euston Road, the Royal Geographical Society in Kensington, and the Royal Botanic Gardens in Kew. For granting me access to Spruce's original notes and journals I am particularly grateful to Kew's archivists, Kate Pickard and Sylvia

Fitzgerald, and for access to Markham's journals to Hugh Thomas, the archivist at the RGS. Thanks also to Lorraine Jones, assistant curator of the Royal Pharmaceutical Society of Great Britain and Diana Wyndham in New South Wales for their help with sources on Ledger, and to Soni Veliz in London for the Spanish translations.

For answering my many questions about the science of malaria and quinine, I am indebted to Professor David Warhurst of the London School of Hygiene and Tropical Medicine and to his colleagues Chris Curtis and Eleanor Riley. Similarly, my thanks to Robert T. Joy of the Uniformed Services University of the Health Sciences in Bethesda, Maryland, for guiding me through the voluminous military bibliography on malaria. All of the above also read early draughts of the manuscript for errors.

In addition, I am grateful for the comments of Dr Fernando Ortiz Crespo of FUNDACYT in Quito, and Jordan Goodman of the University of Manchester Institute of Technology. Although not every suggestion of theirs was adopted, together they saved me from making many embarrassing mistakes (any that remain are entirely my own).

Finally, this book would not have been possible without the expertise of my agent, Derek Johns, the skill of my editor, Jeremy Trevathan, and most of all the unfailing belief and support of my wife, Jeanette, and my parents, Frank and Naomi.

# Contents

# List of Illustrations

The Cinchona Regions of South America

Spruce's Route in Venezuela

Markham's Route in Peru

250 MILES

CARAVAYA

PERU

Caupolicán

Tambopata

R. TAMBOPATA

Sandia

Crucero

Cuyocuyo

Sina

CORDILLERA CARAVAYA

Arapa

LAKE TITICACA

Juliaca

Vilque

Puno

Alto de Toledo

Arequipa

Alto de los Huesos

La Paz

Islay

R. Tambo

PACIFIC OCEAN

BOLIVIA

CHILE

Spruce's Route in
Peru & Ecuador

0                    100
                     MILES

Ventanas
Mocha    Ambato
         Baños
Babahoyo
              Canelos
                    R. BOBONAZA
Guayaquil    Alausi

         ECUADOR                    Andoas
                                         R. PASTAZA
              Cuenca     P E R U

         Loja                                 R. HUALLAGA
Vilcabamba                                         R. MARAÑÓN

                                              Ambato
                                                   R. CHASUAN
                    Limon                     Mocha
                    Ventanas              Mt Chimborazo
                    PASS OF
                    LLULLUNDENGO
                    Guaranda
         Babahoyo
                         Riobamba         Tarapoto

                    0        50 MILES

Guayaquil                     Alausi

# INTRODUCTION

To the amazement of all, she recovered sooner than you can say it.

Sebastiano Bado, *Anastasis Corticis Peruviae Seu Chinae Chinae Defensio*

FOR THE FIRST five thousand years or so of recorded history no one knew where malaria came from or how to cure it. All that was known was that the fever was swift, often lethal, and left survivors weak and debilitated for months. Then, in 1663, a fantastical story began circulating in the salons of Europe. It told of a beautiful woman, Doña Francisca Henriquez de Ribera, the fourth Condesa (Countess) de Chinchón, and her miraculous cure from an intermittent fever in Lima, then part of the Spanish Viceroyalty of Peru.

In 1638, went the story, the Condesa contracted a particularly virulent strain of the parasitic illness at the royal palace. Cold-dry, hot-dry, hot-wet went the cycle of chills and sweats, in a progression that usually ended in death or, very occasionally, the remission of the patient. Her husband, the Viceroy, was beside himself. As the *calentura* – as the Spanish referred to fevers – increased in ferocity the court physicians performed one phlebotomy after another. But the bleeding only weakened the Condesa further and it now looked as though death was inevitable.

There was just one slim prospect. Eight years earlier the Corregidor (governor) of Loja had also been on the point of death from an intermittent fever. On hearing this, a Jesuit missionary had suggested

*1*

the Corregidor might like to try a native remedy that he himself had taken some thirty years previously for a similar fever. The cure was the bark of a tree growing in the Andean rainforests high above Loja, a town eight hundred kilometres from Lima in what is now modern-day Ecuador. The Indians had known the remedy for generations as *ayac cara* – literally 'bitter bark' – or sometimes *quinquina*, the 'bark of barks'. Ground into a powder and taken as an infusion, it had the reputation of being a powerful fever treatment, or febrifuge. Intrigued by the missionary's story the Corregidor had tried the bark and was cured. Now, he suggested, the Viceroy might like to administer it to his wife too.

To cut a long and romantic story short, the Viceroy took the Corregidor's advice, the Condesa was cured and a few years later she made a triumphant return to Spain where she spread the news of the miraculous 'fever bark' far and wide. It was as if, overnight, some-one had discovered a cure for cancer or Aids. By the latter part of the seventeenth century malaria was the scourge of Europe. From Seville to Rome large tracts of countryside had been rendered uninhabitable by the fevers that clung to coastal deltas and swamps. Cardinals feared having to attend Vatican conclaves because of the risk of being struck dead by the 'noxious air' wafting up from the Pontine marshes below Rome. And in 1638 and again in 1658 fever epidemics had swept through England at harvest time, giving the country – as one eye-witness put it – the appearance of a 'public hospital'. No wonder then that within a few years of the Condesa's recovery the Spanish were presiding over a healthy trade in the bark from South America and advertisements for the 'Countess's powder' or 'Jesuits' bark' – as the cure became known – were appearing all over Europe.

Today the cure is better known by its pharmaceutical name, quinine. For years quinine was added to water by British expats in India as a precaution against fever. And long after it was replaced as a prophylactic by new, synthetic drugs like chloroquine, the habit of drinking Indian tonic water flavoured with the bitter alkaloid remained. But while quinine's name endures – without quinine, for instance, Stanley and Livingstone would probably never have penetrated Africa — almost no one today remembers the tree from which it is extracted. That is a pity, for the story of the hunt for red cinchona — as the varieties containing the highest levels of quinine became known — is an epic. What is more, unlike the legend of the Condesa's cure, it has the virtue of being true.

I first heard about cinchona while on a journalistic assignment in Zurich. The working title of the article I was researching was 'The Biggest Robbery in History'. There is no need to go into the details here, merely to say that it involved billions of dollars' worth of American bonds stolen to order by the Mafia, and that the headline, while a bit of a come on, was technically accurate. The point is that in the evening, after interviewing the Zurich police, I had gone out for a quiet bite to eat. To my alarm, however, all the restaurants were packed and I had ended up having to share a table with a Swiss botanist. Anticipating a dull evening but eager to break the silence, I flippantly asked him what he considered to be the most interesting plant in botany. To my surprise he launched into the story of the hunt for cinchona. It was a tale replete with characters every bit as interesting as the one I was working on. What is more it described an act of international skulduggery that was far more deserving of my headline. For if the theft of the most valuable plant ever to come out of the Andes — perhaps the most valuable medicinal plant ever to be found anywhere — did not constitute 'The Biggest Robbery in History', what did?

On my return to London I decided to delve deeper into the history of malaria and cinchona. The first thing I discovered was that the word malaria — from the Italian for 'bad air' — is of relatively recent vintage, only entering the English language in the 1740s when Horace Walpole spoke of 'a horrid thing called the mal'aria, that comes to Rome every summer and kills one.' Before that, the preferred English term was ague. Indeed, many British explorers afflicted with malaria continued to talk of ague well into the nineteenth century.

The second thing I discovered was that the legend of the

Condesa's cure was almost certainly an invention. The source of the story was a book written in 1663 by a Genoese physician, Sebastiano Bado, who was closely associated with the Jesuits. Bado claimed to have heard the story from an Italian bark trader in Peru. Unfortunately, scholars have since shown that the Condesa almost certainly enjoyed rude health throughout her time in Lima and never returned to Spain, dying of a sudden illness, probably yellow fever, before embarking at Cartagena in 1641.

Next I looked up cinchona in the botanical journals. I discovered it was a member of the Rubiaceae (madder) family and a close cousin of coffee. Like coffee, it preferred hot, moist climates and thrived on rich organic soils and well-drained slopes, such as are found on the sheer sides of volcanoes. Like coffee it also often took the form of a shrub or small tree with ovate leaves and fragrant white flowers. However, there the resemblance ended. In flower, cinchonas give off a smell like lilac and attract humming birds in brilliant hues. Older cinchonas grow as high as twelve to fifteen metres and when they are ready to fruit the undersides of their leaves turn a spectacular shade of crimson, making them stand out from the rest of the rainforest canopy. Unlike coffee, which grows anywhere from sea level to eighteen hundred metres, the best cinchonas are found between twelve hundred and three thousand metres. But within this narrow altitudinal band, cinchonas have been discovered as far north as Merida in Venezuela and as far south as Santa Cruz in Bolivia – a distance of nearly three thousand kilometres. More importantly, cinchona is a hybrid. The tree is prone to cross-pollination and comes in so many different varieties that a strict classification is all but impossible.

The inaccessibility of the plant, combined with its botanical complexity, presented a formidable obstacle to early cinchona hunters. But it was only when I began reading about the expeditions to South America in search of red cinchona – the *cascarilla roja* of Ecuador and *calisaya vera* of Bolivia – that I realized just *how* formidable. In order to locate specimens whose plants and seeds were worth cultivating, botanists first had to cross the Atlantic and then either sail around Cape Horn or cross the Isthmus of Panama, to land on the coast of

Ecuador or Peru. From there, they had to mount expeditions that would take them up the western slopes of the Andes, through snow-swept mountain passes and over treacherous glaciers. From as high as three thousand six hundred metres they would then begin the arduous descent to the cloudforests on the eastern slopes of the cordilleras, the Andean mountain ranges, just above the Amazon – a journey that would take them from South American winter to summer in a matter of days. Along the way, they would have to deal with stubborn mules, truculent and untrustworthy guides, and the ever-present threat of death from malnutrition, snakebites and headhunting Indians. Added to this were the instability of the nascent Andean republics, sudden border closings and the risk of detection by native bark collectors keen to protect their livelihood from plundering Europeans. Yet in spite of these obstacles there was no shortage of volunteers. Beginning with a French expedition to Quito in 1735, a succession of European botanists arrived in South America in the hope of seizing the bark and making a gift of it to their sovereigns. But to succeed took knowledge, courage, perseverance and luck. In the absence of one or another of these elements nearly all the early expeditions in search of red cinchona ended either in tragic accidents or the death of the participants.

The result was confusion. Some of the barks coming out of South America were indeed cinchona but others were the medically worth-less Peruvian balsam tree, known locally as 'quina quina' and by Europeans as 'quinquina'. To make matters worse, many unscrupu-lous merchants would stain their bark with aloes to increase its bitterness or substitute cherry bark, which had a similar colouring. When you consider that even genuine cinchona bark could vary widely in purity, colour, taste and weight it is little wonder that physicians had a hard time preparing effective febrifuges. Depending on the variety used, some would contain high levels of quinine, while others would contain none at all. Not only that, for the first two hundred and fifty years after cinchona's discovery no one had the faintest idea how quinine worked, much less that malaria was a parasite transmitted by mosquitoes.

By the middle of the nineteenth century the world's most powerful nations were becoming desperate. Although by the 1840s bark exports to Europe were worth £1 million a year, British and Dutch demand was fast outstripping supply. A series of disastrous expeditions up the River Niger had underlined the fact that without a regular supply of quinine the British would never succeed in colonizing the malarious interior of Africa. Similarly, the British Army in India required seven hundred and sixty tonnes a year just to prevent its troops falling victim to the habitual fevers of Bengal and the Western Ghats. The Dutch were similarly anxious to obtain controlled supplies for their malarious colonies in the East Indies, while in the United States the Union's successful blockade of quinine to the Confederacy had created severe shortages of the bark in the malarious southern states, driving home the drug's importance in warfare.

The British and Dutch decided the time had come to seize cinchona plants and seeds and transport them to their plantations in Madras and Java, respectively, where they could raise sufficient quantities to satisfy the demands of empire. Interestingly, this was not presented as theft but philanthropy. By the 1850s the bark forests of northern Peru and Ecuador had been over-farmed and even in Bolivia the *calisaya* trees were rapidly being stripped to the point of extinction. Clearly it was of urgent importance to 'save' this valuable febrifuge for mankind – or so the imperialists argued – and soon they were actively recruiting men with the necessary qualifications and strength of character for the task.

This was the story that attracted me. It was a tale that pitched Europeans against Indians, botanists against buccaneers and the British against the Dutch, French and Spanish. But most of all it was a story about the courage and determination of a few men – mostly British naturalist-explorers – who set off into the highlands of Ecuador, Peru and Bolivia on not much more than a wing and a prayer. Of those explorers three names stood out: Richard Spruce, a hypochondriac Yorkshireman and moss collector, who despite his fear of disease spent fifteen years wandering the Amazon and Andes on behalf of the Royal Botanic Gardens at Kew; Charles Ledger, a cockney trader who came to Peru to make his fortune at the age of eighteen and left South America broken and penniless after a series of incredible expeditions through Bolivia and Chile; and Sir Clements Markham, the patron of Robert Scott's two expeditions to the Antarctic and the so-called 'father of polar exploration', who in an earlier incarnation as a renowned Inca historian and linguist had coordinated a series of British-sponsored missions to South America in search of cinchona. The question was, how to tell the stories of their epic adventures? Some, like Ledger, had only described their endeavours briefly in letters home, and while Spruce and Markham kept detailed notes and journals, their accounts were often incomplete.

I decided there was only one way to bring their accounts alive and that was to go where they had gone. I would not be following in their footsteps exactly – that would take years, and besides many of the borders they crossed are now closed. Instead I would recall discrete parts of their trails – the ones that led to the heart of their feverish wanderings. In so doing, I would be going not only in pursuit of a plant but also of a riddle. For until the Spanish conquest, South America was almost certainly malaria-free. The conundrum was how cinchona's medicinal properties were first discovered and by whom – the Indians or the Spanish? And if the former, how could they have also known that it would cure malaria, a disease of the Old World not the New?

*Chapter One*

# THE FEVER

He had a fever when he was in Spain
And when the fit was on him, I did mark
How he did shake.

*Julius Caesar*, Act I, scene II

THERE ARE ONLY TWO TOPICS of conversation on the Orinoco during the rainy season: the humidity and the mosquitoes. There are remedies for the former but there is no escaping the latter. Like the Luftwaffe the mosquitoes come in waves, each squadron at its appointed hour.

At first light, and foremost throughout the day, are the *jejens* – small blackflies no bigger than pinheads. Their preference is for the foot and ankle but anywhere will do. In the afternoon, when they swarm from the river, they are so thick in the air it is all that you can do to avoid inhaling them. But though the *jejens* leave a rash of tiny swellings punctuated by angry red dots, they are more annoying for their numbers than for the wounds they inflict.

Their deficiency in that department is more than compensated for by their cousin, the horsefly, known as *motuca*. An inky green with white spots, the *motucas* are the butchers of the jungle. Unlike the *jejens* they bite in light or shade so as to afford the weary traveller no respite from their attentions. Fortunately they are slow and some satisfaction can be had in swatting them.

The tiny sandfly — *flebotomo* — offers no such opportunities. Almost invisible to the naked eye, they come at twilight just as the campfires are being set and slip through the finest mosquito netting. Like the *jejens*, they leave a rash of small bites but the irritation is ten times worse.[1]

However, it is the night bombers that are truly to be feared. The Venezuelans call them *zancudos* — a Hispanic word meaning 'long-legged' (it is a quirk of Latin American Spanish that the word *mosquito* is reserved for day-biting flies) — but in the English-speaking world they are better known as anophelines, the mosquitoes that transmit malaria. To be precise, in the alto Orinoco the vector of the malaria parasite is *Anopheles darlingi*. Like other malaria-transmitting anophelines it has long legs with white socks and a distinctive upward tilt to its abdomen, angled at forty-five degrees when it takes a blood meal. But it is the surgical precision of its proboscis that commands most attention. When the German geographer Alexander von Humboldt visited the Orinoco in 1800, he complained that of all the river's insect tortures it was the *zancudo*'s 'sharp-pointed sucker' that had caused him the 'most acute pain'. And when Richard Spruce, the English botanical explorer, visited the same waters fifty years later he wrote that the *zancudo* was capable of penetrating 'even a sailor's jack-boots'.

For once Spruce was exaggerating, but only slightly. *A. darlingi* can penetrate leather and Gortex and on my first night in the Orinoco it had no trouble biting through the underside of my canvas hammock. Fortunately, I was taking a modern prophylactic — mefloquine — and the next night I slept under mosquito netting. But when Spruce steered his dugout along the Casiquiare canal to the Orinoco in 1853, he had only one defence against malaria: quinine.

By 1853 Spruce had been in South America for four years. He had arrived in Brazil, by steamer from Liverpool, in 1849, gradually working his way up the Amazon to Manaus and from there to the Río Negro. His passage had been arranged by Sir William Hooker, the director of Kew Gardens, and his colleague, George Bentham, and although neither of them knew it at the time, Spruce was to play a crucial role in the quest for cinchona. By the 1850s the Indian government was spending £7,000 a year on imported cinchona bark and £25,000 a year on quinine. In 1852 Dr Forbes Royle, the Reporter on Indian Products to the East India Company – the commercial concern that ruled half of India – recommended raising cinchona in the Nilgiri Hills in Madras. 'Among the vast majority of medicinal drugs produced in various parts of the world there is not one,' wrote Royle, 'with probably the single exception of opium, which is more valuable to man than the quinine-yielding cinchonas.' Indeed, Royle argued that because of the rising demand for quinine and the seeming inability of the Andean republics to conserve their cinchona forests, there was a real danger that supplies would run out unless the British acted quickly. Because of the difficulty of collecting seeds and the Andean republics' 'jealousy' of their bark trade, Royle recommended that the government recruit an experienced botanist who could travel to South America posing as 'an agent who had some other objects in view.' But rather than send a qualified collector to the Andes, the Foreign Office simply wrote to its consuls in South America asking them to forward seeds and plants to India. This was easier said than done. Only Walter Cope, the British consul in Quito, succeeded in getting hold of cinchona, but none of the plants survived the voyage to England.

For the moment none of this was of any concern to Spruce. Although he was first and foremost a bryologist – a student of mosses and liverworts – he had what botanists call the taxonomic eye, and in his voyage through the Brazilian Amazon few new plants escaped his attention. Bentham had agreed to help Spruce finance his travels in South America by selling flora collected in the Amazon to herbaria throughout Europe, and Spruce took every opportunity to add to his botanical presses. In November 1851 he took his piragua – a long canoe made from a hollowed-out treetrunk – from Barra and by the time he reached the falls of Uanauaca, below São Gabriel, his collection was bulging. With characteristic enthusiasm he wrote to his colleague John Smith at Kew: 'Thus far have I advanced into the bowels of the land without impediment, and before adventuring the falls (where I may possibly get a ducking) I seize an opportunity of sending you seed of a beautiful Lythraceous tree which I collected on my way up.'

Yet for all the pleasure he took in collecting, Spruce was ill-suited to jungle labour. Born on 10 September 1817 at Ganthorpe, near Castle Howard, in the North Riding of Yorkshire, Spruce was plagued from a young age with bronchial trouble. An only son, his mother died when he was young, leaving his father, a local school-master, and his stepmother to raise him and his eight stepsisters. Spruce senior taught at Ganthorpe and later Welburn, local schools partially endowed by George Howard, the sixth Earl of Carlisle, and at first it seemed as though Spruce was destined to follow in his father's footsteps. But though he quickly found a position teaching mathematics at Haxby and later at the Collegiate School in York, Spruce never found confinement to the classroom congenial. Inspired by the beauty of the Howardian countryside, he liked nothing better than to spend his spare time wandering the moors and nearby Rye wood, examining local flowers and mosses. His closest friend was a local tinsmith and amateur botanist, Sam Gibson, who kept a copy of Hooker's *British Flora* close by his forge. Encouraged by Gibson, at the age of sixteen Spruce had made a list of all the plants at Ganthorpe and by nineteen he had completed a flora of the whole Malton district, containing four hundred and eighty-five flowering plants.

Thus it was that when, in 1844, the Collegiate School suddenly closed, Spruce seized the opportunity to pursue his real passion. Three years earlier he had found a new sedge, *Carex paradoxa*. The discovery had brought him to the attention of Hooker and Bentham and he now travelled to London to make their acquaintance. The meeting was the catalyst for Spruce's decision to devote the remainder of his life to botany. Bentham suggested he travel to the Pyrenees as a plant collector, funding his expedition by the sale of dried specimens. For someone used to the damp, fogbound Yorkshire hills the Pyrenees were a revelation. Writing to his friend the botanist William Borrer four months after his arrival in the mountains in 1845, Spruce raved: 'I can easily conceive why so few mosses have been collected in the Pyrenees, for the flowers are so numerous and so beautiful, that no person, who was not like myself, quite *en tête* of Bryology, would deign to pick up a humble moss!'

Spruce stayed a year, learning Spanish and setting such a pace he often left his guides gasping for breath. The expedition netted five hundred species of mosses, including seventeen that were new to science, and was so significant that Bentham was soon suggesting the more ambitious collecting expedition to South America. Although Spruce would be dependent for finance on Bentham's skills as his botanical agent, he had little hesitation in accepting.

Spruce's obsession with his own health presents something of a paradox to would-be biographers. By 1849, for instance, he writes that his bronchitis had worsened to the point where he feared it might be tuberculosis. But given that he was to survive for fifteen years in the Amazon and Andes, it is hard not to view these and similarly morbid later diagnoses as the conjectures of a pessimistic, if oddly spirited, hypochondriac. The truth is that throughout his time in South America Spruce was always complaining of catarrh, bilious disorders, gallstones and other diseases, both real and imagined. When forging rapids or climbing mountains he was prone to sudden coughing fits, and when ascending the Ecuadorian Andes he suffered a sudden and mysterious paralysis that left him unable to sit upright at a desk for the rest of his life.

But what he lacked in physical strength he more than made up for in mental endurance. 'I am not one of the fowardest to face perils,' he wrote to his Kew colleague John Smith, 'but once embarked I think no more of the consequences.' Slashing his way through the jungle he was stung by wasps so often he lost count and on another occasion he was attacked by vicious *tucundera* – huge black ants – a pain he likened to 'that of a hundred thousand nettle stings.'

But it wasn't simply his determination that kept him going, it was his curiosity. Whether delayed by the river or the rebellions of his truculent guides, or assailed by insects and suspicious natives, Spruce always found something to occupy his orderly mind. In the course of his travels he collected thousands of botanical specimens, including four hundred plants new to science, made the first botanical study of the *Hevea* rubber tree, found the source of the Indian hallucinogen, *ayahuasca*, and gathered the largest collection of mosses in the world. In addition he was a skilled draughtsman and linguist, drawing innumerable maps of the regions he explored and collecting the vocabularies of twenty-one Indian languages.

Then there was the 'irony' of his malaria. In 1859, while collecting in Ecuador, Spruce was commissioned by the British government to 'proceed' to the bark forests and gather cinchona plants and seeds for export to India with the aim of making quinine freely available to the British empire. As usual Spruce did his duty, but had he not been carrying a bottle of quinine when he was on the Orinoco six years previously, he might never have lived to be of service.

Like his contemporaries Spruce had no inkling of the mosquito's role in transmitting malaria. If he thought about it at all, he would probably have concurred with his friend and colleague, the naturalist Alfred Russel Wallace, for whom malaria – like all fevers – was simply the result of noxious gases emanating from decaying vegetable matter in swamps.[2] Indeed Wallace, who had arrived in South America in 1848, had written to London praising the Amazonian climate, and it was partly as a result of his misleading descriptions that Spruce had booked his own passage a year later. Now he was there, it mattered little that Wallace's reports about the humidity had been wrong, that his neck, arms and legs were a mass of suppurating sores or that for all his colleagues knew or cared he could be dead. For Spruce, the Amazon was the realization of a lifelong dream. Like Wordsworth, whose poetry he often turned to in moments of despair, he was drawn by the 'sounding cataract . . . the mountain, and the deep and gloomy wood.' In his travelling pack he carried a dog-eared copy of Charles Darwin's journals of the voyage of the HMS *Beagle*. Ever since he had first read the book as a youth he had wanted to do for the botany of South America what Darwin had done for zoology. Now, in his letters home, he could scarcely contain his enthusiasm.

> Fancy if you can two million square miles of forest, uninterrupted save by the streams that traverse it . . . The largest river in the world flows through the largest forest . . . Here our grasses are bamboos sixty or more feet high . . . Our milkworts are stout woody twiners, ascending to the highest tops of trees . . . Instead of your periwinkles, we have here handsome trees exuding a most deadly poison. Violets are the size of apple trees . . . Daisies borne on trees like Alders.

If Spruce suffered any dark thoughts amid all this luxuriance he does not record them, but by now he had plenty of reason to be pessimistic, for the fever was everywhere. In 1851 he had passed through Castanheiro, a notoriously malarious region, so deserted, he wrote in his journal, that the river appeared 'dead'. Then, at São Gabriel further up the Río Negro, he learnt that yellow fever had claimed the life of his friend, the entomologist Herbert Wallace, who had sailed to South America with him on the brig *Britannia* two years earlier. Now he learned that Herbert's brother, Alfred Russel Wallace, was also seriously ill – this time with malaria – at São Joaquim, a small settlement on the Río Uaupés. 'I had sad news two days ago from my friend Wallace,' Spruce wrote on 28 December 1851. 'He writes me by another hand that he is almost at the point of death from a malignant fever, which has reduced him to such a state of weakness that he cannot rise from his hammock or even feed himself. The person who brought me the letter told me he had taken no nourish-ment for some days except the juice of oranges and cashews.'

Spruce rushed to his bedside, and after taking quinine for four days and nights Wallace was cured.[3] Incredibly, no sooner had he recovered than he embarked on another expedition, back up the Uaupés and across the Colombian border almost as far as the great falls of Yurupari. At this point, however, his resolve seems to have deserted him and, exhausted, he sailed back downriver with his collection of animal skeletons and artefacts to Manaus, where he immediately set sail for England. Unfortunately, eleven hundred kilometres from Bermuda his ship caught fire, consuming the entire collection. It was not the end of his tribulations. Six years later, this time in Indonesia, he would again be seized with a malarial fever during which he would arrive at the theory of natural selection.[4]

Whether Spruce experienced a similarly blinding revelation when eventually he too became ill is not recorded. By now he was well acquainted with the insect pests on the Amazon, not only the *jejen* and *motuca* but the ghastly *pium-piraga*, known as *mosquito Colorado* in Spanish because of its distinctive red head which, Spruce wrote, 'sucks an enormous quantity of blood, hanging on till its abdomen is extended to twice or thrice its original size and then falling helpless to the ground.' But in passing from the Río Negro to the Casiquiare and Orinoco he found the mosquitoes were more numerous and persistent than anywhere he had previously been. It was Humboldt who first remarked on the phenomenon. 'In the villages on the banks of the river,' he noted in his journal, 'the plague of the mosquitoes affords an inexhaustible subject of conversation. When two persons meet in the morning, the first questions they address to each other are: "How did you find the *zancudos* during the night? How are we today for mosquitoes?"'[5]

Humboldt thought it had something to do with the difference in the colour of the water, and he was right. The iodine coloration of the Río Negro is caused by decaying vegetable matter that turns the water acidic, discouraging insects from breeding. But on the fast-flowing Casiquiare and Orinoco the water is full of silt and suspended solids that make it alkaline, providing the perfect breeding conditions for mosquito larvae.

Spruce's introduction to the mosquito plagues of the upper Orinoco came on Christmas Day, at Esmeralda in the shadow of the Cerro

Duida, a massive granite mountain that rises 2,396 metres, dominating views from the river. In 1853 the village consisted of just 'six miserable huts'. Now it is a military outpost with its own airstrip, mission school and a half-completed museum to Humboldt. But the mud and wattle dwellings, though more numerous, are just as miserable, and despite its magnificent aspect the village is no healthier than when Spruce was there. Ever since reading Humboldt's description of the cloud-encircled Duida, Spruce had wanted to do what no naturalist had done before – conquer the summit and 'rifle its botanical treasures'. But no sooner had he reached Esmeralda than he was overcome by a strange melancholia that drained his spirit.

> You will credit me when I say that to the sight Esmeralda is a Paradise – in reality it is an Inferno scarcely habitable by man. When I stood in the middle of the small square, round which are built the houses – the straw doors all carefully closed and looking as if nothing human ever came forth from them – the warm east wind fanning my face and raising the sand in the plaza but bringing no sound of life on its wings – no bird or butterfly to be seen . . . I thought the scene inexpressibly mournful.

Spruce did not have to search far for the answer.

> . . . Throughout the day the very air may be said to be alive with mosquitoes, from which even with closed doors one can only imperfectly escape. I constantly returned from my walk with my hands, feet, neck and face covered with blood, and I found I could nowhere escape these pests. If I climbed the cerros, or buried myself in the forest, or sought the centre of the savannahs, it was the same, but it was worst of all on the river.

Spruce had arranged to meet Don Gregario, the local *comisario* (commissioner), in Esmeralda's main square. The idea was that together they would journey to the as yet undiscovered source of the Orinoco. But there had just been a change of government in Venezuela and all plans were on hold. Spruce waited for Don Gregario, but when after four days there was still no sign of him he could stand it no longer and 'bade adieu to Esmeralda and its mosquitoes.'[6] Although it was supposed to be the dry season it now began to rain heavily, increasing the insect plagues on the Brazo Casiquiare, and after brief detours to explore Lake Vasiva and the Río Pacimoni Spruce and his Indian porters hurried back to San Carlos.

Then, in May, he headed north. The plan was to explore the Guainía and Atabapo rivers, but the Guainía was navigable by dugout only as far as Tomo. From there Spruce was forced to hire a small canoe and head for Maroa, where there is a road-link to Javita and the Río Temi, which eventually joins the Atabapo. Because of the space restrictions in his canoe and the necessity of his Indians carrying his provisions by foot over Mount Javita, Spruce found himself in a quandary. Should he take two large bundles of papers for his botanical presses, or should he take his medicine chest? He chose the paper. It was very nearly a fatal decision. He set off for San Fernando de Atabapo only with the bare minimum: a small bottle of laudanum, some ipecacuanha root to induce vomiting, and a small vial of quinine sulphate. Emergency supplies.

The town of San Fernando sits on the eastern bank of the Atabapo at the confluence of the Guaviare and the Orinoco. Its broad white sand beach faces Colombia where, thanks to the fighting between Marxist guerrillas and the Colombian government, travel is now dangerous. Little else has changed, however. The town still boasts a Plaza Bolivar, a church and a few stores where vessels replenish their provisions before proceeding north to the cataracts of Maipures. The falls are the magnet. For some twelve kilometres from Atabapo the brown waters of the Guaviare and the lighter waters of the Orinoco run side by side, but as the current quickens they merge until, at Isla Raton, huge granite boulders turn the river into a seething cauldron of dropping channels. The rapids are the end of the road for travellers on the Orinoco. To proceed further you must disembark at Samariapo and follow a single-track tarmac road to Puerto Ayacucho, the capital of Amazonas state sixty-three kilometres to the north.[7] In Spruce's day, however, the disembarkation point was a Salesian mission in the town of Maipures in what is now Colombia.

Spruce left San Fernando on 7 June, one month into the rainy season, accompanied by a local trader, Senhor Lauriano, and several Indian guides. On 18 June they stopped at Marana, a small Indian village, and slung their hammocks in a rum distillery swarming with biting ants. They left early the next morning but owing to Lauriano crossing the river to sell some goods, it was already dark by the time they reached Maipures. The cataracts were treacherous enough in daylight and only Lauriano and one of Spruce's Indians had previously navigated the narrow creek leading to the mission. Now, with the sun setting, they also had to contend with heavy rain and thunder. Lauriano lit a torch and positioned himself in the prow, allowing the current to pull the boat as he scrutinized the way forward. 'Already we could hear the roar of the cataracts mixed with that of thunder and we knew that if we overshot the mouth of the creek the current was so rapid and the fall so near that we were almost certain to be carried away – to certain destruction,' Spruce wrote in his journal. Three or four times the rain and wind nearly extinguished the torches. Finally, after several false alarms, Lauriano found the correct channel and steered the canoe swiftly to the mission post.

The town, however, lay two hundred and seventy metres further on and Spruce and his companions were now forced to cross a marshy savannah traversed by numerous small streams, the classic breeding ground for anophelines. In theory the chances of contracting malaria from the bite of *Anopheles darlingi* in the Orinoco are low – only one in a hundred carry the parasite – but Spruce was now entering a notoriously malarious area where the concentrations of infectious *zancudos* were much higher. Indeed, Humboldt had been well aware of Maipures' reputation for fevers when he stopped at the mission in 1800. And although he had attributed the fevers to a combination of humidity, bad nutrition and 'pestilent exhalations' from the rocks, he observed that the air was 'absolutely filled with venomous insects' and that it was at Maipures that the 'suffering from mosquitoes attained its maximum.'[8]

As a keen scholar of Humboldt, Spruce cannot have failed to have been aware of these passages, but what could he do? In total darkness now, with the torches guttering, and only the canoe to shield him from the rain, Spruce splashed over the marsh for what 'seemed like a mile'. When he eventually reached the pueblo he was exhausted but neither he nor his porters could sleep – the *zancudos* saw to that – and the next night the Indians insisted on sleeping by the river to escape them. Spruce, however, remained in the village. It was the wrong choice.

In Brazil *Anopheles darlingi* are most active in the early part of the evening, but in the alto Orinoco they feed continually from dusk until dawn, reaching a peak of activity in the dead of night when their prey are least suspecting. It is the female who carries the parasite, injecting the protozoan into the blood with her saliva each time she feeds (the male poses no threat, preferring to dine on tree nectar), and like most *Anopheles* she prefers still, dark spaces – caves or the insides of houses.

The parasite takes four forms – *Plasmodium falciparum*, *P. vivax*, *P. ovale* and *P. malariae*. Only one, *Plasmodium falciparum*, is life threatening (in adults at least) but all are hugely debilitating and, in most cases, difficult to tell apart. The Spanish talk of *el paludismo*, from the Latin word '*palus*' meaning swamp. But the local Yanomami word is far more descriptive. To the Indians who live on the Orinoco malaria is simply *prisi-prisi* – 'the fever'.

At first the body displays no symptoms. Having entered the bloodstream, the threadlike malaria parasites (known as sporozoites) make straight for the liver, where they form a cyst and quietly replicate. Then two weeks later the cyst suddenly bursts and the young parasites (now known as merozoites) invade the red blood corpuscles. This is the beginning of the fever cycle. Your first clue that something is wrong is a chill, during which you may begin to shiver and your teeth may chatter – the 'cold-dry' phase. Then, as your white blood cells swamp the parasites in an effort to destroy them, your temperature rises dramatically and the shivering gives way to an extreme sensation of heat. This is the hot-dry phase. Soon you have a raging thirst and headache and, as you slip into delirium, you may literally believe you are burning up. Then without warning your headache and temperature subside and you begin to perspire profusely – the hotwet phase. Even though your bedclothes are now drenched you feel a huge sense of relief and fall into a grateful sleep, only to wake hours later tired and lethargic.

There then follows an intermission, during which you may believe you have recovered. The interval varies according to the malaria parasite. Typically, it lasts twelve to twentyfour hours in the case of falciparum malaria, fortyeight hours in the case of vivax and *ovale* and seventytwo hours in the case of *malariae*.[9] However, the recovery is an illusion: the cycle of shivers and sweats always returns, with more and more red blood cells being parasitized each time. Viewed through a microscope the growing malaria parasites are like a *corps de ballet*: they are all at the liver stage simultaneously and all burst, as merozoites, from the invaded red cells at the same time. It is beautiful and potentially deadly.

At first, Spruce had no inkling of the malaria that was probably already coursing through his system. He spent the first few days after his arrival in Maipures exploring the nearby *cerro*, collecting specimens of wild *Barbacaenia*, *Hypnum* mosses and other species he had not seen before. The greater part of his days, however, were spent turning a side of salted ox in the hot sun so as to stop maggots from breeding in the flesh. With characteristic understatement Spruce later wrote that this gruesome activity, together with the wetting he had sustained on his arrival, 'did not produce any beneficial effect on me.'

The first premonition of ague came during the second week of his stay in Maipures. But it was during the fourday voyage back to San Fernando that Spruce writes that the 'symptoms declared themselves unmistakably'. Spruce's small canoe was so crammed with dried plants and beef flesh that he was forced to sit scrunched up near the entrance to the boat's canopy. Exposed to the sun and rain during the day, and unable to keep warm at night, he was soon 'nearly helpless with continued fever'. When he reached San Fernando he decided that to proceed further was folly and took to his bed.

Spruce made the right decision: judging by his description of his symptoms he had falciparum, the severest form of malaria. For thirty-eight days he lay in a delirious trance. At first the attacks came every twenty-four hours but they quickly increased in length and violence, falling into the familiar cycle of thirty-six hours of fever followed by twelve hours of remission.

> Thus at 4–7 pm began the attack, with *calafrios* and coldness of the extremities, although I had scarcely ever any general shivering of the surface, the cold speedily passing into fever, which continued through the night and through all the next day. Then towards the second night the fever increased in violence – pulse so rapid that it could not be counted – thirst unquenchable – breathing laborious and with great fatigue of chest – mouth constantly filled with viscid saliva, and towards morning the attack would begin to pass off and leave me with forces completely prostrated.

Spruce was now locked in a deadly dance with the parasite. Most forms of malaria result in anaemia but what makes falciparum so dangerous is that torn blood cells can become clogged in the arteries, restricting the flow of blood to the brain. If untreated, the result is cerebral haemorrhaging and death. The recommended cure then, as now, is quinine. But for some reason Spruce refused to dip into his supply. Perhaps he was uncertain that he really had malaria – after all, the fever could have been the result of any number of tropical diseases. Or perhaps the quinine was simply too precious for him to take without sufficient cause.

Whatever, the question was very nearly academic. Spruce's porters had traded all his equipment for rum and were so drunk they were unable to attend to his needs. Sustained only by arrowroot broth, he was at risk of starvation and dehydration. A friend had procured a nurse, Carmen Reya, but she also seemed anxious to speed him to an early grave. According to Spruce, Reya was a *zamba*, a mixture of black and Indian, 'that race by which nine tenths of the most heinous crimes are said to be committed in Venezuela.'

> When young she had not been ill-looking, but when out of temper (which for the most part occurred without any reason that I could possibly assign) her face put on a scowl such as one of Macbeth's witches could not outdo. I was already very ill and almost helpless, and nearly all I could do was to ask for what I wanted, yet my slightest word and action was interpreted into something in her disfavour.

At first Spruce allowed himself to be guided by Reya's advice. During fever fits he drank orange juice and, afterwards, instead of replenishing his strength by eating, he took ipecacuanha and another emetic. But gradually he realized that Reya was trying to exacerbate his symptoms. One evening, when he was very sick, she abandoned him for the night, leaving him with just a few jugs of water by his bed. On another occasion she gathered her friends in an adjoining room, taunting him with 'all the vile names in which the Spanish language is so rich.' According to Spruce her favourite curse was: 'Die you English dog that we may have a merry *velorio* (watch-night) with your dollars!'

Spruce was too weak to reply. Instead, he sent for the local *comisario* so that he could give orders for the disposal of his effects. It was only on the fifteenth day of his illness that he became convinced that the continual purges were detrimental to his health and decided to dip into his precious store of quinine. At first he took 130–195mg (2–3 grains). But as his symptoms improved he upped the dose, until by the nineteenth day he was taking 390mg (6 grains) four times daily. The effect was instant. His fever fell and his appetite returned, and within two days he was able to sit up at the table and drink wine. He continued dosing himself with quinine, coffee and rum until on 4 August he suffered another attack. The next day, however, he felt better and dined on tapir — a reputed local cure for fevers. 'From that day to this,' Spruce wrote on 21 September 1854, 'I have had, thank God, no more fever.'

On 13 August — two days after his last fever attack — Senhor Antonio Diaz, a Portuguese hammock manufacturer, arrived at Maipures. Spruce knew Diaz, having run into him the previous year at Tomo where he had commissioned a rare feathered hammock from him as a gift to the Countess of Carlisle, as thanks for the Howard family's support for his botanizing. Made from the thread of the prickly palm and decorated with feathers of humming birds, toucans, parrots and the *gallop ad serve* (cock of the rock), it took fifteen months to complete and is a rare example of local Indian workmanship.[10]

For Spruce it was a fortunate reunion. Anxious to escape his vile nurse, Spruce asked Diaz to take him upriver. Diaz agreed, transfer-ring him to one of his hammocks for the overland journey from Javita to Pinchin. Seven days later, on 20 August, Spruce reached Tomo, where he was reunited with his large canoe and, more importantly, the medicine chest he had left behind in June. He rested for two days to make sure he had recovered his strength, then he was on his way again, reaching San Carlos on the twenty-eighth. Two weeks later he felt well enough to resume his correspondence with Kew. 'But a few weeks ago I thought I would never write to you more,' he wrote to George Bentham. 'In seeking the wherewithal to sustain life, I came within little of meeting with death ... Even yet at the end of three months from the first attack, I am very far from having regained my strength, and I am unable to work continuously on anything.'

Spruce had had a narrow escape. However, within five years the British government would send him on an even more dangerous mission. It was a task that would test his endurance to the limit. Once again he would be following in the footsteps of Humboldt. But his journey would take him across jungle forges and over mountain passes that even Humboldt had not dared to tread.

*Chapter Two*

# THE CURE

*Amar el árbol es comprender la vida.*

Reinaldo Espinosa, Ecuadorean botanist

FROM THE SUMMIT OF Mount Cajanuma in southern Ecuador the province of Loja resembles the surface of a prune: there is not a flat piece of ground anywhere, just a succession of camel-backed ridges and V-shaped valleys rolling towards the horizon. It is as if when God created Loja He reached down from heaven and gathered the earth into His fist, much as you would clench tight a bedsheet. It has not unfurled yet.

Anywhere else Loja's daunting topography would be cause for commiseration but the Lojans are blessed. Although it is just four degrees south of the equator, Loja's altitude and position at the confluence of two weather systems – that of the Pacific and the Oriente – ensure a perfect year-round climate. Most of the Amazon's heat and humidity never reaches the narrow valley in which the city of Loja nestles but is spilt instead on the eastern slopes of Mount Cajanuma, while to the west the Cordillera de Chilla performs a similar trick with *El Niño* and other, less violent Pacific fronts. The result is a climate that is neither too hot nor too cold and neither too wet nor too dry, but just right for both plant and animal life.

In Vilcabamba, a subtropical idyll a hundred kilometres south of Loja on the way to the Peruvian frontier, it is said that the inhabitants live to be a hundred and twenty. Few birth certificates are available but no one who has spent any time in Vilcabamba doubts that the diet and climate is conducive to long life. The terraced slopes groan with yuca, bananas, fresh corn and San Pedro – a hallucinogenic cactus much in demand on what is left of the hippie trail. Crystal-clear streams – perfect for drinking or bathing in – pour from the verdant hillsides, and you need only walk out of your front door to find oranges, papayas and avocados the size of bells swinging from the trees. It is thought that when the Inca passed through here on their way to Quito they were so struck by the cornucopia that they immediately dubbed it a second 'sacred valley' after the one they had left behind in northern Peru and planted *huilca* trees on the hillsides in veneration.

However, it is not for the sacred tree of the Inca but for another plant that the province is best remembered. Cinchona was Loja's first and greatest gift to the world. Anywhere else that would be an excuse for a whole industry, complete with guided tours and kitsch renderings of the celebrated 'fever tree' in ceramic and plastic. But in Loja there is not so much as a museum dedicated to cinchona, let alone a shrine to the Spanish countess after whom it was named. The only clue to Loja's place in history lies five kilometres south of the city on the road to Vilcabamba. Blink and you will miss it: a crumbling wall, a rusty gate, an overgrown arch and, above it, a simple inscription: *Amar el árbol es comprender la vida* ('To love a tree is to understand life').

The quotation comes from Reinaldo Espinosa, the Ecuadorian botanist in whose honour the gardens were opened in 1949. Driven by a conservationist ethic, Espinosa hoped to restore to Loja many of the native plants and trees like cinchona that had disappeared from the surrounding hillsides in the colonial period. But in a province famed for being the 'bread-basket' of Ecuador his efforts came to naught and today the gardens – home to 839 species of flora – are the only record of Loja's rich botanical heritage.

Espinosa isn't the only botanist memorialized in the gardens. Open the rusty gate, turn left and there above the ticket office you will notice another lengthy inscription, this time from Carolus Linnaeus, the Swedish father of botany. The inscription reads: 'What other scientific investigation is as fatiguing or as difficult as the botanist's endeavours? We know not how to explain the extreme delight of this study [but] it is such that our love of plants surpasses even the love we owe to each other.'

It was Linnaeus who in 1742 decided that the quinine tree should bear the name of its first and most glamorous patient, Doña Francisca Henriquez de Ribera, the fourth Condesa de Chinchón. Enamoured by the romantic story of her cure, his intention no doubt was to immortalize her name taxonomically. Unfortunately, in so doing Linnaeus made an elementary spelling mistake, leaving out the first 'h'. By the time other scholars noticed it was too late and the genus has been known as cinchona ever since.[1]

To be precise, the species that cured the Condesa was *Cinchona officinalis* — *officinalis* being the Latin term for 'storehouse of medicine'. Few have described it as memorably as the German naturalist-explorer Alexander von Humboldt. 'This beautiful tree,' he wrote, when he passed through Loja in 1802, 'which is adorned with leaves above five inches long and two broad, growing in dense forests, seems always to aspire to rise above its neighbours. As its upper branches wave to and fro in the wind, their red foliage produces a strange and peculiar effect, recognisable from a great distance.'

When sixty-six years earlier another explorer, Charles-Marie de la Condamine, had arrived in Ecuador the cinchona tree was the last thing on his mind. A soldier turned mathematician, La Condamine had been had been sent to Quito in 1735 by the French Academy of Sciences to settle a dispute then exercising the best minds in Europe: was the earth, as Sir Isaac Newton asserted, an oblate spheroid — a globe flattened at the poles — or did its diameter lengthen from pole to pole, as the Italian-born French astronomer Jacques Cassini maintained? For largely chauvinistic reasons most Frenchmen sided with Cassini, arguing that the earth lengthened at the poles and was pulled in at the equator, 'much as a pot-bellied man might pull in his girth by taking in a few notches in his belt.' One of the exceptions was Voltaire, who had recently returned from England a convert to Newton's theory and translated his *Principia* into French. The other was Voltaire's young disciple La Condamine.

With the help of a group of mathematician-scientists, and the permission of Philip V, the King of Spain, La Condamine was despatched to the New World to measure one degree of latitude at the equator and thus resolve the dispute once and for all. But no sooner had he arrived in Quito and completed his measurements than La Condamine learnt that a rival French team had already reached Lapland and settled the argument in Newton's favour. Marooned in Spanish South America, surrounded by suspicious and increasingly hostile natives, La Condamine needed to find a new purpose, and quickly, if he was to return to France in glory. It did not take him long to find one. First he would collect plants and seeds of the famous 'fever tree' from the forests near Loja. Then he would sail down the Amazon to Brazil just as the Spanish conquistador Francisco de Orellana had done two hundred years before, hop on a boat to France and present the quinine tree to his sovereign, Louis XIV. In so doing his name would for ever be linked with the cure for malaria – or so he must have calculated.

La Condamine headed straight for Loja and Cajanuma, the mountain on whose slopes the finest cinchonas in the New World then grew – the so-called 'Crown' barks of Peru, whose anti-malarial properties were then in such demand throughout Europe. Since the supposed cure of the Condesa de Chinchón the Spanish had presided over a lucrative trade in quinine from Cajanuma and other nearby mountains like Uritusinga, shipping the bark around Cape Horn to Seville, where it found its way to Madrid and other malarious European cities like Rome, London and Antwerp.[2] But while by the middle of the seventeenth century the powder of the brittle, highly coloured bark was a familiar part of the apothecary's arsenal no European had ever laid eyes on the tree from which it came. La Condamine's eyewitness account, *Sur l'arbre Quinquina*, was the first and it caused a sensation.

La Condamine left Quito on 18 January 1737, following the road that passed directly over the sierra to Cuenca – today's Pan-American Highway – reaching Loja two weeks later. On 3 February he was on his way to the summit of Cajanuma, three thousand metres above the town of Loja, where he passed the night with a local *cascarillero* – an Indian who made his living stripping the bark from the forest – returning the next morning with specimens of the leaves, flowers and seeds. La Condamine explained that 'quinquina' came in three colours, white, yellow and red. The preference was for the red bark, which was bitterer than the others, although the yellow was almost as good. At first glance the trees appeared identical, their leaves, flowers and exterior bark being the same. It was only when you inserted a knife beneath the tree's skin that you could see that the underside of the yellow bark was softer and more brightly coloured.

Not only was La Condamine the first to point to the link between the bark's colour, taste and febrifugal content, but by adopting the Quechua '*quina quina*' – literally 'bark of barks' – he ensured quinine a place in the English language. But La Condamine also could not resist leavening his account with local folklore and half-remembered popular myths. Thus La Condamine accepted the legend of the Condesa's cure as true, giving 1638 as the year of her recovery and adding for good measure that the Indians probably discovered the bark's febrifugal qualities after observing pumas, who suffered their own form of intermittent fever, drinking from a lake that had been suffused with the trunks of fallen quinine trees. Years later, as in a game of Chinese whispers, the same story would re-emerge in subtly different form: the lake was the same but this time the discovery was attributed to a feverish Spanish soldier who had drunk from the quinine-rich waters. The stories, like that of the Condesa's cure, of course, are highly fanciful and informative only in so far as they reflect the shifting politics and prejudices of the early Spanish chroniclers. In all probability it took years for the Spanish to discover the secret of the bark and then only as a result of observations by Jesuit physicians working closely with native Indian healers in the field.[3] But even when the Jesuits began proselytizing in quinine's cause the bark's acceptance was by no means assured.

Quinine had to compete with such well-known and time-tried remedies as viper's broth, crab's eyes and murderer's skulls, and any attempt to proceed by the rational observation of its therapeutic effect was met with incredulity if not outright hostility. For the Galenists all disease was attributable to either 'wet' or 'cold humors'. Thus quotidian fever was caused by an excess of mucus, tertian by too much bile and quartan by black bile, a supposed secretion of the spleen. To expel this '*materia morbi*', debilitating measures were required – hence the passion for bloodletting and the enthusiastic use of purgatives and emetics. Incredibly, the bark's opponents argued that it 'fixed the humours' and thus maintained the symptoms.

We now know that quinine is a powerful antipyretic, which lowers the body's temperature, and blocks the malaria parasite's ability to invade human red blood cells, thus interrupting the cycle of fevers and sweats. More importantly, in stopping malaria, it was the first drug in the medical pharmacopoeia to cure a specific illness. As such it revolutionized the study and treatment of disease, leading to the foundation of chemotherapy and inspiring the study of homeopathy. But that is not how it appeared at the time; 'quinquina', or 'china china' as it was sometimes known, was simply another New World bark of unproven efficacy. Not only were supplies from Peru erratic but the substitution of spurious barks, soaked with aloes to give a bitter taste, was rife. Combined with the uncertainty over the correct dosage needed to break the cycle of fevers and sweats it is hardly surprising that few physicians were willing to stake their reputations on the remedy, and that the few that were preferred to cloak their adherence to the bark in fantastical tales of a beautiful woman's cure in the distant Spanish viceroyalty of Peru.

In fact, the first reference to the tree comes in a long and dense religious chronicle written by Father Antonio de Calancha, a member of the Augustan Order of monks, and printed in Lima in 1633. Most of Father Calancha's thousand-folio treatise consists of accounts of the early missionaries' attempts to convert the Inca in the province of Vilcabamba, Peru, and is hard going. The Yale archaeologist Hiram Bingham, the discoverer of Machu Picchu and Vitcos, who trawled through the text seeking clues to the location of the Lost City of the Incas, describes it as 'an omnigatherum of fact and pious fancy'. In it, Calancha devotes only one tantalizing sentence to the tree, writing: 'There is a tree of "fevers" in the land of Loja, with cinnamon‑coloured bark of which the Lojans cast powders which are drunk in the weight of two small coins, and [thereby] cure fevers and tertians; [these powders] have had miraculous effects in Lima.'

Calancha never explains who discovered the tree, how he heard about it or what the 'miraculous effects' might be. Elsewhere in his treatise he describes the Incas' expertise with other medicinal plants but the quinine tree does not appear to be one of them. Perhaps Loja was beyond Calancha's compass and that is all he knew. But you would have thought that Lima was well within it and had the Condesa de Chinchón been one of the beneficiaries of the tree's 'miraculous effects' he would have mentioned it.

The second reference comes from another early Spanish chronicler, Father Bernabé Cobo. In his *History of the New World*, published in 1653, Cobo devotes a whole chapter to the 'Arbol de Calenturas' (the Fever Tree). Like Calancha he writes that the tree is found in Loja and has a thick cinnamon‑coloured bark. However, while he adds that the bark is 'very bitter' and that the powders must be taken 'a little before the chills begin' to be effective, there is no reference to the Condesa or any other cure in Lima.

It is not until ten years later, in 1663, that we get the first written account of the popular story. It comes in the book *Anastasis Corticis Peruviae Seu Chinae Chinae Defensio* by the Italian physician Sebastiano Bado, and purports to recount a true story as told to him by an Italian merchant, Antonius Bollus, then living in Peru. According to Bado the Condesa had fallen ill in Lima 'thirty or forty years before' – thus placing her malaria in 1623–33, not – as La Condamine maintains – in 1638. On hearing of the Condesa's fever the Governor of Loja had ridden to Lima to inform the Viceroy of how he had been miraculously cured of a similar fever some thirty years previously. Unsure of whether to believe the Governor's story, the Viceroy ordered the court physicians to test the bark on various palace hangers‑on to make sure it was safe. Only then did he agree to administer it to the Condesa. Her recovery was supposedly instantaneous: 'When this was learnt in the City,' writes Bado, 'the people approached the Vicereine by intermediaries, not so much joyfully and congratulatorily, but supplicatingly, begging her to deign to help them, and say, if she would, by what remedy she had at last so marvellously, so quickly, recovered, so that they, who often suffered from precisely this fever, could also provide for themselves.'

Relieved at her narrow escape, Bado continues, the Condesa ordered large quantities of bark to be sent from Loja and began distributing the cure with her own hands to the sick of Lima and later, on her return to Spain, to tenants on her husband's estates at Chinchón, near Madrid. The result was that 'just as she herself had experienced the generous hands of God in that miraculous remedy, so all the needy who took it marvellously recovered their health . . . and this bark was afterwards called *Countess's powder*.'

As scholars have subsequently shown, Bado's story is poppycock. Doña Francisca Henriquez de Ribera, fourth Condesa de Chinchón, died on 14 January 1641 in Cartagena. In other words she never returned from the New World to Spain and thus could not have brought cinchona with her to Madrid. The records do not give the cause of her death but suggest that it was from some epidemic disease then sweeping the Colombian port – most likely yellow fever.

Moreover, it is highly unlikely that the Condesa suffered malaria during her time in Lima. Don Luis Gerônimo Fernández de Cabrera Bobadilla y Mendoza, the Viceroy and fourth Conde de Chinchón, kept a meticulous diary that he himself observed is 'so long and prolix that it will be hard to read'. Yet nowhere in the copious jottings recorded by his secretary and official diary keeper, Antonio de Suardo, does the Viceroy mention his wife's illness. Indeed, in the eleven-year period covered by the diary, there are only two references to her being unwell. On the first occasion, in November 1630, she is suffering an 'inflamed' throat for which 'the doctors order her to be bled twice'. On the second, in October 1636, she has 'flux and cough on the lungs' (again, the treatment is phlebotomy).

The Conde is a far better candidate for the legend. His diary makes it clear that between May 1631 and October 1638 he suffered a number of illnesses which frequently confined him to his bed. The first reference to an intermittent fever comes in his entry for 5 May 1631, where he mentions an attack causing 'great anxiety and grief'. Fifteen days later, on 20 May, he is again 'ill with an attack of chills and fever,' and on 5 June the fever returns 'becoming quartan'. And so it continues right up to October 1638, by which time the Conde is so debilitated by his illness that the Condesa, still apparently in rude health, orders a mass and distributes candles and alms for him throughout the city. On 8 November, however, the Conde suddenly recovers and, according to the diary, 'from this day he steadily improved, having in his illness been in great danger of death.' What caused his sudden remission he does not say. But had it been the bark of a hitherto unknown tree you would have thought he would have recorded it. That he did not is damning evidence against the story related by Bado and all subsequent versions of the legend.[4]

The question then is how were the bark's therapeutic properties discovered and by whom, and did Bado have other motives for spreading such a fanciful and easily refutable legend? The short answer is no one knows for sure. Some medical historians are adamant that the Indians of South America must have known about the quinine tree long before the Spanish arrived in Peru, while others argue just as forcefully that the cure can only have been discovered by the Jesuits.[5] The belief that the Indians got there first is based partly on recent ethnobotanical research showing that the rainforest is a virtual phar-macopoeia to the people who live there. To take just two examples: in the 1940s American botanists were amazed to see Indians treating abrasions with *sangre de drago*, dragon's blood, a natural antiseptic that creates a seal around a wound like a liquid bandage, and toothache with *croton*, a plant in the rubber family.

We also know that Pizarro's soldiers were said to have preferred treatment by the native doctors to their own, and that in the first decades following the conquest of South America innumerable herbs, resins and balsams were despatched by galleon to Spain. Given their acquaintance with the medical properties of other plants it thus seems unlikely that the Indians would have overlooked the virtues of cinchona.

Unfortunately, there are a number of problems with this theory. The first is the complete absence of any references to cinchona bark in the hieroglyphics and archaeological remains left by the Inca, or in the 'medical books' of the great Indian civilizations of North and Central America.[6] The second is that it is widely accepted that falciparum malaria and even other, milder forms of malaria probably did not exist in South America prior to Columbus. No malaria, runs the argument, no need for the bark. The third is that even if the pre-Colombian Indians had a limited acquaintance with intermittent fevers their medical beliefs would have prejudiced them against the bitter-tasting bark.

To this day many South American tribes believe, like the ancient Greeks, that illnesses are either hot or cold and dry or wet, and that the remedy should be the reverse of the condition. Thus if a patient suffers from a hot-dry condition, he or she should be given a cold-wet drink. Quinine – runs the argument – is utterly confusing to the Indian way of thinking since, given at any point in the malarial cycle, it temporarily raises the body's temperature before reducing the fever (hence its relevance to homeopathy). Interestingly, one of the first to accept the conclusion that the Indians could not have known about cinchona was Humboldt. As we have seen, it was while travelling through Loja that Humboldt saw his first cinchona tree. More importantly for the present argument, he also observed that while 'agues are extremely common . . . the natives there . . . would die rather than have recourse to cinchona bark, which, together with opiates, they place in the class of poisons exciting mortification. The Indians cure themselves by lemonades, by oleaginous aromatic peel of the small green wild lemon, by infusions of *scoparia dulcis*, and by strong coffee.'

As against this, some ethnobotanists argue that by the early nineteenth century the Spanish had destroyed most of the Indians' culture and traditions. Thus the medical prejudices Humboldt observed were not the Indians' own but an assimilation from Europe. Nevertheless Humboldt is adamant that it was the Jesuits who discovered the bark. He claims this occurred by chance when they were testing various trees that had been felled in the Loja forest. 'There being always medical practitioners among the missionaries, it is said they had tried an infusion of the cinchona in the tertian ague, a complaint which is very common in that part of the country.' Humboldt concludes: 'This tradition is less improbable than the assertion of European authors . . . who ascribe the discovery to the Indians.'

But is the claim that the Indians knew about the cure really so improbable? La Condamine may have gilded his sighting of the quinine tree with all sorts of fanciful stories but on one point he was adamant: the Indians *had* known about the cure but had deliberately hidden the secret from the Spanish because of their hatred of the conquistadors. What made him so certain?

The answer, I believe, lies in La Condamine's introduction to his eyewitness account, where he makes a passing reference to Joseph de Jussieu, the French expedition's botanist, who he says has furnished him with 'various historical and physical' information on the tree. In fact, it would appear that La Condamine relied heavily on de Jussieu, who was already in the process of completing his own, far more thorough study of cinchona when he set off for Loja. Unfortunately for de Jussieu, La Condamine beat him to publication and by the time he and his manuscript reached Paris in 1771 no one much cared about his insights. This is a pity, for it is de Jussieu who provides the missing link in the story. Like Humboldt, he begins with a moving homage to the tree: '*Le quinquina est un arbre d'une grande hauteur qui domine presque ses voisins. Son tronc est droit et nu, et son diametre depasses parfois neuf ou dix pouces*' ('The quinquina is a tree of great height which dominates nearly all its neighbours. Its trunk is straight and bare, and its width often exceeds nine or ten inches'). Unlike La Condamine, de Jussieu distinguishes four types of bark: red, yellow, white and '*rougesse*'. Agreeing that the red is the strongest, he claims that 'the Spanish don't dare use it, fearing that by the strength of its heat, which they believe to be excessive, it will provoke a burning fever.'

This is a crucial insight – one that suggests that the prejudice against the bark was an imported, not a native, tradition. But de Jussieu goes further, adding a few pages later on that 'it is certain' that the discovery is owed to the Malacatos Indians, a tribe from the malarious coastal region of Ecuador who had settled in the valley of Vilcabamba. 'Since they had endured much suffering from the hot and humid climate and from intermittent fevers,' he writes, 'they were forced to find a remedy against the *maladie aussi importune*. After experimenting on various plants, they discovered that the bark of quinquina was the last and almost unique remedy against intermittent fevers.'

According to de Jussieu, the Malacatos Indians called the cure '*yarachucchu carachucchu*', meaning 'bark of the tree for the cold of fevers', or simply '*ayac cara*', 'bitter bark'. The Spanish discovered the secret only when a Jesuit was passing through Malacatos and fell ill with fever. Taking pity on him, the local *cacique* (chief) offered to cure him and went to fetch some bark from the nearby mountains. On his return he prepared an infusion and the missionary recovered. Accord-ing to de Jussieu the Jesuit later noticed similar trees growing throughout Peru and imported the bark to Spain. Significantly, he makes no reference to the story of the Condesa or the cure of the Corregidor of Loja, suggesting that these details were incorporated into the legend at a later date.

That de Jussieu is a superior and more reliable chronicler than La Condamine is underscored by his warning against the adoption of the word 'quinquina' which, he points out, is used indiscriminately by the Peruvians to refer both to quinine and the medically worthless balsam tree, *Myroxylon peruiferum*. Unfortunately, few people read de Jussieu's sage advice and for many years bark from both trees was distributed under the name 'quinquina' in Europe, fuelling medical scepticism about the efficacy of the cure.

As far as medical scholars have been able to establish, the Jesuits first introduced the bark into Spain and Italy in 1632, in other words around the time that Bado says the Condesa was being treated in Lima. However, the Jesuits only began to experiment systematically with the bark about twelve years later when it was brought to the attention of the influential Spanish Cardinal, Juan de Lugo.

Born in Madrid in 1583 of a noble and wealthy family, de Lugo was raised in Seville, where some of his earliest memories were of the arrival of Spanish galleons loaded with gold and exotic plants and spices from the New World. After studying law at Salamanca, de Lugo entered the Society of Jesus in 1603 where he quickly developed a reputation as a brilliant young theologian with an unrivalled command of jurisprudence. In 1620 he moved to Rome, where he taught for many years at the Gregorian University. Then in 1643, at the age of sixty, he was suddenly elevated to the rank of cardinal. By now the fevers then rampant in the Roman Campagna had seriously undermined his health. Indeed, such was the fear of malaria that when his benefactor, Pope Urban VIII, died, seven months after Cardinal de Lugo's investiture, the other foreign cardinals would not cross the Campagna to attend the conclave. Fortunately, de Lugo survived and when an ally of Spain, Innocent X, was elected Pope, he found his influence in the Vatican greatly increased.

At this point, the bark was still something of an unknown quantity. In 1642 the first references to cinchona — under the name *pulvis indicus* — had appeared in Belgium in the writings of a public health official in Ghent. The bark may have been shipped to Antwerp by Michael Belga, physician to the Marqués de Mancera, who had succeeded the Conde de Chinchón as Viceroy of Peru. But if cinchona was in circulation in northern Europe at this date it had yet to win the approval of leading physicians, as can be seen from the death of Ferdinand Habsburg, Viceroy of the Netherlands, in 1641 from a tertian fever exacerbated by the usual purges and blood-lettings.

However, by now Bado, first as physician to de Lugo and later as head of Genoa's two city hospitals, had become an enthusiastic convert. More importantly, Bado tells us, de Lugo himself had taken the bark and been cured after 'lying at the point of death' with a fever.

In around 1644, spurred by the reports from his missions in the New World and anxious to test the claims of the 'miraculous' cure, de Lugo did something no doctor had hitherto contemplated – he instructed the Pope's physician, Gabriel Fonseca, to subject the remedy to empirical testing. It was a simple idea, but radical at the time: if observation showed that the bark halted the cycle of shivers and sweats then the Church would recommend its use. Fonseca's report must have been favourable because not long afterwards de Lugo began distributing the bark free to the poor of Rome from his house and palace and at the Hospital of Santo Spirito. Streams of pilgrims began flowing to the Eternal City to try the new medicine, where it was known as *pulvis cardinalis* or *pulvis Jesuiticus* – 'Jesuit's bark'.

Despite de Lugo's ministrations in Rome, however, the remedy was still little known outside Spain and Italy. The event which changed this was the death in 1649 of the Father General of the Society of Jesus. At the resultant council in Rome to elect a new head of the Order, de Lugo was able to recommend cinchona to the assembled delegates, ensuring that they would carry the message to their missions throughout the world. The meeting also coincided with the arrival in Seville of large, regular shipments of cinchona from Peru, and under the supervision of the Jesuits it was soon being traded on mercantile exchanges where it acquired the popular name, 'Peru-vian bark'. In no time at all demand was at a fever pitch with everyone from court physicians to the lowliest apothecary clamouring for supplies of the new miracle cure. Interestingly, in a policy mirrored today by the distribution of the latest generation of anti-malarial drugs, de Lugo sold the bark to the rich at high prices in order to give it away to the poor.

Not everyone jumped on the bandwagon, however. Although by the 1650s Belgium and Holland had become major centres for the bark, physicians – particularly in Puritan England – remained deeply suspicious of a cure so closely associated with Rome. Partly this was political expediency on the part of the medical establishment. In 1649 Charles I had been executed and his Catholic wife sent into exile. Now Oliver Cromwell, Lord Protector and guardian of the Protestant faith, was determined to banish the last vestiges of Catholicism from English life. His timing could not have been worse. In the autumn of 1638 there had been an outbreak of 'harvest ague', and by 1658 the fever epidemic raged so fiercely in southern England that it was said there were 'scarce hands enough to take in the corn'. No one was safe, not even in London where the river at Westminster and Lambeth had the reputation for being particularly malarious. Perhaps that explains why in July and again in the autumn of 1658, a small advertisement for the bark appeared in the *Mercurius Politicus*. The advertisement spoke of 'the excellent Powder known by the name of Jesuit's Powder, which cureth all manner of Agues, Quotidian, Tertian and Quartan.' Imported from Antwerp, 'it is to be had at the Black-Spred-Eagle over against Black and White Court in the Old Baily, or at the shop of Mr John Crook, at the sign of the Ship in St Paul's Churchyard, a Bookseller, with directions for using of the same.'

Ironically, one of those most in need of treatment was the Lord Protector himself. Born in 1599 in Huntingdon and raised on the Cambridge fens, Cromwell had been a malaria sufferer all his life. He had frequent bouts of fever as a young man and there is evidence he suffered repeated relapses both during and after the Civil War. In 1647, for instance, during the crisis between the army and parliament, he was taken seriously ill, and following the Scottish campaign in February 1651 he suffered three fever attacks in as many weeks. Three months later, in May, he was stricken with fever again, this time in Edinburgh, leading his valet, Charles Harvey, to conclude that 'this [Scots] air is not so suitable to his temper as that of England.' As before Cromwell recovered, in time to subject the royalist forces to another humiliating defeat, this time at Worcester. The next seven years appear to have been malaria-free — instead Cromwell had to endure the agonies of a kidney stone, gout and a painful boil. But with the hot summer of 1658, fevers raged once again throughout the island and on 24 August Cromwell fell ill with what his physician, Dr George Bate, termed a 'bastard tertian ague'. On 27 August Cromwell had severe cold and hot fits. Then on the night of 30

August a tremendous storm swept the country, uprooting many large trees in St James's Park and blowing the roofs off houses. With Cromwell's condition deteriorating, his political secretary, the usually unflappable John Thurloe, wrote to Henry Cromwell, his son:

> This is the thirteenth day since the ague took him, havinge been sicke a fortnight before of a generalle distemper of the body. It continued a good while to be a tertian ague, and the burninge fits violent. Upon Saturday it fell to a double tertian havinge two fitts in twenty-four hours; one upon the heeles of another, which doe extremely weaken hym and endanger his life; and truly since Saturday Morning he hath scarce been perfectly out of his fits. The Doctors are yet hopefull that he may struggle through it, though their hopes are mingled with much feare.[7]

The doctors were right to be fearful; within four days Cromwell was dead. It is not known whether or not they offered to treat him with cinchona bark. According to popular legend, they did and he refused it because it was a 'Popish remedy'. Even if he had agreed, it is far from certain that it would have worked. In previous malaria bouts Cromwell had recovered, suggesting that he had the relatively benign vivax strain of the disease. Falciparum, unless imported by sailors returning from Jamaica, was unknown in England. Indeed, the post-mortem carried out after Cromwell's death suggests that the immediate cause of death was probably septicaemia brought on by a urinary infection – although malaria, by weakening his immune system, could have been a contributory factor.[8] More likely, Bates and the other physicians attending Cromwell never offered him cinchona, either because of their own religious prejudices or their suspicions, to some extent justified, of the many bogus powders and preparations on the market.

Ironically, it was thanks to the success of one of these supposedly bogus preparations that the bark finally began to win the confidence of the wider medical profession. The catalyst was Robert Talbor, an unqualified quack from Cambridge who had settled on the coast of

Essex — a major smuggling centre and then one of the most malarious regions of England — so as to be closer to the seat of the disease. There he experimented with different combinations of bark, eventually perfecting his own mysterious mixture of powders, which he advertised as 'Talbor's Wonderful Secret'. One of his favourite sales pitches was to tell patients that his elixir would help them expel their 'ague cake' — the English term for the enlargement of the spleen that follows infection with the malaria parasite (apparently they were to accomplish this remarkable feat through their mouths). In fact, Talbor's success was more likely due to his assiduous observations of his patients, and soon his reputation was such that his fame had spread to London.

The turning point came in 1672 when Charles II was visiting the coastal fort of Sheerness on the Thames estuary in Kent. One of the members of the King's party was a French nobleman who had previously been treated by Talbor in the Essex marshes. When the Frenchman related the story of Talbor's cure to Charles the King was intrigued and insisted on meeting the so-called 'quack' in person. Impressed with Talbor and anxious to discover the secret of his remedy, in July Charles made him a physician to the royal household and brought him to London. Styling himself a 'pyretiatro' — literally, a feverologist — Talbor began practising in the metropolis and in no time his cures were the talk of the town. The same year he published a book, *Pyretologia, or a Rational Account of the Cause and Cure of Agues*, prefacing it with the verse:

> The Learned Author in a generous Fit
> T'oblige his Country hath of Agues Writ
> Physicians now shall be reproacht no more
> Nor Essex shake with Agues as before
> Since certain health salutes her sickly shoar.

Talbor boasted that he had developed a secret remedy for tertian and quartan agues consisting of four ingredients, two of which were native to England, the other two from abroad.[9] Disingenuously, he cautioned against *Jesuit's powder*, warning that while it was an excellent cure when properly administered it could also lead to convulsions. In fact the bark was the key ingredient – the others being wine and opium – and the basis of his success.

By now, Talbor was not the only person in England experiment-ing with the bark. Jesuit's powder had also caught the attention of more respected, establishment scientists, such as the physician Thomas Sydenham. Born in 1624, Sydenham had served as a captain under Cromwell during the Civil War – a cause that led him to miss most of his university work – and later became a doctor. A friend of the philosopher John Locke and a disciple of Bacon, he was a convert to the novel concept in medical circles that the same sort of empirical observations should be applied to disease as to any other physical effect. He was the first to describe scarlet fever and added much to the knowledge of gout, from which he suffered. Bringing the same painstaking methods to bear on intermittent fevers, he observed that while the bark did not always cure the ague, it was certainly the only remedy he had seen which managed to halt its progress. In 1666, in his *Methodus Curandi Febres*, he cautiously recommended the bark, but only between paroxysms and not at the height of the attack. By 1676, however he had a better opinion of the treatment. This was partly a result of further experimentation, but also because by now he could not ignore Talbor's growing success. Sydenham now recommended the bark unequivocally for the treatment of quartan fevers and no longer suspected it of exacerbating the cycle of fevers and sweats. In his private letters he was even more confident, writing 'I have had but few trials but I am sure that an ounce of bark, given between the two fits, cures.'[10]

Sydenham had to be cautious, not least because rivalry at court between pro-Spanish and anti-Papist factions still made advocacy of the bark dangerous. The event which changed this was Charles II's recurrent malaria. In 1679, at the very moment that pro-Spanish elements were plotting at court to poison him, Charles summoned Talbor to Windsor Castle to treat his ague. Whether this was because he had received news of the plots or feared being bled to death in the name of science is not known. The point is Talbor administered his quinine mixture and the king recovered. Next Charles recommended Talbor to his friend Louis XIV whose only son, the dauphin, was seriously ill with fever. To the consternation of the French medical profession once again Talbor worked his magic and soon *le remède anglais* was the talk of *tout* Paris. Louis was so grateful he awarded Talbor a royal pension and paid him two thousand *louis d'or* for his proprietary 'secret' on condition that it not be published until after his death. So it was that with the new title of Chevalier, Talbor began travelling the courts of Europe, curing amongst others Louise Maria, the Queen of Spain, and – as he put it – 'a large number of lesser personages.'

Talbor did not enjoy his fame and fortune for long. In 1681, aged just forty, he died and was buried at Trinity Church, Cambridge where a family monument describes him as 'Febrium malleus'. The following year Louis published his secret formula with an introduction by his chief surgeon, Dr Nichola de Blegny. The revelation that Talbor had been using Jesuits' bark all along did not go down well with the medical profession, particularly as, according to de Blegny, Talbor had bought up all the best bark to prevent others discovering his secret, probably via his smuggling contacts in Essex. Nevertheless, the publication of the formula made the case for Jesuits' bark irresistible and *le remède anglais* was swiftly incorporated into the London Pharmacopoeia under the name *cortex Peruianus*. Twenty years later, in his monumental *Therapeutice specialis*, the Italian physician Francesco Torti confirmed through exhaustive observation of fever cases that quinquina – or 'china china' as he styled it – was the sole remedy for intermittent fevers, and the popularity of cinchona bark was secured.[11]

One of the results of Talbor's deception was to underline the importance of travelling to South America to study the trees from which the best bark was taken. 'Some authors make two kinds of quinquina, one which they say is wild and of little value, and another which they think is cultivated,' he wrote. '. . . To make a true estimate of their quality, it were fit one should be upon the place where they grow.' This was the task that La Condamine had begun, but the French Academician's description of *Cinchona officinalis* was only the first stage of what would prove to be a complex botanical and pharmacological riddle.

Broadly speaking, cinchonas are distinguished by their ovate or lanceolate leaves arranged in pairs at right angles to one another and by their pretty terminal flowers and seeds. The problem is that, as in the case of the colour of the bark, these morphological characteristics are not sufficient to distinguish one species from another. Neither do they necessarily provide a good indication of the level of quinine in the bark. To complicate matters further cinchona is a hybrid. In the wild the trees are apt to cross-pollinate, making it difficult to say where a variety ends and a new species begins.

When you consider that cinchonas tend to be found in the most inaccessible parts of the Andes, in forests cloaked for nine months of the year in impenetrable mist, and that the local names for the trees are often at variance with those assigned to them by botanists it is little wonder that the result has been taxonomical confusion. To this day some botanists argue there are twenty-three species of cinchona while others maintain there are just fifteen, the remaining eight simply being subspecies or varieties of the others. Nevertheless, this is a vast improvement on the position in 1867, when one botanical collector listed 143 species.

But the greatest challenge of all facing collectors was not the plant but the land and its people. To reach the cinchona forests on the eastern slopes of the Andes botanical explorers faced daunting natural obstacles: precipitous mountain passes and impassable rock faces; rainforests thick with hornets, mosquitoes and vicious biting ants; and rushing torrents that could sweep the earth and rocks from beneath a man's feet. Then there was the risk of ambush by head-hunting Indians or by *cascarilleros*, who were dependent on the bark for their livelihood. Nevertheless, in spite of all this, the Spanish had succeeded in removing other botanical treasures, such as the potato, from the Andes. Why should cinchona be any more formidable?

*Chapter Three*

# THE CURSE

Good God, when I consider the melancholy fate of so
many of botany's votaries, I am tempted to ask whether
men are in their right mind who so desperately risk life
and everything else through the love of collecting plants.

Carolus Linnaeus, *Glory of the Scientist* (1737)

WHEN LA CONDAMINE arrived in the New World with his party
of earth-measurers in 1735 there were only two ways to reach the
Viceroyalty of Peru. One was to disembark at Cartagena on the
Caribbean coast of the New Kingdom of Grenada (Colombia), and
raft six hundred and fifty kilometres up the Magdalena River to Santa
Fé de Bogotá, from where you could proceed along the spine of the
Cordillera Central to Popayán and on to Quito. The other was to
sail with the Spanish fleet as far as Puerto Bello, where you could
cross the Isthmus of Panama to the Pacific and catch a ship direct to
Guayaquil.

As it happened, La Condamine was so keen to see Cartagena –
no Frenchman had been inside the famous walled city since its
foundation – he stopped there first before proceeding across the
Isthmus to the coast of Ecuador. Nevertheless both routes were equally
gruelling and, from a health point of view, both were equally dangerous. The reason was the mosquito.

No one knows when malaria and other mosquito-borne diseases, notably yellow fever, reached the Americas but the Condesa de Chinchón was by no means their first victim. Six weeks after sacking Cartagena in 1586, for instance, Francis Drake had seen fit to flee the port because of a mysterious disease that visited his guards during *la serena* or 'evensong'.

'They say and hold very firme opinion,' wrote Drake, 'that who so is then abroad in the open ayre, shall certainly be infected to the death, not being of the Indian or naturall race of those countrey people: by holding their watch, our men were thus subjected to the infectious ayre.'

Although it is impossible to be certain, this reads very much like malaria, which is only transmitted at night when anophelines take their blood meals. Similar accounts of deadly fevers crop up time and again in the records of the early Spanish explorers. For instance, when Vasco Núñez de Balboa crossed the jungles of Darién to become the first European to see the 'southern sea' he lost seven hundred and twenty men to fever. And during his exploration of the Orinoco in 1534, Diego de Ordaz recounts how he lost more than three hundred men '*enfeebled by fever* and other diseases induced by the hot, damp atmosphere of the lower stretches of the river.'

The Spanish word for the fevers they encountered in the Carib-bean was *calentura* – a catch-all term that could apply to a plethora of diseases beside malaria, including cholera, typhoid fever and amoebic dysentery. The accepted view today is that if any of these diseases were malaria – and it is a big if – the disease probably arrived with the Spanish conquest. The reason is that the first inhabitants of South America were the Indian descendants of Asiatic peoples who migrated across the 'ice bridge' from Siberia to Alaska and through Central America and the Isthmus of Panama. Malariologists argue that such a migration would almost certainly have resulted in falciparum, and most likely other strains of malaria too, being 'frozen out'. And while it is possible that malaria could have been introduced to the coast of Chile by Polynesian peoples crossing the Pacific, such a migration is unproven.

In contrast, we know that by the time of Columbus's first voyage vivax malaria was endemic to Seville, Lisbon and the Tagus River, on whose banks the Conde de Chinchón had his estates. In addition, the holds of the ships that brought the early Spanish and Portuguese settlers to South America contained a natural repository for both yellow fever and the falciparum parasite – namely, the blood of black African slaves.

Unlike South America, Africa has almost certainly been malarious for several million years. Indeed, our apelike ancestor, *Homo erectus*, was probably already carrying *Plasmodium falciparum* in his blood when he emerged from the jungle one million years ago and began his long march across the African savannah to the Fertile Crescent and into Asia. The result is that many black Africans and blacks of African descent enjoy natural immunity against malaria thanks to genetic traits, such as sickle-cell anaemia, that have evolved in response to their long exposure to the disease. And even those who do not enjoy such genetically conditioned immunities often acquire limited immunity as a result of repeated exposure to the disease in childhood.

From the Spanish point of view, this resistance to malaria and other tropical diseases made black Africans the ideal labourers to replace native Amerindian populations who, ironically, had been decimated by the importation to the New World of Old World diseases such as smallpox and measles. Indeed, Father Las Casas, one of the early Spanish chroniclers, observed that white settlers believed that the only way a black would die was if they hanged him.

The result was that as early as 1502 the Spanish Crown gave the Governor of Hispaniola permission to import *ladinos* – African slaves who had been two or more years in Spain. And by 1518 the demand for black slaves on Hispaniola was so great that Charles I was persuaded to allow blacks to be imported direct from some of the most malarious regions of Africa – notably, the Gold Coast and the Bight of Benin.

From the plasmodium's point of view this was excellent news, as it created a group of human carriers capable of transporting the disease overseas. Beginning with the slave trade in the sixteenth century this is exactly what happened: slaves were brought from Africa to the Caribbean and the West Indies, turning previously healthy islands into breeding grounds for malaria and yellow fever.

Once the diseases were established in the Caribbean, trade and the imperatives of conquest rapidly spread them to the South American mainland. The Spanish renegade Pedro de Heredia might well have been the first to introduce malaria and yellow fever to Colombia when he set sail from Santo Domingo with several slaves in 1533 and landed at Santa Marta, where he immediately put them to work as *macheteros*, clearing the underbrush. Soon afterward he founded Cartagena and began importing more black labourers, this time to replace Indians who were reluctant to work in the Spanish gold mines.

As the Spanish thirst for gold intensified so the demand for slaves increased. In the first two decades of the eighteenth century alone the English brought seventy-five thousand slaves to Latin America – the majority destined for the gold mines in the Choco, Colombia, and the coast of Ecuador. The result was that by the early eighteenth century Cartagena had been transformed into a major centre of Caribbean slavery.

The legacy of these successive, enforced human migrations can still be seen in Cartagena today, not only in the Plaza de Coches, the old slave market, but in the bewildering array of skin tones on display in its narrow, cobbled streets. Retracing La Condamine's steps through the old walled city – past the pretty colonial-era houses of the Spanish nobility with their massive iron-studded doors and wooden balconies reminiscent of Seville – you are presented with every shade of the human palette, from black to white to tobacco.

But if racial miscegenation is the most obvious legacy of the slave trade, it is not the only one. Just as malaria and other tropical diseases retarded European colonization of Africa, so the slave trade, by bringing malaria and probably yellow fever to South America, acted as a brake on European ambitions to overturn the 'fact' of the Spanish conquest.

This lesson was dramatically brought home to me at Cartagena's Museo Naval de Caribe by Iris Londono, an ex-merchant navy seaman who supplements his meagre pension by offering bilingual tours of the museum. Having served on British ships for many years Londono told me he was proud to speak the Queen's English, but even prouder of the fact that *cartageneros* still spoke the King's Spanish – a fact he attributed to Don Blas de Leso, a one-armed, one-legged Spanish naval officer, and the mosquito. As we weaved through the display cases littered with the detritus of corsairs and cannons recovered from bottom of Cartagena's bay, Londono warmed to his theme.

On 15 March 1741, he explained, the Spanish, African and *mestizo* citizens of Cartagena had awoken to a fearsome sight. Spread out across the bay beneath Cartagena's bastions were fifty British warships accompanied by seventy-four transport and supply vessels – the largest armada ever assembled in anger by one nation against another. The fleet contained 6,000 marines, 8,000 infantry, four companies from Jamaica and four battalions of raw American recruits. In all, a force of 18,760 fighting men.

Led by Brigadier-General Wentworth and the English Admiral, Sir Edward Vernon – or 'Old Grog' as he was affectionately known by his men[1] – the task force's aim was to sail into the bay and sack the city, then the wealthiest on the Spanish main.

England had been itching for an excuse to invade Spain's colonial possessions for some time. For decades English buccaneers had been raiding ports and shipping lanes on the Spanish Main, egged on by a British public eager for the latest instalment of their piratical adventures while Parliament turned a blind eye. Sometimes the Spanish intercepted them but more often than not they escaped. Then in 1739 a Spanish coast guard stopped an English merchant ship allegedly loaded with illegal contraband. The captain of the ship was Robert Jenkins and his ear – or rather what was left of it – was to go down in history.

Every schoolboy used to know the story of the War of Jenkins's Ear: how the honest master mariner had protested his innocence to the *guardacosta* only for the dastardly Spaniard to cut off his ear in a fit of pique and then spit in what was left of it, 'Go tell your King that I will do the same to him should he dare to act as you have.' Whether

Jenkins was quite as upright or innocent as he subsequently made out, or the coast guard officer quite so despicable, is unclear. But what is indisputable is that when Jenkins limped back to Britain carrying the remains of his ear in a jar and told his story to Parliament there was uproar. Inflamed by English commercial interests, and spurred on by the hawkish Vernon, the Prime Minister, Robert Walpole, reluctantly revived Cromwell's 'Western Design' — the blueprint for the break-up of Spain's colonial possessions. Two armadas were assembled: one to sail around Cape Horn under the command of Admiral Anson and attack the Spanish in the Pacific; the second, led by Wentworth and Vernon, to assault Cartagena. Once Cartagena had fallen and the task force had knocked the commercial stuffing out of the Spanish empire, the English reasoned it would be a simple matter to sail up the Magdalena river and take the rest of Colombia too.

In theory, the only thing that stood between the task force and success was San Felipe de Barajas, the huge fort guarding the land entrance to Cartagena, and Blas de Leso, the veteran Spanish naval officer in charge of the city's defences. But, as Londono now explained — pausing by a grimy display case marked with numbers delineating the course of the naval engagement — Wentworth and Vernon had forgotten to factor for the bay's formidable outer defences and, equally importantly, the mosquito.

After raising the British ensign in front of the walled city, Vernon had skirted Cartagena's ramparts and positioned his fleet in front of Boca Chica — the smaller of the two entrances to Cartagena's bay. Having previously taken Puerto Bello with just six ships, Vernon was probably anticipating a short naval engagement, followed by a triumphant entrance to the city. But de Leso had been warned of the task force's arrival and had reinforced the batteries on Tierra Bomba, the island that guarded the narrow channel, delaying the cocksure Admiral's advance for fifteen critical days.

In truth, the decisive factor was not so much the Spanish defences as Wentworth's indolence and incompetence. Not only were his gunners useless, but he put his camp in line with his batteries so that shot from San Luis de Bocachica that flew over the English artillery landed amongst his men. Although Vernon repeatedly urged him to storm the fort and put an end to the confrontation, Wentworth demurred. The delay gave Cartagena's mosquitoes an opportunity to go to work on his troops.

It just so happened that Tierra Bomba was peppered with cisterns in which the local inhabitants kept their drinking water. The cisterns provided the perfect breeding ground not only for *Anopheles* but also for *Aedes aegypti*, the mosquito that carries yellow fever. Unlike malaria, yellow fever is a viral infection that is transmitted rapidly from ship to shore and vice versa. The onset of the disease is sudden – the first fever attack usually occurs within five days –and typically results in black vomiting, haemorrhaging and yellow discoloration of the eyes and skin. In contrast to malaria, which typically has a two-week latency period and is not always fatal, yellow fever is also characterized by a high initial death count.

From the descriptions left by observers of the battle it is not clear whether the troops and marines were attacked by yellow fever, malaria or both. Some observers mention black vomit, which occurs only with yellow fever, but others mention only fever. And since most of the men did not begin displaying symptoms until at least two weeks after the initial attack some epidemiologists believe that malaria must have been the main cause of death. Whatever vector or vectors were involved, however, the effect on the health of the English force was catastrophic.

On 5 April Wentworth finally gave the order to storm San Luis de Bocachica. The Spanish fled without firing a shot, proving that Vernon had been right in urging him to mount an attack earlier. Nevertheless, at this stage Vernon was still confident of victory. Indeed, no sooner had he entered the bay and landed his marines at Manzanillo than he despatched a courier to London, announcing the fall of Cartagena.

However, the British had reckoned without disease and the determination of Blas de Leso. Although the army had suffered relatively few casualties in the assault on Tierra Bomba, by 14 April 'general sickness' had reduced Wentworth's force to 3,500 and he was pressing to abandon the attack. Vernon, however, was determined to continue. He peppered Cartagena with shell and grapeshot. Then on the night of 20 April he launched a frontal assault on San Felipe de Barajas. It was a disaster. The fortress was too strong and as the British struggled to gain a foothold the Spanish launched a bloody bayonet charge. By dawn 800 English dead lay strewn about the ramparts and some 1,000 troops had been taken prisoner.

The force had no choice but to retreat to the harbour. It was now that yellow fever and malaria began to take hold and by 7 May many of the transports had been converted into hospital ships. According to Smollett, the naval surgeon, the scene was horrendous. 'Nothing was heard but groans, lamentations and the language of despair invoking death to deliver [the men] from their miseries,' he recalled. When men died, there were too few hands to prepare the corpses for a proper sea burial. The result was that soon the bay was strewn with shark-torn bodies floating on the surface.

The final casualty figures make sober reading. Having made an inglorious retreat from Cartagena, it was decided to redeem English honour by attacking Jamaica and Cuba. But here the depredations of the *Aedes aegypti* and *Anopheles* mosquitoes were as great as before, and by the time the task force limped back to England, the army had lost 6,500 men to fever and disease, and the marines reported only 3,500 men fit for duty.

The humiliating defeat underlined as never before the military necessity of having a prophylactic against malaria and other tropical diseases. But it would be another thirty years before the Scottish naval surgeon James Lind would recognize the importance of Peruvian bark in preventing fevers when, in 1771, he persuaded the Admiralty to introduce cinchona in wine to crews on 'ships of war on the Guinea station'. By the turn of the century the practice had also spread to other theatres. In December 1803 when Admiral Nelson, on the recommendation of Dr Snipe, Physician to the Mediterranean Fleet, directed that 'a dose of Peruvian-bark, in a preparation of good sound wine or spirits' be given to sailors in the morning before going ashore in marshy areas, 'and the same in the evening on his return on board.'

By 1808 this regimen had been refined, and it was found in Article 24 of the Instruction to Surgeons:

> The Peruvian Bark with wine having been found useful as a preventive, the Surgeon is, when his ship shall be in such tropical climates, to request the Captain a list of men who are to be sent on shore on wooding or watering duty, and to administer to each man, previous to his leaving the ship in the morning, a drachm of Bark in half a gill of sound wine, and he is also to give each man the like quantity of wine after he shall have taken the Bark; and a like quantity of Bark and wine proportioned in the same manner is to be given to each man in the evening of the same day on his return to the ship, particularly observing that the Bark administered for this purpose is always to be given in substance, and not in tincture.

Nevertheless, it was not until 1847 that the Lords of the Admiralty issued a directive allowing surgeons to lay in provisions of the prepared quinine wine 'in such quantities as their respective complements may seem to require', and then only as a result of the navy's experience off the coast of west Africa and in the notoriously malarious seas of the Bight of Benin.[2]

Ensconced in Ecuador, La Condamine had plenty of time to mull over Vernon's defeat. One of the ironies was that Puerto Bello was then a major trading post for cinchona. The bark would come from Paita and other Peruvian ports to the Pacific coast of Panama, from where it would be carried across the Isthmus by slaves – a gruelling four-day journey. The Academicians had had reason to be grateful for this traffic when, shortly after leaving Cartagena, de Jussieu had fallen ill with fever at Puerto Bello and prepared a decoction from the bark to cure himself. If only Vernon had seized the opportunity of provisioning his ships with cinchona when he sacked Puerto Bello history might have turned out differently.

Now the War of Jenkins's Ear began to have repercussions for

La Condamine's work too. After sending his description of the cinchona tree to the French Academy of Sciences, La Condamine had returned to Quito to continue plotting one degree of latitude at the equator. But following Vernon's assault on Cartagena the whole Pacific coast was up in arms in expectation of an imminent attack by Admiral Anson. As the Peruvians nervously waited for the English to strike from the south they turned a wary and increasingly suspicious eye on the foreigners in their midst. For six years the Academicians had been measuring, drawing maps and experimenting with strange instruments. The Frenchmen claimed they were measuring the arc of a meridian but what was their true purpose?

At least one resident of Quito thought he had the answer: the Academicians' collection of triangles and theodolites was really a new method for divining gold. 'For what could induce gentlemen,' he asked rhetorically, 'well born and of high station, to lead such a dismal life, uncouth and uncomfortable, climbing mountains, passing over celestial deserts, looking at the stars, for any other reason than earthly profit?'

When it was learnt that La Condamine had built a pyramid near Quito, at the point where he had first measured his base line, suspicion turned to anger. Anson's attack on Colombia never came but for the next two years La Condamine found himself embroiled in his own war, the War of the Pyramids. The central issue was whether he had the right to erect a pyramid bearing the French coat of arms on Spanish soil. Did this mean he was laying claim to Peru on behalf of the King of France?

After interminable legal wrangling it was decided he was not making any such claim and that the pyramid could stay on condition that the Bourbon coat of arms was obliterated and the name of La Condamine's Spanish explorer colleagues inserted instead. The decision was a diplomatic triumph for La Condamine but he was now exhausted and anxious to return to France. First, however, he had to fulfil the second part of the vow he had made when he had visited Loja five years earlier: to gather plants and seeds of cinchona and transplant them to Europe, associating his name forever with the cure for malaria.

As he climbed Mount Cajanuma a second time La Condamine must have thought his fame was assured. Accompanied this time by two Indian porters he gathered nine young saplings, together with their seeds, placed the plants in an earthen box and descended the eastern slopes of the Ecuadorian Andes to Borja. The idea was to paddle down the Amazon to Cayenne, on the coast of French Guiana, where he would place the trees en dépôt for transportation to the Jardin des Plantes in Paris. Incredibly he succeeded in recreating Orellana's epic journey, but at Belém a wave washed over the boat, carrying away the boxes and plants. 'Thus,' wrote La Condamine, 'I lost them after all the care I had taken during a voyage of more than 1200 leagues.'

His attempts to cultivate the seeds fared no better. At Cayenne he had taken them to a plantation run by a community of Jesuits. But the soil and climate were not the same as at Loja and they failed to germinate. By now La Condamine had had enough of South America and was ready to return home, but his trials were far from over. He had to wait five more months in Cayenne before finding passage on a Dutch vessel to France. On the way he was twice attacked, once by a British ship and the second time, oddly enough, by a French.

It is hard to feel sorry for him, however. When he finally arrived in Paris in 1745 there was not a savant in Europe who did not wish to speak with him. In the course of his travels La Condamine had not only made the first description of cinchona but had become the first European to describe the Hevea rubber tree, fashioning a bag from the latex to keep his scientific instruments dry in the Amazon. He had also conducted experiments with curare that foreshadowed its later use as an anaesthetic and became a convert to inoculation against smallpox – a practice he had seen the Carmelite friars apply with success in Belém (La Condamine went through life with pockmarked skin, the result of a childhood bout of the disease).

Far more deserving of our sympathy is de Jussieu. Born in Lyon in 1704, he was the fourth son in a family of sixteen. Although he studied medicine in Reims and Paris, he also excelled at mathematics and engineering – indeed, the other Academicians often called for his help in making geodesic calculations. But de Jussieu was first and foremost a botanist and in 1737 and again in 1739 he had also gone to Loja to study the tree. Unlike La Condamine, de Jussieu experimented with the bark, preparing infusions and testing them on himself to see if the Spanish were correct to fear the 'heat' of the red variety. In 1740, he proved that the Spanish prejudice was nonsense when he took *cascarilla roja* to cure himself of a fever at Quito. After practising medicine there for several years he then set off, via Lima, for the cinchona forests of Bolivia, presumably with the intention of seeing whether the yellow *calisaya* barks were equally efficacious. I say 'presumably' for he left no account of his travels. We know from the Spanish records that his wanderings took him to Santa Cruz de la Sierra as well as to the silver-mining centre of Potosí, and that while in Bolivia he investigated the cultivation of the coca shrub, becoming the first botanist to record the use of the revered stimulant of the Inca.

His intention had been to continue to Buenos Aires and on to France. By now he had a huge collection of specimens all carefully stored away in boxes. But just as he was about to return home to what should have been a hero's welcome fate intervened. De Jussieu had entrusted the boxes to an Indian servant with strict instructions that he should watch over them night and day as they contained objects of the greatest value. Believing they must be stuffed with gold – for what else was more highly prized by Europeans? – the servant disappeared with the lot.

The boxes were never recovered. In his despair de Jussieu turned his back on botany and Europe, returning to Lima to set up a medical practice. In his spare time he consoled himself with geometry, the only study which, in his own words, '*le satisfaisant par l'évidence de ses démonstrations.*' By the time he eventually returned to Paris in 1771 his memory was gone. He could recall nothing of the earlier hunt for cinchona in Ecuador or what exquisite varieties of *calisayas* he had collected during his wanderings in Bolivia. All that remained was the unedited manuscript he had written on the cinchona tree in 1737. He had kept it with him the whole time and was still clutching it when he was confined to an institution for the mentally insane in Paris. In 1777, de Jussieu's description was finally published in a concise report in the *Histoire de la Societé Royale de Medicine.* Two years later, on 11 April 1779, he died.

It is tempting to view de Jussieu's and La Condamine's failures as more than bad luck. Indeed, those of a superstitious bent remarked that it was as if the tree was protected by some ancient Indian curse. The Spanish had succeeded in stealing the Incas' gold but it seemed that those who attempted to remove cinchona – a far more valuable product of the Andes – were doomed. There were good reasons why the attempts to steal cinchona were so fraught – not least the botanical complexity and inaccessibility of the tree and the huge distances involved in transplanting it to Europe. Indeed prior to La Condamine there is evidence that the Spanish believed that cinchonas did not produce seeds at all but were sterile. The reason for their mistake was simple: cinchona, like coffee, has a short and unpredictable flowering and fruiting season. They need only have arrived in the bark forests too early – or too late – and they would have missed the seeds entirely.

Luckily, Charles III, the King of Spain, now had a man in South America well equipped to succeed where the French had failed. He had a heavenly name – José Celestino Mutis – and he had come to the New World expressly to gather cinchonas. Born in Cadiz in 1732, Mutis had studied medicine in Seville and Madrid. There his prowess as a doctor had brought him to the attention of the newly appointed Viceroy of New Grenada, who asked him to join him in Bogotá as the court physician. Mutis readily agreed, believing that the appointment would allow him plenty of time to indulge his passion for botany and astronomy, but when he reached New Granada in 1760 he found his duties were so onerous he had little opportunity to stray beyond the confines of the palace. In his frustration, in 1763, he wrote directly to Charles III urging him to let him form a botanical expedition to collect cinchona. His royal plea would prove prophetic.

For many years the Jesuits had been nagging the *cascarilleros* to replace felled or dying trees with five more planted in a quincunx – the sign of the cross. But the bark cutters had ignored the Jesuits' commonsense injunctions and by the 1760s the forests in Loja where the best trees grew were nearly exhausted. Now, in a letter that anticipated the philanthropic arguments of British cinchona hunters a century later, Mutis reminded Charles that he had a duty to his subjects to secure affordable supplies of the febrifuge. 'America,' he wrote, 'is rich not only in gold, silver, precious stones and other treasures but also in natural products ... there is quinine, a priceless possession of which Your Majesty is the only owner and which divine Providence has bestowed upon you for the good of mankind. It is indispensable to study the cinchona tree so that only the best kind will be sold to the public at the lowest price.'

Mutis received no answer. He sent another petition. Then he sent drawings and dried specimens of cinchona flowers gathered in Loja to Linnaeus. The Swedish botanist replied immediately – they were the first examples he had seen since La Condamine's twenty-five years previously and they enabled him to complete his classification.[3] But still Mutis heard nothing from Charles III. The silence was doubly frustrating as Mutis had now discovered another variety of cinchona on his doorstep. One day, while riding through the mountains of Bogotá, he had spotted the characteristic rustling of red leaves. He would later claim that the tree, which he christened *Cinchona bogotensis*, was the first cinchona found north of the equator. In fact, by now two other far more valuable species – *C. lancifolia* and *C. cordifolia* – had also been found in Colombia, but it was certainly true that Mutis was the first to classify them, describing all the new Colombian species in a paper, *El Arcano de la Quina*, written by his nephew, Sinforoso, and published in 1793.

The discoveries were important for two reasons: firstly, it meant that cinchonas could now be harvested in Colombia and transported straight to Spain via Cartagena, rather than having to come around Cape Horn from Peru's Pacific coast or across the Isthmus of Panama. Secondly, it raised the intriguing possibility that the geographic distribution of cinchona was far wider than had previously been suspected. If it could grow in the Colombian Andes what valuable varieties might exist at the southern limits of the same mountain chain?

In an attempt to answer that question in 1777 Charles III sent two botanists –Hipolito Ruiz and José Pavon – to hunt for cinchonas in the forests of central and southern Peru and Chile. Accompanied by the French naturalist Joseph Dombey, the Spanish botanists left Cadiz in November 1777 and arrived at Callao in Peru five months later. For seven years they explored Peru and Chile, penetrating the forests of the central Andes, and discovering seven new species of cinchona. By the time they returned to Lima in 1785 they had fifty-three boxes packed with specimens. They despatched them to Spain on the *San Pedro Alcantara* then resumed their collecting in the Peruvian Andes. But if Ruiz and Pavon thought they had outwitted the curse they were wrong. In July 1786, while collecting in the forests of Huánuco, the house where they kept their journals and specimens accidentally caught fire. Ruiz reached the hacienda just in time to see the flames engulfing his precious manuscripts. Without regard for his safety he dived into the inferno and had to be dragged out kicking and screaming by his peons. That was not the end of their misfortunes, however. Six months later, within days of reaching Cadiz, the *San Pedro Alcantara* was wrecked off the coast of Portugal, taking Ruiz and Pavon's remaining boxes of specimens with it.

Mutis was spared a similar fate but even worse was to befall his followers. In 1783 Charles III finally acknowledged Mutis's entreaties and appointed him chief botanist and astronomer to the 'Real Expedición Botánica del Nuevo Reino de Granada'. Gathering around him a group of talented young naturalists and artists, he scoured Colombia's mountains and river valleys for new species of cinchona and other flora, eventually amassing a huge collection that was stored in a specially constructed library, the grandly titled Instituto Botánica del Nuevo Reino de Grenada (Botanical Institute of the New Kingdom of Granada). By 1791 Mutis's staff consisted of some ten scientists and fifteen artists. The most talented of all was Francisco José de Caldas. Born in Popayán, in southern Colombia, in 1770, de

Caldas was endlessly inquisitive. A student of botany, he was also adept at mathematics, meteorology and geography. While crossing the Andes, he constructed his own barometer and sextant, and – ignorant of discoveries already made in Europe – independently arrived at the method for gauging altitude with a boiling-point thermometer. Next he visited Loja and conducted a thorough survey of the cinchona forests of Ecuador and Colombia together with a map showing cinchona's geographic distribution. By the time he was finished he had described twenty-two separate species – far more than anyone hitherto. More importantly, Caldas kept a careful note of the altitudes and climate and soil conditions in which the trees were found. From this he was able to establish that the most valuable species of cinchona rarely grew below twelve hundred or higher than three thousand metres. He also noticed that they were most abundant on the eastern slopes of the Andes, where the Amazon and its effluents had their sources, and tended to cluster on the sides of river valleys and in the crevices of mountains, rather than on more open ground. The red barks, in particular, seemed to prefer areas of steady year-round rainfall and loamy, alluvial soil – such as are found near volcanoes.

These insights would later prove crucial to the success of trans-planting cinchona overseas, but at the time it seems they were ignored by Mutis, as Caldas was soon complaining that he was not being afforded the recognition he was due. Worse, Mutis made a funda-mental error by claiming that *Cinchona lancifolia* and *C. cordifolia* – respectively, the orange and yellow-coloured Colombian barks – were identical to the valuable red and yellow barks described by La Condamine. In fact, as Caldas must have known since he had visited Loja and Mutis had not, this was false. Thus it was that when in 1808 Mutis died, having published just two short papers on cinchona, Caldas seized the opportunity to put the institute's massive collection in order and correct his master's errors. Unfortunately, he had just begun on this immense task when he was interrupted by an independ-entist revolt against the Spanish government. Caldas promptly joined the rebels, eventually rising to the rank of captain in Bolivar's army.

In between the fighting he returned every now and then to the institute, but by 1816 the rebels were in retreat and Caldas had been taken prisoner by the Spanish. Tried as a traitor, he pleaded for his life to be spared so that he could finish his taxonomy of cinchona, but his pleas were rejected and on 29 October 1816 he was executed by firing squad. The result was that for all Spain's efforts the world's understanding of the relationship between the different species of cinchona and the febrifugal properties of the barks had advanced little since the time of La Condamine and de Jussieu.

By the turn of the century this failure had become a source of irritation not only to pharmacists but also to the military. Advances in chemistry meant that pharmacists were at last in a position to identify and isolate the key alkaloids in the bark – the so-called 'febrifugal salts'. The problem was they still did not know the correct botanical classification for the barks containing the highest levels of quinine. In addition, the practice of adulterating cinchona bark with 'false' quinas to boost profits was widespread among merchants and apothecaries, further undermining medical confidence in the remedy. As Mutis had pointed out in his deposition to Charles III: 'Such quina tends to be the remedy in which a doctor vainly trusts in the most desperate moments and such finally is the antidote which a poor sick man buys for greater harm to himself. How sad and lamentable would be the spectacle, which a lively imagination could call forth, of a limitless army of loyal subjects tragically lost and abandoned at the foot of your throne!'

In fact it was not Charles III who had to witness this pitiful spectacle but George III and, once again, the lesson came at sea.

In 1809, encouraged by victories over the French in Portugal and Austria, the British decided to stage a raid against Napoleon in northern Europe. The site chosen was Walcheren in northern Belgium, an area of low-lying marsh that lies in the Scheldt, the estuary that flows from Holland into the North Sea. But as Lord Chatham, the eldest son of William Pitt, assembled an armada on the south coast of England in preparation for the assault, Napoleon remained unimpressed. 'We must stop the English with nothing but fever, which will soon devour them all,' he predicted, adding that, 'in a month the English will be obliged to take to their ships.'

Napoleon did not have to wait long to see his prediction dramatically fulfilled. Unlike at Cartagena, the navy had taken the precaution of provisioning their ships with 'Peruvian bark'. But it appears that they had bought the wrong type of bark or else that, in the absence of any advice from the Army Medical Board, no one had thought to provide sufficient supplies for the army too. Whatever the case, Walcheren was a disaster.

With the French fleet anchored at Antwerp, the English landed easily in the Scheldt. But on 10 August, as Chatham sought to invest Flushing, Napoleon cut the dykes, and by the middle of August 40,000 English troops were camped on a flat plain surrounded by pools of stagnant water and swarms of mosquitoes.

The first cases of 'Walcheren Fever' appeared at the end of the month. By the end of September deaths on Walcheren and the neighbouring island of South Beveland had reached 1,000, and several thousand more troops lay sick on hospital ships just as Napoleon had foreseen. By the end of October the situation was even worse, with deaths running at 20–30 a day.

The army was wholly unprepared for the crisis. Regimental surgeons warned the healthy not to sleep in the open air, distributed extra rations of rum and urged troops to smoke cigars in order to 'purify' the atmosphere. But when the Scottish regimental surgeon James McGrigor arrived to take command of the medical disaster he found men sweating on the open decks of ships, unattended save for pails of bark. The problem was that the demand for bark far exceeded the supply and it was only by chance that he was able to purchase fresh stocks from a Yankee clipper that had just docked at Flushing.

By the end of the expedition more than 4,000 men were dead and another 11,500 lay ill in hospital. Although some of the casualties were undoubtedly attributable to other diseases such as typhoid and cholera, there is little doubt that the main cause of death was malaria. So intense was the public reaction that a committee of the entire

House of Commons conducted a two-month investigation into the failure of the administration. The inquiry resulted in the dismissal of the Medical Board and a complete reform of the army's medical department.

If the British had any lingering doubts about the military value of cinchona Walcheren erased them, but from a clinical point of view identifying which barks contained active levels of the febrifuge was still very much hit and miss. Following the discovery of cinchona in Colombia, the Spanish had begun exporting bark direct from Cartagena. By 1792 the bark shipped from the Caribbean port had reached three hundred and sixty-five tonnes a year, far surpassing exports from Peru and encouraging the British and Americans to open a contraband trade with Colombia. But while the Colombian grey and orange barks were far cheaper, doctors soon noticed they were not nearly as effective against intermittent fevers as the more highly valued red and yellow barks. Dramatic confirmation of this came in 1799 when the British intercepted a Spanish frigate sailing from Lima to Cadiz loaded with red Peruvian bark. At first druggists in London and Ostend were unable to dispose of the cargo, but when doctors began testing the red bark on their patients they discovered it was much better at clearing agues and the price shot up. Within a few years, every major teaching hospital in London had acknowledged the bark's superiority, prompting widespread demand for it from country practitioners, particularly in malarious areas of England like Kent and Essex. However, it was only when chemists began isolating the essential 'febrifugal salts' in the barks that they were at last able to distinguish which types were more effective.

The first to succeed was Bernardino Antonio Gomez, a Portuguese naval surgeon. In 1812 he mixed powdered grey bark with a precipitant and succeeded in extracting an alkaloid to which he gave the name cinchonino. But the real breakthrough came in France. Pierre Pelletier and Joseph Caventou were brilliant young pharmacists who had already made a name for themselves in 1817 by isolating emetine, a cure for amoebic dysentery, from ipecacuanha – the plant Spruce had taken at Maipures to purge himself in the belief that it would also rid him of fever. The following year they isolated strychnine. Then, in 1820, they subjected the yellow and red cinchona barks to similar analysis. They discovered that the febrifuge was actually seated in two alkaloids that occurred separately or together in different kinds of bark. The first they called cinchonine, the second they called quinine. The red bark, they found, contained both. But the yellow bark was abundant chiefly in quinine.[4]

Pelletier and Caventou's discovery was hugely significant, not only from a clinical point of view but also from a commercial one. At the time, 1lb of bark fetched £1 at auction in Amsterdam and London – a not inconsiderable sum of money. To treat a case of malaria, a patient would need nearly 2lb of bark as a first dose, and 1lb a week thereafter – in other words, as much as £5 worth in total. But because of the variations in quality, one patient's £5 investment might not be equivalent to another's. Clearly, the first company to succeed in extracting controlled doses of the key alkaloids would be in a position to reap huge rewards. The race was on, but which alkaloid was the most effective against malaria and from which variety of cinchona did it originate? The first part of that question was easily answered; it was the second that would prove problematic.

Within a year of Pelletier and Caventou's discovery, a number of French doctors had begun testing the 'salts' on their patients. Nearly all of them reached the same conclusion: namely, that quinine sulphate was the most effective. Incredibly, Pelletier and Caventou had not applied for a patent to safeguard their discovery. The news of quinine's superiority quickly spread overseas. In 1823 a Dublin doctor tested quinine sulphate on thirty patients, including four who had not responded to treatment with cinchona bark. The treatment succeeded in every case. Around the same time American physicians began similar experiments and by 1825 quinine sulphate was the recommended treatment for intermittent fevers in Philadelphia – then the centre of American medical teaching.

Then came the surprise. When chemists tested the barks again they discovered that the ones with the highest quinine content of all were not the red cinchona barks from Ecuador and Peru, but the *calisaya* barks from Bolivia. Confusingly, the bark of these trees was yellow – although they were known as '*roja*' by the *cascarilleros* because of their deep reddish-purple leaves. The value of *calisayas* had long been recognized in Madrid, where their bark fetched some of the highest prices of all, but aside from de Jussieu and the Indians of the Bolivian highlands no one had ever seen the tree in the wild. In addition, botanists still had to answer the vexed question as to whether the red bark tree of Loja – the *Cinchona officinalis* of La Condamine – was one species or several. But at least botanists now knew roughly where to look. Slowly the mists were beginning to clear, and once again it was a generalist – admittedly the most brilliant scientific all-rounder of his day – who showed the way.

When Baron Alexander von Humboldt set sail for South America in the summer of 1799 accompanied by the French botanist Aimé Bonpland, he boasted to a friend that he intended to 'walk from California to Patagonia'. 'I'll collect plants and animals, I'll analyse heat and electricity, and the magnetic and electric content of the atmosphere . . . I'll measure mountains, but my true purpose is to investigate the interaction of all the forces of nature.' Such a feat was well within his abilities. Part geographer, part naturalist and engineer, it is said that Humboldt's intellect encompassed every branch of the known sciences – hence his soubriquet as 'the universal man'.

Disembarking at Cumaná, in Venezuela, he and Bonpland were soon about their work. First they investigated the famous 'oil birds' of Caripe – prized by the Indians for their fat – then they paddled up the Orinoco River in a dugout, gathering plant specimens and conducting bizarre experiments on, among other things, electric eels. Next, having reached Esmeralda – the site of Spruce's travails fifty years later – they retraced their steps and proceeded along the Brazo Casiquiare. It was here that they came face to face with the full horror of the biting insects. More importantly, in navigating the natural canal Humboldt not only proved that the Orinoco and Amazon river systems were linked but that the Brazo Casiquiare flows south across

the continental divide into the Río Negro – a hydrological phenomenon that European geographers had previously considered impossible.

Having completed their investigations in Venezuela, Humboldt
and Bonpland then set sail for Cuba and, after a long delay,
Cartagena, with the intention of circumnavigating the globe.
Humboldt's idea was to proceed by sea to Guayaquil and then on to
Lima where he hoped to hitch a lift on a passing French schooner.
But hearing that the winds were unfavourable and the journey might
take two or three months, he opted instead for the more arduous
overland route via the Magdalena River to Bogotá and from there to
Quito. Not only would the journey enable them to pay their respects
to Mutis but also it would take them directly through the cinchona
forests of Colombia and Ecuador.

The first leg took eight weeks and, for all but Humboldt, the
journey was an ordeal. Bonpland had only recently got over a bout of
typhus fever on the Orinoco. But now as they poled slowly up the
Magdalena River he began to feel ill again. This time he had malaria
and as he shivered and sweated it became clear he was not alone:
seven of their rowers were also showing signs of the illness. At Honda,
where the Magdalena runs swift and narrow, three of the party were
so sick they had to remain behind. But Bonpland struggled on,
climbing with Humboldt over the Andes and across the chill
savannah of Bogotá at two thousand six hundred metres. Fortunately
they had sent letters ahead warning Mutis of their imminent arrival
and a party of dignitaries accompanied by the archbishop's six-horse
carriage rode out to welcome them.

Mutis – then sixty-nine years old – received the European
explorers in his library with great ceremony. Tall and heavy set, with
dark, piercing eyes, grey hair, and a series of chins that cascaded over
his clerical bands, he cut a majestic figure. By now his fame was
celebrated throughout Europe. Linnaeus had bestowed on him the
accolade 'Nomen immortale, quod nulla aetas numquam delebit.' His herbarium housed twenty thousand plants and a team of thirty draughtsmen. Under his direction they had executed six thousand botanical
illustrations. However, he was not so famous that he had forgotten

how to be a physician and hearing that Bonpland was ill his first act was to administer a decoction of one drachm (60 grains, or 3,900mg) of powdered bark dissolved in half a cup of hot water. Having cured Bonpland's malaria he then invited him to tour his institute. Bonpland and Humboldt were suitably impressed. So impressed in fact that they remained in Bogotá examining the collection for five months and later inserted a portrait of Mutis, together with a grateful inscription, in their *Plantes Equinoctiales*. The result was that it was September before they were ready to leave for Quito.

The journey took four months and the conditions were appalling. Rain and sleet assaulted them on their climb up the through the pass of Quindiu, and on the way down their feet became covered in *niguas* – tiny parasites that burrow into the soles of the feet and toes. Christmas was spent camping at three thousand metres. Cold and hungry, Humboldt for once lost his equanimity, commenting that 'it would hardly be possible to picture a more horrible road.' Then, when they limped into Quito, there was more depressing news: the French schooner they had been hoping to sail in would not be calling at Lima after all.

Geography's loss was botany's gain. Humboldt had no choice but to remain in Ecuador and apply his body and mind to other challenges. The first was to conquer Chimborazo, the 'monarch of the Andes', which rises to 6,310 metres – then thought to be the highest mountain in the world; the second was to travel to Loja and examine the tree whose febrifugal bark had proved such a boon to mankind.

Today, only Humboldt's conquest of Chimborazo is remembered. He and Bonpland ascended to 5,878 metres – a feat that was not surpassed until the development of Himalayan climbing. But in visiting Loja they also cleared up some important misconceptions about cinchona's taxonomy. First, they showed that the Colombian *Cinchona lancifolia*, described by Mutis in 1793, was a completely different species from the *cascarilla roja* of Loja. Second, they proved that Linnaeus' description of the species, which he called *Cinchona officinalis*, was a composite, based upon the sample La Condamine had sent him and another completely different specimen that Mutis had sent years later from Colombia. According to Humboldt, the reason for Mutis's mistake was that he had paid insufficient attention to the forms of cinchona's leaves. In fact, as Humboldt observed, these varied considerably even in plants of the same species, the length and shape depending as much on the climate, elevation and whether the trees grew in isolation or in clumps.

This was an important insight. It was later shown that the colour of cinchona leaves varied at different heights even on the same plant, and the shape of the leaves could also be different depending on their position on the same branch. But the most important characteristic of cinchonas – which was only discovered in 1948 – is that their flowers are heterostylous, making self-pollination extremely improbable. The result is that hybridization is extremely common. Indeed, it was only by trial and error – principally by comparing the alkaloids in the bark and further expeditions to the Andes – that botanists were eventually able to narrow down the distinctive characteristics of the genus.[5] This process would take a further forty years and even then it would not be complete. But after Humboldt botanists could have little doubt about the complexity of the task facing them.

To recap, cinchonas grew thousands of metres above sea level in some of the most inaccessible ranges of the Andes. On one side they were protected by the Amazon, on the other by precipitous mountain passes and near-impenetrable rainforest. And to top it all, the trees producing the most valuable bark varied in size, shape and colour depending on the climate, altitude, soil and their propensity for cross-pollination. No wonder it was so difficult to work out which were the *true* cinchonas. The Indians could hardly have devised a more fiendish defence if they had tried.

Now there was another complication: politics. Spain's South American empire was breaking up. The nascent Andean republics were at war with each other and themselves. Travel in the highlands of Ecuador, Peru and Bolivia – treacherous at the best of times – was becoming positively dangerous. Militias under the command of tinpot generals roamed the countryside, press-ganging men and supplies into their makeshift armies. To complicate the botanists' task further, in 1844 Bolivia passed laws establishing a national cinchona bank and banning the export of cinchona without a licence. The idea was to protect their monopoly by regulating the trade to discourage smugglers and the reckless stripping of the forests. But this is not what happened. Instead, the company to which the government had granted the monopoly paid the *cascarilleros* such pitifully low prices for their bark that they had even less incentive to practise good husbandry than before. The result was that by the 1850s the cinchona forests were slowly but surely being raped to exhaustion and no one seemed to be able to stop it.

Curse or no curse, something had to be done. Mutis had first identified the issue when he submitted his request to Charles III for a botanical expedition eighty years previously. Now another warning echoed across the Andes, this time from the summit of Chimborazo. 'If the governments in America,' wrote Humboldt, 'do not attend to the preservation of the quina either by prohibiting the felling of the trees or by obliging the territorial magistrates to enforce the cutters to guard them from destruction, the highly esteemed product of the New World will be swept from the country.'

*Chapter Four*

# THE VISION

The blows of the axe revived our strength as by enchantment and very soon we were near that great and magnificent tree which I was seeing for the first time, and which
for so long had been the object of my dreams.

M. Delondre, French quinine hunter,
on reaching the *calisaya* forests of northern Bolivia

IT IS ONE THING to attempt to steal a nation's botanical property
but quite another to transport it across jungle and oceans to a continent
ten thousand kilometres to the east. Rogue waves and jealous Indians
are only the beginning of one's problems. To succeed, the cinchona
hunters first needed to find a sure way of preserving the young plants
during the arduous sea crossing to Europe – a voyage that involved
fluctuations in temperatures from well below freezing at Cape Horn
to more than 100 degrees Fahrenheit at the equator.

Until the early nineteenth century the standard method for moving
botanical specimens from one continent to another was to pack them
in crude wooden boxes fitted with hoops and loops over which a
rough canvas was stretched to shield them from the sun. Usually the
boxes were lashed to the deck or, if the captain would allow it, in his
cabin. But the boxes had to be continually monitored to ensure that
the plants had sufficient moisture and were free of mould and it was
usually a toss-up whether or not they made landfall alive.

Dr Nathaniel Bagshaw Ward, a general practitioner from the East End of London, hit on a completely new method of plant transportation in 1829. A member of the Linnean Society and an amateur naturalist, Ward made his discovery by chance when he buried the chrysalis of a sphinx butterfly in a moist mould at the bottom of a bottle and covered it with a lid. A week later he was surprised to notice that a seedling fern and grass had sprouted in the mould. He observed that during the day when sunlight heated the mould the moisture, unable to evaporate, condensed on the side of the glass, then towards evening when the glass cooled ran back down the bottle to the mould, maintaining a constant humidity. Incredibly, the fern and grass lived for four years until the lid finally rusted and rainwater got into the bottle while Ward was on holiday.

Ward had stumbled on the principle of a unique specialized environment: during the day, the soil produces moisture through evaporation, and the plants absorb the carbon dioxide and photosynthesize it with the help of the sun; during the night they emit more carbon dioxide and vapour. As long as there are sufficient nutrients in the soil and sufficient light, the conditions are perfect for plant life.

Ward had often spoken with William Hooker and members of the Horticultural Society about the problems of transporting plants from the colonies. In 1833 he decided to try an experiment. Taking the old wooden cabins, and using his bottle as a model, he manufactured two cases with glass sides and tops that could be hermetically sealed. He then filled the cases with ferns and grasses and sent them to Sydney.

The plants arrived in perfect condition. The real test, however, came on the return journey. This time the cases were filled with native Australian ferns and despatched to London via Cape Horn and Río. The temperatures on board fluctuated from 100 degrees at Sydney to 20 degrees at Cape Horn, where the decks were covered with snow, to 120 degrees crossing the equator. Nevertheless on reaching the English Channel the plants, which had been placed on deck and never watered, were perfectly preserved.

News of Ward's invention fired collectors' imaginations. Now any plant or flower, no matter how fragile or exotic, could be transported from the tropics and raised in greenhouses in England. One of the first to exploit the new invention was the Duke of Devonshire. In 1835 his gardener, Joseph Paxton, sent a young man from the Duke's estate at Chatsworth to India to gather orchids and *Amherstia nobilis*, a tree famed for its startling blood-red flowers. On his return, the collection caused a sensation and soon royals and aristo-crats throughout Europe were ordering Wardian cases for their own greenhouses.

The real impact, however, was on economic botany. One of the first to use the Wardian cases in a systematic way was the Horticultural Society. In 1843 Robert Fortune, a Scottish horticulturalist on secondment from its Hothouse Department in west London, sailed for China with orders to bring new plants and seeds to enliven its collections – in particular Chinese orchids, aquatics and plants with 'very handsome flowers'. Braving hostile mobs and suspicious customs officials, in 1846 he succeeded in sending eight Wardian cases from Canton packed with the sweetly scented winter-flowering honeysuckle, *Lonicera fragrantissima*, lace bark pine and the graceful bleeding heart, *Dicentra spectabilis*.

Two years later he was back in China, this time as an employee of the East India Company. Not satisfied with forcing the Chinese to partake in its opium trade, the company now wanted Fortune to smuggle 'the finest varieties of the Tea-plant, as well as native manu-facturers and implements, for the Government plantations in the Himalayas.' Disguising himself as Chinese, Fortune gathered up his Wardian cases and set off for the Hwuy-chow district, three hundred kilometres inland from Ningpo. Staying at rudimentary Chinese inns or in Buddhist temples so as not to arouse suspicion, he rapidly amassed a collection of plants from the three main tea-growing districts of China. Sowing two hundred and fifty seedlings in the cases, Fortune then set off for the Himalayas. The teas sprouted en route and on arrival two hundred and fifteen of the plants were found to be in perfect condition, laying the foundations of the Assam and Sikkim tea industry.

Interestingly, it was the Dutch – always more commercially minded than the British – who first attempted to use the new technology to solve the fraught problem of transporting cinchona overseas and, coincidentally, their effort came at the very moment that Spruce was lying ill with malaria on the Orinoco.

For many years, Dutch botanists had been urging their government to introduce cinchona to their colonies in south-east Asia. But it was not until 1852 that Charles Pahud, the Dutch Minister of the Colonies, was authorized to employ an agent. The man he selected was Justus Charles Hasskarl, a botanist and the former superintendent of the Dutch gardens at Buitenzorg in Java. Armed with twenty Wardian cases, Hasskarl set sail for South America in December 1852 with orders to collect as many valuable species of cinchona as possible. His original orders were to land at Guayaquil and proceed first to Loja, but Hasskarl changed his mind en route, landing at Lima instead and crossing the cordilleras in May 1853.

His first stop was Uchubamba in northern Peru, where he collected a number of plants of a species he called *Cinchona ovata*. But his real goal was the *calisaya* forests of southern Peru and in September he made his way south via Cusco to Sandia, a town near the border with Bolivia. So as not to arouse the suspicion of the *cascarilleros*, Hasskarl posed as a nature lover, saying he liked nothing better than wandering in the cinchona forests contemplating the unspoilt beauty of the eastern Andes. Unfortunately, Hasskarl arrived too late in the *calisaya* flowering season and, finding the seed panicles burst, returned to Lima to bide his time until the following year.

Hasskarl was next seen at Sina, a tiny village on the frontier between Peru and Bolivia, in April 1854. This time he had assumed a false name, Dr José Carlos Muller, and was posing as a businessman of German extraction. Presenting Muller's card to the local governor, Hasskarl had a proposal: would the governor be willing to help him procure a supply of *calisaya vera* – the so-called 'true' cinchona of Bolivia? The governor declined, probably out of fear, for the Bolivians were notoriously protective of their bark trade and willing, if necessary, to defend their monopoly on *calisayas* by force. Instead he introduced

Hasskarl to a Bolivian, Clemente Henriquez, a dishonest and unscrupulous local fixer. For a down payment of $50, Henriquez agreed to procure four hundred *calisaya* plants with a further $100 to be paid on delivery thirty days later. But soon after arriving in the Bolivian bark forests Henriquez was arrested for illegal collecting and fled back to Sina. There he employed a local Indian to gather plants on the Peruvian side of the border while he confined his own collecting to an area near the Bolivian frontier.

In June he presented the fruits of his labour to Hasskarl. There were some *calisayas* but of the wrong Peruvian variety, and all sorts of other cinchonas besides. Hasskarl, however, did not know this. Instead, he paid Henriquez the balance of the money he owed him and set off across the cordillera to Arequipa and to the port of Islay where he loaded the plants onto a waiting Dutch frigate, the *Prinz Frederik der Nederlander*, and resumed his real identity.

No sooner had he set sail than news of his deception reached the *cascarilleros* in Sandia. Believing their livelihoods were about to be destroyed by the transplantation of the *calisayas* to Java, they threatened to cut off Henriquez's feet, forcing him to flee a second time – this time back to Bolivia.

They need not have worried. Unknown to Hasskarl, Henriquez had taken the precaution of mixing arsenic with the earth in the Wardian cases. The result was that by the time Hasskarl reached Batavia on 13 December only two of the plants were still alive. Luckily for him, he had also obtained some seeds and when these were planted in Tjbodas, a range of mountains south of Batavia, they germinated. Pahud was so delighted he made Hasskarl Knight of the Netherlands, Lion and Commander of the Order of the Oaken Crown, and nominated him director of the cinchona plantations, which were to be expanded.

Such are the rewards of crime when it is carried out in the name of the state. But fortunately for the Bolivians the Dutch celebrations were premature. Not only was Tjbodas unsuitable for cinchona cultivation but subsequent analysis of the bark from the plants – named *Cinchona pahudiana* in the minister's honour – showed they contained hardly any quinine at all. Hasskarl's fate was sealed. In 1856 Pahud, now Governor-General of Netherlands India, relieved him of his duties and handed the direction of the gardens to a more experienced botanist, Dr Franz Junghuhn.

It had been an audacious attempt by the Dutch, but not for the first time a scheme to steal cinchona from South America had failed due to human error.

Few men had the perspicacity or patience to learn from such blunders but it just so happened that one such man was in Peru now. What is more he had run into Muller/Hasskarl at Cojata, a town on the shores of Lake Titicaca, shortly before the Dutch botanist had returned to his rendezvous with Henriquez at Sandia. The man's name was Charles Ledger. Unlike Hasskarl he was not a botanist but a merchant. But by the time of Hasskarl's arrival in South America Ledger had already spent seventeen years in Peru and knew more about the famous *calisaya vera*, or yellow bark of northern Bolivia, than any European alive.

Born on 4 March 1818 in Stockwell, south London, Ledger was just six months younger than Spruce. He came from a large, upwardly mobile working-class family. His father was a mercantile broker and although Ledger described himself as 'a real cockney' there was French blood in the family. His father's ancestors had been Huguenots – Protestant refugees from religious persecution in France – and as a boy Ledger's uncle's house in Smithfield had been a popular meeting place for exiles fleeing the revolution. After apprenticing as a silver-smith, Ledger had set sail for Peru in 1836 on the steamship *Swallow*, with the aim of making his fortune from the growing trade in cinchona bark and Peru's other great export, alpaca wool. Working his own passage, his only possessions were a box of steel pens, a prized novelty that he intended to sell in South America, and a letter of introduction to several British trading firms in Lima. His investment in the pens paid off as soon as he landed at Buenos Aires, where he sold them for a small profit. Then the *Swallow* proceeded to Lima, where Ledger found a job as a clerk at Naylor's, a respectable British merchant house. Englishmen of Ledger's education were rare in Peru at that time and after learning the Spanish language and Naylor's administrative procedures he was put in charge of one of its branch offices in Tacna. Located between Lake Titicaca and the coast, it was one of the firm's most important trading outposts and it was through here that all the best quality Bolivian bark and alpaca wool flowed. Ledger quickly realized that to the untutored eye all the barks looked the same reddish-brown – to succeed he would have to become as expert as the Indians at telling one from the other. He threw himself into the study, learning to distinguish the Bolivian *roja* from the inferior *calisaya* barks from Peru. He also learned how to select only the bark from the *tabla*, or trunk of the tree, ignoring the bark from the small branches, and how to prepare the *serons*, the hides used to transport the bark in a dry condition to England.

By 1842 Ledger decided he had learned as much as he could at Naylor's and set up on his own. He at once recruited a Bolivian Indian, Manuel Incra Mamani, who he had met the year before at La Paz. Very little is known about Mamani other than that he was from the highlands of northern Bolivia, was either of Quechuan or Aymara Indian descent and possessed a phenomenal knowledge of cinchonas. Like the best *cascarilleros*, he could spot the trees simply by surveying the rainforest canopy. Nothing escaped his attention – a handful of brightly coloured leaves carried by the wind into his path, the peculiar lustre of a leaf tip; either was sufficient to warrant further investigation. Gradually, during their long rides together into the Peruvian interior – Ledger on his mule and Mamani on foot chewing coca – the Indian began to impart his deep love and affection for the tree to his master. It was a profound friendship and one that would bestow incalculable benefits on mankind.

Ledger quickly realized that Mamani had a better grasp of cinchona than any European botanist. During one journey he distin-guished twenty-nine different varieties, pointing out the ones likely to contain the highest amounts of quinine. He was also deeply religious. Every now and again they would come to a group of five cinchonas, planted as per the Jesuits' instructions in the sign of a cross, and he would fall to his knees in order to pray for the departed souls of the 'buenos padres'. In this way Ledger's appreciation of the tree began to grow and it was not long before he too was imbued with respect for the valuable calisayas.

By now good quality bark was becoming increasingly hard to find. The idea behind the Bolivian cinchona bank had been to regu-late the supply of bark and so protect this valuable natural resource for the future. But the monopoly measures simply encouraged a black market trade in calisaya bark. The result was that, despite Humboldt's warning, by the 1850s the cinchona forests were slowly but surely being raped to exhaustion. It was against this background that the Dutch and British began to argue that it was their humanitarian duty to 'save' this valuable plant before it disappeared.

Meanwhile in Peru the Bolivian monopoly had brought the authorities to a different conclusion. Worried that they were not exploiting the full potential of their own forests, the Peruvians invited Ledger to lead a fifty-six-man expedition to locate new supplies of Peruvian calisaya in Huánuco, a region north of Carabaya. Although Mamani was sceptical of discovering cinchona there, Ledger was convinced his fortune was made. 'I, with many others,' he later recalled, 'entertained no doubts but that we should succeed in dis-covering large quantities of the best calisaya making rapid fortunes.' Each man put up five hundred silver dollars of his own money and on 16 March 1845 the expedition started from Puno.

Mamani was right. They did not find one genuine calisaya, returning three months later empty-handed. Ledger was bitterly dis-appointed. But there had been no deaths or accidents and during the long and often arduous expedition Mamani had given Ledger an important insight into the distribution of cinchona.

The key conversation took place one night on their way back to Puno. Ruminating on the failure of the expedition, Ledger suddenly turned to Mamani and asked: 'Do you think we shall find the true bark?' Mamani's reply was instant: 'No, Señor, the trees here about do not see the snow-capped mountains.'

'I could hardly contain my laughter at the moment,' Ledger later recalled in a letter to a friend in London, 'but when in bed about an hour after I could not sleep for thinking of Manuel's answer.'

The next day, Ledger unfurled his map and began examining Mamani's proposition. He was right. The cinchona forests stretched from Bogotá, Colombia, in the north to Santa Cruz, Bolivia, in the south. But the best red barks were found in Apolo, Sorata and Coroico – the forests dominated by the peaks of Akamani and Illimani in northern Bolivia – or in Loja, Cuenca and Alausí, in Ecuador, which were overlooked by the volcano Chimborazo.

It was a crucial discovery, one that would hold the key to the success of future cinchona missions. However, Mamani's insight would not be fully appreciated until years later when the British and Dutch began testing the bark of different varieties of cinchona collected in South America in their plantations in India and Java. For the moment, botanists were a long way from appreciating the relationship between the quinine content of the bark and the climatic, topograph-ical and other environmental conditions governing where the best trees grew; and the reason, once again, was the curse.

In 1843 another group of scientific explorers set sail from France, under the ensign of King Louis Philippe. The expedition was led by the Comte de Castelnau, an indefatigable traveller and sophisticated man of letters, and included two botanists, the Vicomte d'Osery and Dr Hugues Algernon Weddell. Unlike Ruiz and Pavon, Weddell did not plan on stopping at the borders of Peru. Inspired by Joseph de Jussieu, he would penetrate the cinchona forests of Bolivia and make a thorough study of the trees from which the most valuable bark of all came – the *calisayas*. This was no longer considered folly but a matter of commercial and political necessity.

By the 1840s France had a colonial empire in north and central Africa and Indo-China that was also plagued by malaria. Like the British and Dutch, the French wanted to transplant cinchonas to their colonies so that they would be assured of a steady supply of quinine.

And like the Dutch they had set their sights on the Bolivian *calisaya* barks. Thanks to the advances in pharmacology, chemists now knew that the *calisayas* contained the highest levels of quinine of all, but besides de Jussieu no qualified European botanist had ever set eyes on the tree. Ignorant of Ledger and Mamani's expertise, this was now one of the main goals of the Castelnau expedition. Weddell and d'Osery would enter Peru and Bolivia, collect as many plants and seeds as possible and then return to Paris. From there it would be a simple matter to send the *calisayas* to north Africa to be raised in plantations in Algiers – or so the French calculated.

Sailing from Brest, the expedition stopped briefly at Senegal, before landing in June at Río de Janeiro. They spent two years in Brazil, exploring the forests of the Amazon, and then headed for the Urubamba River in Peru. It was at this point that the first in a series of disasters befell them. Castelnau was leading Weddell and d'Osery through an area inhabited by wild forest Indians when they awoke one morning to find that their guides had deserted them and they were headed towards a dangerous waterfall. Fearing they were about to be murdered or that their baggage would be swept overboard, Castelnau decided to divide the party. D'Osery was sent to Lima with their precious manuscripts while Castelnau and Weddell continued down-river. Incredibly, d'Osery reached Lima safely and then set off back to the Amazon to rejoin the expedition, which by now had emerged from the forest unscathed. Unfortunately, the authorities in Lima had supplied him with the wrong sort of guides – four headhunting Jivaro. Somewhere on the Río Marañón, d'Osery disappeared. He was never seen again.

At first Weddell had better luck. In early 1845 he returned to Brazil with Castelnau and headed for the Mato Grosso. Then, in May, he parted from Castelnau and set off alone for Bolivia via Paraguay. He entered Bolivia at Campos in August and after passing through the country of the Chiquito Indians travelled south to Tarija. It was here, in January 1846, near the nineteenth parallel, that Weddell established the southernmost limits of the cinchona zone, naming the local species *Cinchona australis*. Next he headed north, via Potosí and

Cochabamba, until he reached the Yungas, the chain of subtropical valleys that roll east and north of the Bolivian Andes. Here, Weddell writes, 'the different species of cinchona multiplied before my eyes' and when he stopped at Enquisivi he got his reward: the tree that yielded the precious *calisaya* bark.

Weddell spent several months in the Yungas gathering information on the collecting of *Cinchona calisaya*, as he christened the tree. The *cascarilleros*, he observed, worked in teams, the most experienced of whom were known as *diestros*. It was the *diestros'* job to make a preliminary survey of the forest, penetrating the woods in several different directions to establish where the greatest concentrations of cinchonas were. This took great skill, as *calisayas* are rarely found growing in patches or clumps, but are more often found singly, lost in a sea of green. 'It is by the slightest indications that he recognizes the object of his search', wrote Weddell. 'The smallest glint of light peculiar to the leaves of a species, the particular colour of the leaves, the peculiar character of a mass of inflorescence . . . Often dead leaves which he may encounter on the ground indicate the neighbourhood of cinchonas, and if they have been swept to the spot where he finds them by the wind, he knows from what direction they have been blown.'

Once the *diestro* had located the most promising area of the forest, the other *cascarilleros* would cut a path to it and then begin clearing the ground to make room for a drying hut. The smallest sheets of bark, from the branches or the small trunks, yielded the *canuto* – thin cylindrical pieces that curled up in the sun, hence their colloquial name, 'quilled bark'. The larger strips from the trunk of the tree provided the *tabla* or *plancha* – the slabs of bark that, once dried and pressed in the sun, formed the most valuable material for export. Despite the skill needed to spot the cinchonas, Weddell was hopeful of discovering many more species as he travelled north. But as he passed through the gold-mining area of Mapiri and headed to Apolobamba, near the border with Peru, Weddell was alarmed to discover that the forests had been stripped to such an extent that it

was necessary to journey for between eight to ten days to find a tree
still standing.

Eventually, in 1847, he crossed into Peru. After surveying the
forests in the province of Carabaya, he journeyed to the ancient Inca
city of Cusco where he was surprised to meet another Frenchman,
a M. Delondre, also interested in *calisaya*. Delondre had set up a
rudimentary plant for manufacturing quinine using machinery based
on Pellettier and Caventou's extraction method. Unfortunately the
Bolivians had just sold their entire quota of bark to a manufacturer
in New York and he had no material to process (the local bark,
of course, did not contain sufficient quinine to make commercial
extraction profitable). Desperate to obtain his own source of *calisaya*
Delondre decided to set up a smuggling operation. But the two men
he recruited died, one murdered by Indians, the other a suicide. With
nothing further to lose, Delondre agreed to join forces with Weddell
and together they set off for the *calisaya* forests of Santa Ana in Bolivia.

It was an awful journey. First they had to climb over the
mountains through sheets of freezing rain; then they plunged down
through the humid cloudforest. The only thing that lifted their spirits
was the clunk of an axe — a signal from their guides that they had
found the *calisayas*. 'We were exhausted,' Delondre later wrote, 'but
the blows of the axe revived our strength as by enchantment and very
soon we were near that great and magnificent tree which I was seeing
for the first time, and which for so long had been the object of my
dreams. I remained in ecstasies, gazing at its beautiful silvery bark, at
its large leaves of a greenish-brownish colour, and its flowers with the
sweetish perfume, slightly reminiscent of the lilac.'

Weddell's description, published in 1849 and in which he listed
nineteen different varieties of cinchona, was more sober and scientific.[1]
But Delondre's poetic tribute must have broken the curse, at least
temporarily, for both men returned safely — Delondre to his factory,
and Weddell to France. In so doing, Weddell succeeded where La
Condamine and de Jussieu had failed, for in his bags he carried the
first cinchona seeds ever to be exported from South America. Some of

those seeds germinated in the Jardin des Plantes in Paris, while others were given to the Horticultural Society in London and one to the Dutch in Java. However, the spirits that protected the tree had simply been toying with Weddell, for subsequent assays on the bark showed they contained very little quinine. What is more, when he returned to Bolivia a second time his luck deserted him and, on this occasion, Ledger was a witness.

By 1851 Ledger was becoming increasingly aware of the value not only of cinchona but also of alpaca. A miniature cousin of the camel, alpaca was first domesticated by the Inca and grazes on the slopes of the Andean highlands. Graceful and docile, its wool has a beautiful sheen that is highly prized both for its warmth and lightness. In 1836 the Bradford mills had overcome the problems of spinning alpaca wool and high prices were being paid for the fleeces in Europe. A number of attempts had been made to introduce the animals into England and other countries but few survived the sea voyage. In 1845, for instance, the *Sir Charles Napier* had left the coast of Peru with four hundred alpaca on board but on reaching the Thames only three were still alive. To the Indians, for whom the alpaca was sacred, the news was a bad omen. 'I shall never forget the commotion among the Indians on the news of this disaster,' wrote Ledger. 'Every misfortune that had happened in the district for the year past was attributed to these animals being sent out of the country.'

Nevertheless, Ledger — who had given up on cinchona for the moment — was convinced alpaca held the key to his fortune, and began crossing them with llama to increase their size. Next he began making enquiries about the climate and terrain in New South Wales with a view to exporting them to Australia from where, he calculated, he would be able to raise herds to supply the British Empire.

There was just one problem: just as the Bolivians had set up a national bark bank to preserve their *calisaya* forests so the Peruvians had banned the export of alpaca in a bid to protect their monopoly on the supply of wool. Penalties for those breaking the law were harsh – ten years hard labour on the guano islands.

In 1851 the Lima authorities turned away an Australian ship chartered for the express purpose of conveying a cargo of live alpaca to New South Wales. Ledger noted the incident with interest. He knew the Indians who bred the alpaca in the highlands better than any man. He also knew the country. Now, during his travels to the Bolivian frontier, he formulated an audacious plan. It was illegal to drive alpaca within sixty-five kilometres of the coast of Peru but there were no such constraints against their export from the coast of Chile or Brazil. The reason was that only a madman, or someone as determined as Ledger, would consider attempting such a feat. In order to reach Chile the alpacas would have to be driven across the Bolivian border, south through Bolivia into Argentina, and then over the Chilean Andes to the Pacific coast. The only other possibility was to drive the alpaca over the eastern range of the Bolivian cordillera down to the Amazonian plain, from where he could transport them by river to the Atlantic.

Of the two, the second option was probably the less likely to succeed. Even if the alpaca survived the treacherous descent to the Beni River, there was no guarantee they would survive the heat and humidity of the jungle. However, this is the route Ledger and Mamani now decided to explore. Ironically, in so doing, they would answer a question that had so far eluded Weddell: namely, what was the variety of cinchona with the highest level of quinine of all?

In 1851 Weddell had returned to South America with the intention of entering the Bolivian cinchona region of Tipuani and gathering plants and seeds of *roja*. After descending the eastern slopes of the Andes, Weddell sailed down the Tipuani River to Guanay, a mission of Lecos Indians, and then ascended the Coroico in a canoe. The riverbanks were crowded with grey cinchona and *Cascarilla magnifolia*, an allied genus with deliciously fragrant flowers. But the bark hunters considered both varieties 'carhua-carhua' – worthless. To find the true *calisaya* they had to venture deep into the forest, an undertaking that Weddell now discovered was fraught with danger.

Weddell had landed on a beach on the Coroico with the intention of camping for the night when he chanced upon the hut of a *cascarillero*. He had only taken a few paces when he spotted a man stretched out on the ground. Nearly naked, and covered with insects, the *cascarillero* was in his death throes. He had been stung all over his body and his face was so swollen that to Weddell it 'no longer appeared human'. On the roof of his hut were his only belongings: a straw hat, some ragged clothes, a knife and an earthen pot containing a little maize and two or three *chunus* – his last supper.

The image of the dead *cascarillero* haunted Weddell all the way back to Peru. It must have been an omen. Certainly that is the way it looked to Ledger when, for the first and only time, he met Weddell at Islay as he was about to embark for Europe. Ledger helped Weddell load two Wardian cases packed with *calisayas* he had collected in Bolivia onto the ship. But when they opened the cases to check the plants' condition, Weddell burst into tears. All the best specimens were dead. Only five small plants were still alive, but they were so sickly they stood little hope of surviving the voyage. 'After five months of immense anxiety, hard work, personal dangers and great expenditure, I could well understand how a strong man could be so affected,' wrote Ledger.

Weddell was too distraught to return to the forest. His mood was not helped by Ledger's description of a huge old *roja* tree that he and Mamani had seen growing at the house of an Italian curate in Apolobamba, in northern Bolivia. Feeling sorry for Weddell, Ledger agreed to collect some seeds from the tree during his next visit and forward them to him in France but, incredibly, no sooner had Ledger gathered the seeds and given them to a friend in Arequipa for safekeeping than the friend's house burnt down. Even so simple and innocent a request, it seemed, was doomed to failure. Weddell had promised to return to Peru in 1853 and go with Ledger to Caupolicán, but after this incident his spirit was broken and, as Ledger writes, 'I heard no more from him.'

Ledger was not so easily discouraged. Moreover, he knew the Indians. He had previously noted how Mamani had been reluctant to collect seeds for export. Now, sitting around the campfire, he questioned him more closely. To protect their livelihood, Mamani explained, the *cascarilleros* would often appear to do the gringo's bidding while secretly sabotaging the operation. A favourite trick was to expose the seeds to heat so that they became sterile; another was to mix the soil in the Wardian boxes with arsenic so that they would die on the voyage home.[2] Sensing Mamani's inner conflict Ledger did not pursue the subject, but the warning was noted. No wonder it was so difficult to smuggle cinchonas out of South America. Even if European botanists worked out which were the most valuable varieties and arrived at the right time to collect the seeds, the *cascarilleros* would be on hand to sabotage them.

Whether out of superstition or fear of his true intentions being discovered, Ledger now began to exercise extreme caution. In 1842 he had married Candelaria Ortiz, a woman from an influential local family in Tacna, and by the summer of 1851 she had borne him three daughters, Elena, Eliza and Isidora. In addition, his younger brother, Arthur, had joined him from England. If Ledger's plans for the export of alpaca or cinchona became known not only his life but also those of his family and even Mamani's could be in danger. Perhaps that is why Ledger's notes from this period suddenly become sketchier and less precise and why, when he wrote to friends in London, such as John Howard, a prominent quinine manufacturer in Tottenham, he left blank the names of people and locations.

From piecing his letters and journals together, however, it appears that Ledger and Manuel set off to explore a Bolivian passage for alpaca in October or November of 1851. Starting from Puno on the west side of Lake Titicaca, they followed the same route as Weddell, through the province of Caupolicán and down to the Bolivian Amazon. Even for two such hardy travellers, it was an arduous journey. The banks of the Amazon's upper effluents were already dangerously swollen, and even small mountain streams had been transformed into violent watercourses. Ahead of them lay a succession of almost impassable steep rocks and forests tangled with roots and vines. The route was so overgrown it was impossible for Ledger's mule to find a way through and soon he and Manuel were walking side by side, both of them chewing coca to keep up their stamina and to steady their heads from the dizzying altitude. After days of hacking through the forest they were about to give up hope when they reached a point where the headwaters of the Beni and Mamore rivers run close together. Suddenly on a slope behind a bend of one of the rivers – from Ledger's notes it is not clear which – they stumbled on a group of fifty huge *roja* trees in full bloom. Usually *calisayas* were found intermixed with other types of cinchona around a bigger and older *tata* (father) tree, but these were all alike and clustered together. Brilliant-coloured humming birds flitted in and out of the branches, savouring the delicate lilac-scented flowers. Combined with the scarlet of the leaves the sight must have been dazzling. Never had Manuel, let alone Ledger, seen such a magnificent group of cinchonas.

Because the trees were in bloom it was too early to collect their seeds and in view of the near-impassability of the terrain it was also impossible to harvest the bark. Besides Ledger had the more pressing business of the alpaca to attend to. Nevertheless, he would never forget the image of those *calisayas*. The vision would stay with him for eleven long years – a period during which no one would lay eyes on cinchonas of their equal again.

Unfortunately the exploratory route for alpaca proved a failure. The only other way of getting the animals out of Peru was to avoid the Bolivian cloudforest and take them across the altiplano to Argentina and then over the cordillera into Chile instead. But it was a long, difficult and dangerous route – a last resort at best. The only other possibility was illegal: driving the alpaca from the highlands across a forbidden sixty-five-kilometre strip of land direct to the Peruvian coast. Normally, this would be out of the question but it now appears that Ledger received encouragement from an unexpected quarter: the British government. I say 'appears' because the records are fragmentary and, according to Ledger, the impetus came from Mr Pitt-Adams, Her Majesty's chargé d'affaires in Lima. Given that Britain and Peru were at peace this was highly improper. According to Ledger, the reason was an Australian protest to British ministers in London about the recent expulsion of one of their vessels. However, there is no record of Pitt-Adams' having put anything in writing and Ledger's claim of official involvement may simply have been a fabrication to cover his subsequent actions. If so it would not be wholly out of character – Ledger's later career and writings indicate he was given to grandiose ideas and sweeping statements.

At this point Ledger's diary becomes even more vague. All that is known is that in March 1853 he left Tacna for Chulluncayani, the estate where he had been raising the alpaca, and began 'putting in motion' – as he put it – part of his herd. Avoiding the road that runs between Tacna and the coast, Ledger rode up the western cordillera towards the border with Bolivia. Presumably he was still exploring possible routes, but here his plans must have been betrayed or else something else went wrong for his diary records that he was detained at the frontier until September – in other words, for six months. It seems that it was during this period that he ran into Hasskarl at Cojata. Incredibly, despite the lengths he had taken to conceal his identity, Hasskarl dropped his pretence and, according to Ledger, confided the true purpose of his mission. Although Ledger was preoccupied with the alpaca that conversation rekindled his interest in cinchona. For Hasskarl confided that the Dutch had been willing not only to underwrite all his expenses but also to provide him with a frigate for the return journey. Years later Ledger's memory of that conversation would become a source of bitterness – one more debit to be added to his tally against the Dutch and British.

The seeds of Ledger's resentment had been planted in 1845 after the failure of the expedition to Carabaya. Realizing that supplies of cinchona were increasingly in short supply, he had written to his father in London 'urging him to solicit the attention of the East India Company or the Government of Great Britain' for a plan to raise *Cinchona calisaya* in India, Jamaica and Ceylon. At the time imports of quinine to India totalled some eight tonnes a year. Indicating how the plants and seeds could be obtained, Ledger had pointed out that all it would take to cut Britain's supply line was 'a miserable war between Peru and Bolivia.'

Ledger had not even received the courtesy of a reply. Marooned in Peru eight thousand kilometres from home, with neither connections nor influence, he was a nobody, just another distant subject of the great British Empire. Perhaps that is why he latched onto the alpaca. The Australians were interested and, if he is to be believed, so were the British. But before gambling everything on such a risky venture he had to be sure that conditions in New South Wales were right for breeding the animals.

He spent the next year at Tacna planning his trip to Australia. His mind was made up: the way to fortune lay in alpaca, not cinchona. Ironically, his obsession with the revered animal of the Inca would lead him to miss the arrival in Peru of an ethusiastic young Inca scholar, a man who would soon be in a position to provide Ledger with the very entrée into the British establishment he so desperately craved.

Chapter Five

# THE PHILANTHROPIST

The almost inappreciable value of the cinchona, commonly called Peruvian bark ... is universally acknowledged. Hence it becomes a duty to humanity ... to
increase the supply of the cinchona trees which yield such
valuable barks.

Memorandum from Dr Forbes Royle to
East India House, March 1857

AT THE HEADQUARTERS of the Royal Geographical Society in
Kensington, London, hang portraits of its distinguished past presidents: Earl Curzon of Kedlestone, Lawrence Dundas, second Marquess of Zetland, and Sir Clements Markham. The paintings are for
the most part dull and uninteresting – oils so darkly rendered they
strain the eye. However, the one of Markham repays scrutiny.

Markham was an explorer of the old school. When he sat for the
artist, George Henry, the year was 1913 and 'Clemmie' – as he was
known to his family and friends – was eighty-three. The Society's
longest-ever serving president, Markham had been geographer to the
Abyssinia Expedition of 1868 and the guiding light behind Scott's
two expeditions to the Antarctic. It is the last for which he is best
remembered, his patronage earning him the reputation as the 'father'
of polar exploration.

But surprisingly his portrait contains only one allusion to the poles

– a small silver sledge – and none to Scott's ship, the *Discovery*, which he both fitted out and brought back after it became trapped in the ice. Instead, on a wall beside the chair in which he is pictured the artist has rendered a painting of '*Cinchona Uritusinga*'. The species is credited to 'Pavon' – the Spanish botanist who accompanied Ruiz on the tragic expedition to Peru and Chile in 1778. But it is by its original name *Cinchona officinalis* or, more colloquially, '*cascarilla fina*', that it is better known.[1] It is of course the famous red bark tree of Loja, the one that supposedly cured the Condesa and whose seeds – along with those of the *calisaya* – were deemed so valuable by the British and Dutch.

The reference is no accident. Although his role in the quest for cinchona is all but forgotten today, Markham considered it his finest hour. He may not have possessed Spruce's botanical expertise, or had Ledger's local knowledge of Peru and Bolivia, but he more than made up for it with his vision and will to succeed. More importantly, Markham had the right political connections. It was those connections that made him the focus – at least as far as the public was concerned – of the quest for quinine. Markham was both the lightning rod and facilitator of that hunt. His genius was to present the plot to steal the seeds and plants from under the noses of the nascent Andean republics not as theft but as philanthropy. To some extent his argument was justified, for by the 1850s the South American bark forests were rapidly being stripped to exhaustion. More importantly, it was Markham who brought Spruce into the hunt. He could have advanced Ledger's cause too but though they shared similar aims their paths never crossed. And by the time Markham learned of Ledger's expertise it was too late.

Born on 20 July 1830 at Stillingfleet in the West Riding of Yorkshire – no more than forty kilometres from Spruce's home town of Ganthorpe – Clements Robert Markham came from a long line of churchmen. His great-grandfather, Dr William Markham, had been Archbishop of York and tutor to both King George IV and William

IV. In 1827 the royal connection had brought Clements' father, the Reverend David Markham, the canonry at Windsor. The post required him to spend two months of the year at the Castle, where he was expected to dine every Sunday with the king and queen. The result was that as a boy Markham often found himself playing with more privileged children from Eton, an experience that no doubt gave him certain expectations in life.

His key role model, however, was his father. Tall, handsome and a keen cricketer, the Reverend Markham was not your stereotypical country vicar. He excelled at carpentry and was a keen student of both medicine and numismatics and it is from him that Markham seems to have acquired his love of academia. Educated at Cheam and later at Westminster, Markham was a precocious student. By the age of eleven he had written histories of England and all the ancient civilizations of the world, and a year later his interests had expanded to include historical biography, astronomy, geography and natural history. But it was in the navy that Markham acquired his lifelong passion: exploration. And his entrée came about because of family connections.

In 1844, after only two years at Westminster, Markham was invited to dinner at the house of his aunt, the Countess of Mansfield, in Portland Place. Either by luck or design he found himself seated next to Rear-Admiral Sir George Seymour, one of the Lords of the Admiralty. In the course of the conversation, the Admiral innocently asked whether Markham would like to join the navy and come out with him to the Pacific in his flagship, HMS *Collingwood*. Not realizing the full import of the offer, Markham said yes. Thus it was that at the age of fourteen he found himself enrolled as a navy cadet and setting sail for Peru, via Madeira, Brazil and the Falkland Islands. It would be the first of three visits to the land of the Inca, and on each occasion he would be drawn deeper and deeper into the country and its history.

Markham quickly proved himself an able cadet as well as something of a favourite with the officers. This, it seems, was due to both his looks and personality. He had fine delicate features, and according to one officer was easily 'the most engaging boy on board the ship'. But Markham found adjustment to the harsh naval regime, with its strict rules and regulations, difficult. Raised in a spirit of Christian forgiveness, he sometimes found the insistence on discipline and punishment at sea cruel and barbaric. And when, in 1845, a lieutenant to whom he had become particularly close was suddenly transferred to another ship he wrote that his heart was 'like lead' and he 'shed bitter tears'.

But for all his misgivings about the navy, Markham loved the sense of adventure that went with seafaring and wrote that his first sight of Lima had filled him with 'delight'. As soon as his naval duties allowed he set off on a tour of the Peruvian capital, visiting the crypt where Pizarro was buried and immersing himself in the histories of the conquest. HMS *Collingwood* sailed on but Markham left his heart in Peru, vowing to return one day to Cusco, the ancient Inca capital, and write a history of its people.

Although he now wanted to leave the navy his father was against it and Markham dared not go against his wishes. Besides, the navy still offered the consolation of travel and in 1850 he found himself in HMS *Assistance* as part of an expedition to the Arctic in search of the English explorer Sir John Franklin. Franklin had set out five years earlier to attempt to find the North West Passage linking the Atlantic with the Pacific. He had not been heard from since. In fact, it was later discovered, Franklin and his crew had frozen to death in 1847–8. Markham would later draw on his experiences in pursuit of Franklin to further the cause of polar exploration but for the moment it was not the poles but South America that obsessed him. Stuck in the Arctic ice during the winter of 1850–51, Markham seized the opportunity to reread W. H. Prescott's classic history of Peru until he knew it 'almost by heart'. He also began studying a Quechua grammar, which he had picked up in Lima. By the time he returned from the Arctic in September 1851 Markham's mind was made up. Telling his parents that 'all my wishes, hopes and aspirations are entirely apart from the Navy', he resigned his commission. However, it was not until the following summer that he plucked up the courage to tell his father of his new ambition, namely 'to go again to South America and search the interior for Peruvian remains.' The Reverend had set his sights on his son studying the law and at first opposed the plan, fearing that 'Clemmie' would not be able to support himself as a writer. Eventually, however, he relented, giving Markham £500 towards his expenses and using his influence to help him obtain letters of introduction to various dignitaries and officials in Peru. Thus it was that on 20 August, Markham left Windsor for Liverpool, crossing the Atlantic with two former messmates from the *Collingwood*. He would never see his father again.

Markham did not head straight for South America. Instead, he crossed to Halifax and proceeded along the coast of North America to New Brunswick and Boston in order to call on Prescott, the Inca historian. They spent ten days together. Between hands of whist, Prescott unhesitatingly approved Markham's expedition to Cusco, the 'navel' of the Inca Empire, saying that unless he was personally acquainted with the places and people he sought to describe he could not expect to write an informed history. However, the delay meant Markham did not set sail from New York until September. It was the beginning of a ten-month visit that would take him not only to Cusco but as far east as the cinchona forests of Urubamba on the Madre de Dios River. Unlike Ledger, Markham at this time knew little of the history of cinchona. He was also wholly ignorant of the importance that the India Office was beginning to attach to the seeds and plants. Later, after he became a part of what he fondly called the 'great work', it would strike him as ironic that at the same time that Britain was making its first efforts to obtain cinchona seeds he had been riding through the very valleys where some of the best trees grew.[2]

Markham's aim in visiting Peru was to survey the seat of Inca civilization and so elucidate the Incas' history by interweaving it with a narrative of his own travels – a very 'modern' ambition. This project would take him along Peru's narrow coastal strip as far as Nazca, site of the famous Nazca lines, over the Andes to Cusco and down the eastern slopes of the cordilleras to the Peruvian Amazon. During his journey Markham was received by past, present and future presidents of Peru and mixed with Peruvians of all classes and racial back-grounds. The trip resulted in two books, *Travels in Peru in 1853*, a two-volume account of his travels complete with drawings and watercolours, and *Cuzco and Lima*, a pedagogical introduction to Peruvian history. More importantly, from the point of view of his later role in the hunt for cinchona, it would give him an insight into Peruvian politics and the highland Indians, many of them descendants of the Incas, and a people for whom he felt a particular affinity.

Markham began his descent of the eastern Andes at the end of April, the beginning of the dry season, reaching Paucartambo, just above the Peruvian Amazon, on 2 May. Intent on following an old Inca trail, Markham first climbed to four thousand metres and then began a difficult zigzag descent to the rainforest. It was here that he saw his first *cascarilla* tree – *Cinchona ovata*, the same species that Hasskarl would later import to Java with such disastrous results. Ignorant as he was of botany, even Markham realized that this was 'not a valuable kind'. However, it was only when he reached the Madre de Dios River, an upper tributary of the Beni and, ironically, the same river on whose banks in Bolivia Ledger had spotted the rare group of *calisayas* the year before, that he had his first inkling of cinchona's potential.

Markham had gone to a hacienda in San Miguel to make the acquaintance of a Carmelite friar, an Italian by the name of Father de Revello. De Revello had spent six years in Paucartambo and as well as being an authority on the Inca was intimately acquainted with the *montaña*. Eight years previously a priest had been murdered at a farm overlooking the Madre de Dios – stuck through with arrows by wild Chucho Indians. The tale so alarmed Markham's guide that he refused to continue. But Markham was determined to see the river for himself and set off with Father de Revello alone. By the time they reached the farm where the priest had been murdered it was noon and the sun was 'scorching'. In order to view the Madre de Dios they had to cut through the jungle between the farm and the river with their machetes. It was worth the effort. The river, writes Markham, was a 'grand sight' and in the evening when they returned to the farm Father de Revello talked about his recently published pamphlet, *El brillante porvenir del Cusco*, 'The Splendid Future of Cusco'. 'He spoke of cinchona trees yielding quinine . . . of the Indian rubber trees, a source of boundless riches, of the balsam trees, the chonta palms, and bamboos and their many uses . . . Then in imagination he called up before his mind's eye the thousands of square miles that might be cultivated with coca, maize, coffee, cocoa, bananas, sugarcane and cotton and the happy Christian population such crops would sustain in comfort.' Father de Revello's agricultural utopia would never be realized, of course – that dream had disappeared with the Inca. But long after Markham returned to England he would recall the 'wealth of the *montaña*'. Father de Revello had planted a germ in Markham's mind –of the potential not only of cinchona but of rubber. That germ would grow and grow.

Markham returned to Cusco on 16 May and four days later reached the coast at Islay, where he boarded a steamer for Callao. A few days later he reached Lima. It was there he learned his father was dead. He heard the news in the cruellest way, through an obituary in *The Times*, and hurried back to England to be with his family. The homecoming brought Markham back to earth with a jolt. His father had been both a friend and mentor. Although he had never stopped him from pursuing his bliss, he had always urged on him the importance of a proper vocation. Now that the exhilaration of the Andes was over Markham had to face reality. He was broke. In order to have time to write his histories he would have to find a paying job, and quickly.

Fate now conspired to place him in one of the few places where he could be both financially secure and realize his wider ambitions. At first glance the Legacy Duty Office of the Inland Revenue where Markham was offered the post of junior clerk looked like a dead end. The job required him to spend his days in the gloom and dust of Somerset House, filling out ponderous registers and preparing indexes. But due to a bureaucratic anachronism the Inland Revenue was also responsible for the department of the Board of Control, an office that worked closely with the East India Company in administering the government of India. After just six months at Somerset House Markham was offered the chance to transfer to the Board's Secret and Confidential Branch. It was the perfect posting for him. Here Markham would be responsible for copying letters and despatches from India, Persia, Syria and the Orient and still have free time to write his histories. More importantly, he would also come to the attention of the officials who ran the India Office.

By the 1850s as many as two million adults a year were dying of malaria in India and a further twenty-five million had been afflicted with the disease at one time or another. Partly this was a result of the East India Company's disastrous 'land tax' policy, which had mired the peasantry in debt and led to the neglect of roads, canals and river works essential to controlling mosquito larvae. By the middle of the decade the Company was spending £100,000 a year on importing bark from South America for its employees, but it was not simply a question of cost, it was also a matter of supply. Writing to India House in 1852 Forbes Royle, the Reporter on Indian Products to the East India Company, had warned that Bolivia's national bark bank, rather than stabilizing the price of bark and protecting its monopoly, was leading to rapid inflation and the destruction of the *calisaya* forests.

At the same time, the British were also beginning to realize the value of quinine in furthering their wider colonial ambitions. Nowhere was this truer than in the 'white man's grave' of west and central Africa. From the Scottish shipbuilder MacGregor Laird's disastrous 1832 expedition up the Niger — when all but nine of his forty-nine crew members died of malaria — to the Niger Expedition ten years later (forty-two deaths out of a hundred and forty-five), British ambitions of penetrating the continent's 'dark' interior had been impeded by tropical disease.

Interestingly, the first person to apply the medical lessons of these expeditions was the missionary explorer David Livingstone. While practising medicine in Botswana, he had obtained a copy of the medical report of the 1842 Niger Expedition and noted the high incidence of malaria and the failure to administer quinine early enough. The result was that when he set out with his family for Makolo country in 1850 he made sure he brought ample supplies of quinine – a fact that almost certainly saved the lives of his son and daughter when they were suddenly stricken with malaria at Lake Ngami in northern Botswana. Two years later, travelling alone this time, Livingstone also contracted malaria and cured himself with quinine. The following year, in May 1853 – a few months before Spruce contracted malaria in Venezuela – he suffered another bout of fever at Luanda. From then on he took quinine regularly, both as a curative and a prophylactic, enabling him to survive the malaria-infested Zambezi and numerous other expeditions to central and southern Africa over a further period of twenty years.[3]

Livingstone was not the only medic to laud the prophylactic benefits of quinine. Although the importance of administering quinine wine to sailors *before* disembarking for work ashore had been recognized for some time, it gained new urgency from the West African squadron's experience on the Gold Coast and in the Bight of Benin, the notoriously malarious seas surrounding the vast Niger delta that inspired the sailor's refrain: 'Beware and take care of the Bight of Benin/There's one comes out for forty goes in.'

In 1854 William Balfour Baikie, a Scottish naval surgeon in charge of yet another expedition to the Niger, instituted a strict regime of quinine prophylaxis. The result was that his vessel, the *Pleiad*, made it to the confluence of the Niger and Benue rivers, from where he was able to chart a further three hundred and eighty kilometres of passable river to the east, and back again without a single loss of life (indeed, only two Europeans fell ill). Although Baikie – like all doctors at the time – remained ignorant of the connection between the mosquito and malaria, his conclusion was unequivocal: 'In no essential does African endemic fever differ from the fever of Hindustan, of Borneo, of the

Spanish Main, of the West Indies, or of fenny and marshy countries in Europe.' Moreover, in each case Baikie believed there was only one treatment – quinine.

In 1848 the army's medical department had also taken the first tentative steps towards quinine prophylaxis, directing its governors in West Africa in the use of quinine to prevent fever. And by the time of the Crimean War five years later quinine had become a standard precaution for both cavalry and infantry.[4]

As quinine's value became more and more obvious, Royle warmed to his theme. In March 1857 he wrote again to India House, arguing that it was now the government's 'duty to humanity' to gather cinchona seeds before the forests were stripped bare and raise the plant in India. 'The subject is yet of such great importance, both in an economical and philanthropic point of view, that every exertion should be made to ensure its accomplishment.' It was a clever argument. Anxious to maintain its reputation as the powerhouse of British botany, Kew Gardens had been campaigning for some time for the collection and cultivation of all the varieties of cinchona growing in the Andes. By recasting the theft as philanthropy Royle had provided the bureaucrats at the India Office with the perfect justification for putting Kew's plan into action.

It was against this background that the Court of Directors of the East India Company approved Royle's proposal to send an experienced plant collector to the cinchona forests. But Royle died before his plan could be activated. Then in May 1857 came the Indian Mutiny, plunging the British administration of India into crisis. Responsibility for the governance of India passed from the East India Company to the Crown and Royle's scheme was momentarily forgotten in the reshuffle of responsibilities. In November 1858 Kew's director Sir William Hooker tried to inject new urgency into the plan, writing to the India Office to warn, 'the Dutch have already got plantations of cinchona trees in Java 30 feet high, and we not a live plant in India for want of some energetic practical men to direct such operations.' The implied criticism of the Foreign Office's earlier lackadaisical approach was clear. The task was now too important to be left to the

South American consuls. But it was only with the appointment of Royle's successor, Dr Forbes Watson, that in March of the following year Lord Stanley, the Secretary of State for India, was persuaded that an expedition to South America for the sole purpose of obtaining cinchona was essential. The question was, who was to lead it?

By now Markham had spent five years as a clerk in the Special Department. He had used the time profitably, completing his history *Cusco and Lima* and contributing papers to the Royal Geographical Society, establishing his reputation as a Peru expert and explorer. In the summer of 1856 he had also met the love of his life, Minna Chichester. The daughter of the Reverend James Chichester, Rector of Arlington, Minna shared Markham's ecclesiastical upbringing and, like him, was a skilled linguist. They were married within a year and became lifelong companions, Minna accompanying Markham on many of his travels and helping him with his translations.

It is not clear when Markham first became aware of the importance of cinchona to India. It would be surprising if through his position in the Special Department he was not familiar with the growing correspondence on the subject between the India Office and the home government. However, it was only when Henry Deedes, Assistant Secretary in the India Office's Public Department, approached him with the proposal that he should lead the expedition that Markham became an enthusiastic convert to Royle's arguments. 'I gave the subject most careful consideration,' Markham later recalled, 'and being convinced that this measure would confer an inestimable benefit on British India, and on the world generally, I resolved to undertake its execution.'

It wasn't quite that simple, of course. Markham had no botanical qualifications and first had to convince the Council of India he was the right man for the job. In April he began a determined letter-writing campaign, reminding the Council's Chairman of Revenue and the Under-Secretary of State for India of his facility with Spanish and Quechua and his familiarity with the bark forests of Peru, as well as with the landowners of the eastern cordilleras. He argued that failure in the past had been due to leaving the work to agents and that great care and personal attention was needed during the collection and transportation of the seeds and plants to ensure they survived the journey and propagated. It was 'necessary', wrote Markham, to select someone 'whose heart is really in the business', adding that he was prepared to receive only his salary as a junior clerk (£250 per annum plus expenses).

Not everyone was convinced of Markham's suitability for the task. The *Gardener's Chronicle* predicted that his efforts would fail because of his ignorance of botany and science in general. But Markham's enthusiasm overrode any doubts his superiors may have harboured about his lack of qualifications and on 8 April Lord Stanley entrusted him with the commission.

It was a daunting responsibility for one so young. Markham was still just twenty-nine. Sure, he had visited one of the areas in Peru where cinchonas grew but his familiarity with the trees was cursory. Unlike Ledger he had never been to Bolivia and he certainly could not tell the difference between the red bark from Ecuador and the more valuable *calisayas* from Carabaya and Apolobamba. More importantly, Markham was a novice in the art of deception. During his visit to study the Inca remains the Peruvians had gone out of their way to welcome him. This time, however, they would put every obstacle in his path. In short it was the sort of commission that could make or break a man's career. Succeed and he would be elevated to the ranks of the great and the good. Fail and he would be consigned for ever to the dustbin of botany.

If Markham was worried about the consequences at this stage, however, he kept his concerns to himself. Instead, he threw himself into the study of cinchona. In the archives of the Royal Geographical Society two of Markham's notebooks from this period have survived. Lovingly bound in leather and labelled 'Cinchona Notebooks I and II', the pages are crisp and yellowing but the ink has hardly faded. Their contents attest to Markham's enthusiasm and thoroughness. There are extracts from letters to Weddell, notes of his conversations with John Howard, the Tottenham quinine manufacturer, and extracts from the archives at Kew. Markham noted down every variety of cinchona then known to botanists, beginning with their Linnean classification and followed by their commercial name, bark type and location. There are sketches of the leaves, styles and anthers, details of the climate and soils in which the cinchonas grow, and notes of the latitudes and elevations at which the best varieties are found. But most impressive of all is Markham's scholarship. He has read La Condamine in the original French, been to Madrid to examine for himself the writings of Ruiz and Pavon, translated Hasskarl's expedition from the Dutch. And, of course, he has consulted Humboldt.

Although it is true that Markham lacked the 'right' botanical qualifications, it is clear from his notebooks that he worked hard to correct that deficit. More importantly, he had a firm grasp of cinchona's medical and commercial importance and, as a Christian with a strong humanistic streak, was able to embrace the philanthropic argument seemingly without cant. Markham claimed that his aim was nothing less than the introduction of a cheap form of the cinchona febrifuge into every pansari's shop in India at a cost of one farthing or less. 'Thus,' he wrote, 'countless multitudes will be saved from death or grievous suffering.'

With this goal in sight, Markham was determined to leave nothing to chance. The Ecuadorian government had recently granted four and a half million acres of land between Loja and Cuenca to a private company in an attempt to reduce its foreign debt. But when the company had tried to interest the French and British in an exploratory mission aimed at transporting cinchonas from Ecuador to the East Indies and Algiers, Forbes Watson had rejected the plan, arguing that the best cinchonas grew in Bolivia. Markham now boldly insisted that if his mission was to succeed the collecting should not be confined simply to Bolivia but should extend throughout the whole cinchona range as far north as Colombia. Rather than sending just himself, he proposed that the India Office fund four separate but coordinated expeditions aimed at gathering the eight most valuable varieties of cinchona growing in the Andes. These included both the Bolivian *calisayas* and two varieties of red bark in Ecuador. In addition, collectors should be sent to Huánuco, the area in Peru that Ledger had explored unsuccessfully in 1845, for the so-called 'grey barks' and to Popayán for the Colombian barks. 'If the thing is worth doing at all, it is worth doing well,' he wrote to the India Office in July.

> It is now merely intended to send me to Peru, with a gardening assistant, to procure plants and seeds, and to convey them to India in the best way I can. The dangers, accidents and hindrances which might thwart me at every turn decrease the chances of success, because the whole thing would depend entirely upon the luck of one individual. In my opinion four separate expeditions should be sent in four different directions, their collections should be received on board one vessel, and taken direct to India; and thus all eight more valuable species of cinchona would be obtained.

In the end Markham only received permission for three expeditions: his own, another to Huánuco and a third to Ecuador. His aim was to penetrate deep into Bolivia and Carabaya in Peru in search of *calisayas* while his 'fellow-labourers', as he put it, mopped up the other cinchona species, much as assistant gardeners might rake up leaves. But Markham misread the political situation in Bolivia and had it not been for the success of the Ecuadorian expedition there would be little reason for associating his name with cinchona. That there is is due almost entirely to the labours of one man: Richard Spruce.

After his near-death experience with malaria at Maipures, Spruce had waved goodbye to the insect plagues on the Orinoco and returned to San Carlos. But, while he was now back on the mosquito-free waters of the Río Negro, he faced new threats.

In November 1854 Spruce began working his way downriver to São Gabriel with the intention of continuing his botanizing in Brazil. But on the journey to the Amazon his Indian guides hatched a plot to steal his money and murder him, reasoning that no one would be surprised to hear that a man as ill as Spruce had been had died. Fortunately, Spruce overheard their conversation and foiled the plot by lying awake all night in his canoe with one arm around his money chest and a double-barrelled shotgun propped on his knee. Reaching São Gabriel safely, he then descended the Amazon to Manaus and Santarém, where he caught a steamer back the way he had come to Peru. By the summer of 1855 he had established a collecting station at Tarapoto on the Marañón River and was busy acquainting himself with the local flora, including cinchona. It was his first chance to examine in nature the tree that had saved his life and he seized every opportunity to do so.[5]

By now Bentham and Hooker would have been aware of the importance that the government was beginning to attach to cinchona in India. As director of Kew, Hooker may not have had direct access to the India Office's reports, but through his many government contacts he would have known of its growing interest in the cinchona trade and would have been anxious to find a role for Kew in the developing enterprise. Who better than Spruce, a qualified botanical collector familiar with Spanish and the other Indian dialects and already in the Peruvian Amazon, to volunteer for the task? For whatever reason, however, his name was not put forward. Perhaps Hooker's influence did not extend as far as he would have liked, or perhaps he and Bentham feared for their friend's health. By 1856 Spruce had already endured six hard years in the jungle. As he would later bitterly recall, much of the time had been spent scrunched up in a dugout ankle-deep in water, his head and body exposed to the elements. His diet was monotonous – manioc, yams, smoked fish, sometimes if he was lucky a little beef or pork. He often had to do without sleep due to the heat, the attacks of venomous insects or, what was even more dangerous, the threats posed by his fellow man. And as he now reminded Hooker: 'The Venezuelans say very expressively that however completely a man may think he has thrown off the ague, there always remains a bit of it sticking to his backbone.'

There may also have been more practical reasons for Kew's hesitation. Although as the crow flies Chimborazo is only eight hundred kilometres from Tarapoto it is a far from easy journey. Today, it is possible to drive from Tarapoto to Jaén and then proceed north by road along the spine of the Andes to Ecuador's avenue of volcanoes. By 1857, however, Peru was in the throes of a bitter civil war and travel by road was impossible. This meant that the only way to reach Ecuador was by river. From Tarapoto Spruce would have to descend the Marañón to the Huallaga and then ascend the Pastaza to the Bobonaza, before proceeding by foot to the cinchona forests on the slopes of the Ecuadorian Andes. This would entail fighting his way up a series of rapids and whirlpools, forging rivers swollen by rain and cutting his way through dense jungle inhabited by head⁄hunting Jivaro Indians. In short, the terrain was so inhospitable that it would have been far simpler for him to return to Brazil via the Amazon and then take a ship around Cape Horn to Guayaquil. But in that case why not simply send a fully fit and healthy collector by steamer from England?

Spruce, however, was determined to reach Ecuador if for no other reason than that he was broke. Although he had more than £100 on account with Singlehurst & Co., the company that processed his botanical collections, the money had yet to arrive and he was tired of living on a shoestring. In December 1855 he wrote to Bentham from Tarapoto that he had met a traveller from Quito who had already ascended the Pastaza several times and was planning to return by the same route the following autumn. Recognizing that he would be risking 'a painful and dangerous voyage', Spruce told Bentham that he was inclined to accompany him. Quito, he had heard, was 'the most splendid station for a botanist in South America.' Besides, after so many years on the Amazon scrabbling for food and botanical paper, it would be 'such a fine thing to have headquarters where every necessary care be promptly obtained.'

Interestingly, the only mention of cinchona at this stage came not from Bentham or Hooker but from a London druggist, Daniel Hanbury. The Hanburys had long had an interest in medical botany, establishing a physic garden on the Italian Riviera, and together with their nephews the Allens ran a successful pharmaceutical manufac⁄

turing business in Spitalfields. On hearing of Spruce's arrival in Tarapoto, Hanbury had asked Bentham to pass on a letter introducing himself as a potential client. It was the beginning of a lifelong friendship. Between 1856 and 1875 Spruce and Hanbury exchanged more than five hundred letters, and towards the end of his life Spruce used the correspondence to give vent to what he saw as his mistreatment by the India Office and his bitterness at his poverty and ill health.

On 10 May 1856 Hanbury prepared a memorandum, reminding himself to draw Spruce's attention to cinchona, 'a group of plants, whose importance to medicine, we are all aware.' The memorandum urges Spruce not only to collect specimens of young cinchona but of the 'old bark rich in alkaloids', which owing to an 'absurd prejudice' was being all but ignored by European traders. 'Botanical specimens of Cinchona & its allies, accompanied by small, authenticated specimens of bark, could not fail to meet with some demand here and on the continent in quarters where the general herbarium would not be subscribed . . .'

Unfortunately, his letter to Spruce has been lost, but it must have contained very similar wording. In enclosing the letter to Spruce, Bentham writes that Hanbury 'is a young man of great abilities who has devoted himself much to pharmacology and is anxious on the question of cinchonas etc upon which he writes to you.' And in a followup letter in July, Bentham adds: 'I am very desirous to do anything to assist him – and he is very ready to give any fair remuneration.'

What effect, if any, this had on Spruce's thinking is unclear. As far as Spruce was concerned, Hanbury was just one more collector. Besides, he had no reason at this stage to believe that cinchona was going to prove more lucrative than any other plant. His motives were purely practical. He had money in the bank, but because of the war in Peru it was impossible to get his hands on it. In Ecuador, however, Bentham had arranged for him to pick up a draft from the local Lloyd's agent. If he could only get to Quito he would have the freedom to work on his collections in a climate agreeable to his health.

So it was that on 23 March 1857, Spruce set off from Tarapoto on an epic three-month journey to Baños in Ecuador via the Huallaga and Pastaza rivers. Teaming up with two Peruvian businessmen, Spruce hired twelve Indians, five for the Peruvians and seven to crew his twelve-metre mahogany dugout. It was a journey that no one has attempted before or since and was so arduous that, even when Spruce reached Baños three months later, he could 'hardly bear to think of it'.

The voyage began, as it would continue, with a rainstorm. The first stage, to Chasuta, was overland. In the dry season such a trek takes no more than a day, but it was so wet that it took Spruce and his party two. The storms had deepened the potholes in their path and the track was so muddy that Spruce was obliged to walk barefoot to preserve his shoes. The result was that by the time he reached Chasuta he was both lame and suffering from fever.

At Chasuta Spruce provisioned canoes for the descent of the Huallaga. The boats had to be open so as to be able to pass safely under the many waterfalls en route but no sooner had they begun descending the river than they faced a far more serious danger: whirlpools. It was all Spruce's crew could do to keep the canoe from capsizing. Unfortunately Spruce had his dog, Sultan, whom he had reared from a pup, with him in the boat. According to Spruce 'the horrid roar of the waters' drove Sultan mad, and from then on he would neither drink nor eat. For six days Spruce watched over him in the hope that he would recover. But when Sultan, almost worn to a skeleton, began snapping at people and bolted for the woods 'uttering the most unearthly sounds', Spruce wrote: 'I saw all hope of saving him was vain, and was obliged to shoot him.'

Sultan's death seemed to drain the life from Spruce. Sultan had accompanied him all over the Amazon. Now he was alone with only his Indian porters and the Portuguese for company. To make matters worse, the Huallaga was infested with *zancudos* and his skin was soon pockmarked with bites and ulcerations from the constant scratching.

The next few days passed in a monochrome blur. The river was flat and monotonous. Coupled with the absence of human habitation,

Spruce found the journey 'heart-sickening'. Eventually they reached the mission at La Laguna, near the mouth of the Marañón, where La Condamine had stopped on his way down the Amazon a century before. Although it was two weeks before Easter, Spruce's porters were intent on performing their penitence for Holy week before journeying further upriver. Accordingly, while Spruce bought fresh provisions, the Indians prepared whips dipped in pitch and embedded with bits of broken glass. On the Saturday before they were due to embark the 'penitents' assembled in the main street. Spruce writes he had never seen a more 'horrible sight'. The Indians applied the straps 'unceasingly', flagellating themselves until their backs were 'one mass of gore' in the belief that it would ensure their safe return from the perilous journey ahead. Noticing they were drunk, Spruce doubted the value of their penitence. However, at noontime on Monday each man was seated at his oars, ready to row, without showing any outward sign of discomfort.

It is only eighty kilometres from the Marañón to the mouth of the Pastaza but the river was so low, and food so scarce, it took Spruce five days. On 9 April, three days out from La Laguna, he reached a small village, deserted save for a dozen cane houses and several sacks of rice. It turned out the men had been murdered by wild forest Indians while cutting cane and their wives and children had had to flee for their lives. From then on, the Indians refused to sleep on shore and Spruce never left the canoe without his gun.

Once they had entered the Pastaza it took a further fortnight to reach Andoas. The village, on the border of Ecuador, lay three hundred and twenty kilometres upriver. The Pastaza was practically deserted and the only settlement they passed was infected with leprosy. Although it rained continually, the water was low and at several points the porters had to leap out of the canoes and drag them over the shallow beds by hand.

On 29 April Spruce finally reached Andoas. It took him five days to lay in fresh provisions and engage a new crew to take him up the Bobonaza River to Canelos. Then, on 5 May, he was off again. With its narrow, winding course, the Bobonaza reminded him of the

Casiquiare. The water was muddy and sluggish and once again progress was slow. It was only when they reached the village of Sara-yuca that the vegetation began to change and the scene became more picturesque: waterfalls, and cliffs clad with ferns and mosses and 'a Helicomia with . . . pendent scarlet and yellowish spikes'.

Now the going became tougher. The river was swollen by melted snow cascading off the distant volcanic peaks of the Ecuadorian Andes, and the Indian rowers had to paddle against a six-knot current. On 21 May they reached Puca-yacu, a village perched seventy-five metres above the river. They tied the canoes to lianas overhanging the narrow sandbar then climbed up to pay their respects to the governor. But when they returned to the boats at sundown the sky began to darken ominously and at 9 p.m. the heavens opened. The storm caused the level of the river to rise rapidly, swamping the beach 'in a roaring surge which broke under the canoes in whirlpools'. Fearing the boats would break their moorings, the Indians leapt into the trees to secure the lianas higher up. But the surging waters now threatened to dash the boats against one another and it was all the Indians could do to hang on in the hope of averting disaster. 'Assuredly I had slight hopes of living to see the day,' writes Spruce, 'and I shall for ever feel grateful to those Indians who, without any orders from us, stood through all the rain and storm of that fearful night, relaxing not a moment in their efforts to save our canoes from being carried away by the flood.'

It was only at 10 a.m. the following morning that the waters abated sufficiently for them to unload the boats and haul the sodden cargo up the cliff-face. 'Wearied to death', Spruce spent that night in the village. But the following day he was well enough to explore the plateau above the river. At his feet stretched the valley of the Bobonaza. Looking north and west was the deep gorge of the Pastaza and rolling away from it, at sundown, 'the lofty cordillera . . . in cloudless majesty.' Looking from south to north he could just make out the volcanoes Sangay and Altar and the bluff peak of Tungura-hua. And there, 'peeping over its left shoulder', was Chimborazo, 'the monarch of the Andes'.

Spruce was so taken with Puca-yuca he stayed three weeks, gathering mosses in the nearby woods and making a collection of the local beetles. Then on 10 June, to the accompaniment of the distant rumble of Sangay, he set off on the final leg of his epic journey.

Spruce reached Canelos in two days, but from here on the gradients of the Bobonaza valley became steadily steeper and more dangerous. The only way of proceeding was on foot, and to have any chance of reaching Baños he had to lighten the loads as much as possible. Accordingly he entrusted his drugs, barometer and other valuables to the Portuguese, and packed his remaining belongings, including some precious drying papers, into five small boxes. From here on in, he would have to confine himself to pressing mosses and lichens.

Spruce set off early in the morning of 14 June, accompanied by eight Indian porters. There were no paths as such, just a series of slippery ascents leading up and over the ravines of the Bobonaza valley. To reach Baños, he would have to ford a series of streams separating the Bobonaza and the Pastaza, each one more swollen and treacherous than the last. The rain and mud were constant companions and only a pair of rubber boots purchased from a German traveller in Canelos kept his feet dry. From the outset, his porters complained bitterly and insisted on frequent rest stops. Passing through Jivaro country, his annoyance at the delays was lessened, however, by the discovery that he was now in the mossiest place on earth. 'Even the topmost twigs and the very branches were shaggy with mosses,' he enthused. 'Whenever rains, swollen streams, and grumbling Indians combined to overwhelm me with chagrin, I found reason to thank heaven which had enabled me to forget for the moment all my troubles in the contemplation of a simple moss.'

The Indians, however, did not share his enthusiasm and by the twentieth were fed up with struggling under the weight of the loads. Spruce had been forced to pay them in advance and, fearing they would mutiny and desert him in the middle of the night, he now had no choice but to get rid of all the drying papers that had not yet been used for pressing.

The next few days were sunny for once and soon they came out on a plateau above the Pastaza. A series of steep ravines intersected by rushing mountain torrents now lay in their path. Using bamboo poles as bridges, they inched their way across each impediment until, finally, they reached the largest one of all – the River Topo. Here, Spruce writes, his worst fears were realized. It had been raining steadily for two days and for as far he could see the Topo 'was one mass of foam'. The thunder from the water was so great it 'made the very ground shake to some distance from the bank'. They were less than two hundred metres from the junction with the Pastaza but there seemed no way across. The rocks that provided the usual support for the bamboo poles had been washed away. The only possibility was a group of three rocks higher upstream but these too were now partially submerged beneath the surging waves. The only choice was to wait and hope that the river would fall, but after two days there had been little change. Spruce now faced a stark choice: send his porters back to Canelos for fresh provisions and risk their deserting, or risk a crossing. He called a council by the riverside and put it to the men that if they were game there was a possibility of creating a bridge at the new group of rocks. The only problem was that because of the distance and difference in height between the rocks the bridge would necessarily slope and bend considerably in the middle.

The Indians agreed to give it a shot. Four bridges would be needed in all. The bridge from the bank to the first stone was short and completed with relative ease, but the second strained their ingenuity to the limit. Normally, a bamboo would be levered from one rock to another and, once in place, a man would crawl along it dragging another bamboo secured with a liana to lie alongside it. Once four bamboos had been laid in this way, they could be lashed together and the construction of the next bridge could begin. In the case of the second bridge, however, the bamboos were too short and only reached the side of the rock. To add to the difficulties, the roar of the water was so deafening that Spruce could only communicate by means of hand signals. Eventually, the Indians succeeded in laying four bamboos, but by the time they had completed the third and

*Above, left:*
1. One of the earliest illustrations of the 'Peruvian tree of fevers', from Jonston's *Dendrographias*, published in 1662.

*Above, right:*
2. Charles Marie de La Condamine's sketch of *Cinchona officinalis* from a 1745 Amsterdam edition of *Sur l'arbre du quinquina*.

*Right:*
3. By 1801, when this watercolour was painted, *Cinchona officinalis* was known as the 'true Jesuit's bark'.

*The Officinalis, or true Jesuits Bark.*

PERUVIA COLLECTA NOVIS CHINCONIUS ORIS
ACCIPIT A SERVIS PHARMACA FEBRIFUGA

POTAT LIMA CONIUX CHINCONIA FEBRIM
ANDO POCULA TINCTA FUGANT

PURPUREUS PATER HIS SOLATUR IN AEDIBUS AGROS
MA CORTICE FEBRIFUGO

4. Oil on canvas triptych, after frescoes in the Santo Spirito hospital in Rome. Entitled 'Episodes in the history of cinchona', the panels recount the legend of the Condessa's cure and show: (1) The Conde de Chinchon instructing an Indian servant to collect cinchona bark for the royal pharmacy; (2) the presentation of the 'miraculous bark' to the Condessa; and (3) Cardinal de Lugo distributing the bark in Rome.

5. A woman gripped by the rigor of a malarial chill warms herself by an
open hearth while the ague 'monster' creeps up behind her, in this 1788 coloured
etching by Dunthorne and Rowlandson.

6. Richard Spruce, shortly after his return from South America in 1864.

7. Clements Markham, date unknown.

8. Charles Ledger, circa 1880.

9. Manuel Incra Mamani, date unknown.

10. José Celestino Mutis, examining a flower petal in a 1930 portrait.

11. Alexander von Humboldt, pressing flowers in an 1806 portrait.

12. Chimborazo, the 'monarch of the Andes'.

13. Author's pack horses being loaded on the sierra prior to his trek over Chimborazo. Transportation in the Andes has changed little since Spruce passed this way in 1860.

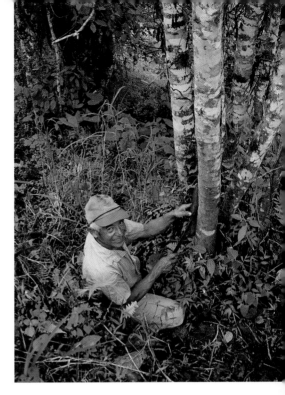

14. A young *Cinchona succirubra* tree, growing from the stump of an old, felled trunk on a mountain ridge beneath Chimborazo.

15. A *cascarillo* stips bark from a stand of cinchona trees on 'Spruce's ridge'.

16. Gathering and drying cinchona bark in a Peruvian forest, circa 1867.

17. Coloured lithograph of *Cinchona succirubra* from John Eliot Howard's *Illustrations of the Nueva Quinologia of Pavon*, London, 1862.

18. Sir William Denison, Governor of Madras, and others, planting the first cinchona tree in the Nilgiri Hills, India, circa 1861.

fourth bridges it was noon and the water level had started to rise again. If they were to cross they would have to be quick, but no sooner did they venture out onto the second bridge than it began to bend under the weight of Spruce's heavy boxes. Spruce had no choice but to abandon them by the riverside, trusting that he could send someone from Baños to retrieve them later. Even so, he barely made it. As he inched across the bamboos, a wave wet him 'to the knees', washing away the bridge soon after.

Spruce's ordeal was almost over. The next day they waded for a kilometre and a half through 'fetid mud' before descending to the shores of the Pastaza via a wooden ladder attached to the sheer cliff-face. From here on in it was simply a matter of following the course of the Pastaza north until they reached the falls of Agoyan. Normally, the falls are crossed via a stout bridge suspended twelve metres above the river, but the rains in the Sierra had been so great that the bridge had been washed away. All that remained were three or four trunks, of which only one was unbroken. Gingerly, they inched their way safely across. A few hours later they arrived at a farm and Spruce procured a horse. It was now just a short twenty-five-kilometre trot to Baños.

Spruce reached the pretty spa town nestled beneath the Tungura-hua volcano the same afternoon. It was 1 July. In all, the journey from Tarapoto had taken a gruelling 102 days. By now Spruce's features lay shrunken behind a three-month-old beard. He was emaciated from lack of food and desperately needed to recuperate. But Baños was not what he expected. Located nearly two thousand metres above sea level, the air was so cold it immediately set his teeth chattering. Then came the catarrh, 'with a cough so violent as often to bring up blood from both nose and mouth.' He was disappointed to discover there was no drying paper to be had in the town, and that in addition the house he was renting had been destroyed by an earthquake seven years previously. Nevertheless, he spent the next six months collecting ferns and mosses on the wooded slopes below Tungurahua, and in October made a return trip to the Topo River and the forest of Canelos (earlier he had sent his porters back to the

Topo to recover his belongings; they found them crawling with maggots but otherwise undisturbed).

Ecuador, like Peru, was now in a state of political turmoil. War between the neighbouring republics was imminent and the Ecuadorian army was roaming the countryside pressing men, money and horses into its ranks. Despite these difficulties, at the beginning of 1858 Spruce moved to Ambato, a town strategically located on the high sierra midway between Quito and Guayaquil. This was to be his collecting station for the next two and a half years. Soon afterwards, he made an important acquaintance: Dr James Taylor, the former medical attendant to General Flores, Ecuador's ex-president. Born in Cumberland, Taylor had married the daughter of one of Bolivar's generals and was well placed to help Spruce. His relationship with Flores would prove particularly useful as Flores was a substantial landowner and one of his estates, on the western slopes of Chimborazo, was in the heart of the red bark region. For the moment, however, Spruce and Taylor confined themselves to discussing Ancient Greek, Spruce coming away with the opinion that Taylor was 'a very kind-hearted, honourable man, which can't be said of many Englishmen I have met in South America.' Through Taylor, Spruce also met the American Ambassador to Ecuador, Philo White. Whether Taylor and White also introduced Spruce to Walter Cope, the British Consul in Quito who had gathered cinchona plants for the Foreign Office in 1852, Spruce does not say. But it seems that it was following a conversation with Cope that Spruce finally realized the importance to the British government of procuring cinchona.

Spruce stayed a month with Taylor, and then headed for Riobamba, where he visited a spectacular waterfall on the southern side of Tungurahua. However, the effort of wading up to the waist in the icy snowmelt under a hot sun took a predictable toll. Finding himself confined to bed for four days with fever and 'rheumatic pains from head to foot', Spruce wrote Bentham a long, self-pitying letter. It is worth quoting in full, if only to underline his straitened circumstances, his continued ignorance of the cinchona effort and the depth of his hypochondriac self-doubt – somewhat ironic given the Herculean task he was about to undertake on behalf of Her Majesty's government.

> I should be very glad to return to England as you recommend me, to distribute my mosses, but I am fearful of again falling into delicate health if I go there. I have, besides, no funds beyond what are in your hands; these would soon be exhausted, and poverty is such a positive crime in England, that to be there without either money or lucrative employment is a contingency not to be reflected on without dread. On the other hand, I already feel myself unequal to the painful mountain ascents, exposed at the same time to a burning sun and a piercingly cold wind. The eastern slopes of the Andes no doubt contain much fine ground, but for want of roads they can scarcely be explored, except by one to whom the pecuniary value of his collections would be no object, and who could go to any amount of expense. I have often wished I could get some consular appoint-ment here, were it only for £150 a year; but I have no powerful friends, without which a familiarity with the country, the inhabitants, and the languages go for little.

'Poverty is such a positive crime in England . . .' Plus ça change. In spite of Bentham's urgings, and in view of his 'delicate health', it is not hard to see why he would have preferred the eternal spring of Ambato to the anonymity of damp, rain-swept Yorkshire, and why in probing for some means of financial security he would have sought a meeting with Cope in Quito. Not long after this meeting, in September 1858, Spruce wrote what can only be described as a 'begging' letter to Cope's superior, George Lenox-Conyngham, chief clerk to the Foreign Office. A note of the letter is buried in Markham's Cinchona Notebook I. Markham never alludes to it, either in his published works on cinchona or in his later correspondence with the India Office on Spruce's behalf. Perhaps he thought it was too embarrassing – an individual of Spruce's qualifications touting for work – or perhaps it interfered with the image he wanted to project of himself as the architect of the quest. In the letter, Spruce writes that

Cope informed him that 'for want of some trustworthy person' familiar with cinchona the Foreign Office had been unable to procure the specimens requested. Spruce continues that should the government so wish then he could 'undertake to supply them' and 'speedily transport myself' to the cinchona forests. Echoing Royle's arguments, Spruce continues: '. . . the bark trees are rapidly verging to extinction, and it is therefore of the first importance that steps should be taken for their cultivation on a large scale, in some country where there is no lack of industrious hands. I will therefore venture further to observe that should HM government think proper to employ me in this matter, they will have the advantage of a person already on the spot, and familiar with the country, the people and the language and (what is of more importance) with the plants whose products are sought.'

Spruce's letter reached Lenox-Conyngham in December. It must have triggered an immediate enquiry to Kew along the lines of 'Who the hell is Spruce?', for in January Hooker wrote directly to the Foreign Office in support of his wayward botanist. 'I will venture to say without hesitation if the Government ever makes an attempt of the kind there is no man so competent to the work as Mr Spruce.'

But the Foreign Office was not calling the shots, the India Office was, and it was only with Markham's appointment in April that the wheels were set in motion. By now the Ecuador Land Company, in its desperation to interest the British in its cinchona forests, was claiming it had recruited Spruce. Markham quickly established this was not true and in May was authorized to open negotiations directly with the Yorkshireman. Used for so long to botanizing on a shoe-string, Spruce priced himself far too cheaply, asking only £30 a month – £10 more than he normally received from his subscribers. Unsurprisingly, the India Office leapt at the proposal. When the plant collector Robert Fortune had brought tea plants from China he had been paid £500 for a year's work. Although transporting cinchona would entail the India Office in greater outlays, given the hardships involved Spruce's offer was a bargain. Later this would become a source of some resentment to him; as usual, however, he was more preoccupied with his present health than his future livelihood. 'I have been entrusted by the India Government with the charge of obtaining seeds and young plants of the different sorts of cinchona found in the Quitonian Andes,' Spruce wrote to his colleague John Teasdale in April 1859. '. . . This task will occupy me (if my life be spared) the greater part of next year.'

Spruce was right to be apprehensive. Because of the huge demand for cinchona, the more accessible forests had already been stripped bare. In order to find virgin trees he would have to ride along the central cordillera and then descend either the eastern or western Andes and penetrate deep into the cloudforest. In the case of the eastern cordillera – where the climate alternates between spring and summer – this was relatively pleasant. But in the case of the western foothills of the Andes, where the Pacific weather system rules, the forests were subject to almost continual rain. The best time to approach them was between June and September – the South American winter, when the rains eased off. But these were also the coldest months on the Paramo de Puenevata, the plain on the southern side of Chimborazo, whose shoulder Spruce would have to skirt near the snow-limit before dropping down to twelve hundred metres. The difficulties involved in such an expedition, wrote Spruce, 'were not slight ones'. Nevertheless, he decided that if he was to succeed he needed to acquaint himself as soon as possible with the different varieties of bark. So, with Ambato as his base, he began making a series of excursions, first to Riobamba, and then to Alausí south of the volcano Sangay, running the gauntlet of the army and deserting troops on the way.

Meanwhile, back in London, Markham was making preparations for his own expedition. One of his first stops was the home of the renowned English quinologist, John Eliot Howard. A staunch Quaker, Howard had been interested in cinchona ever since apprenticing in the family pharmaceutical business at the age of twenty. Quinine was fast becoming one of the firm's most important manufactures and, encouraged by his father, Howard began cultivating cinchona seeds in a greenhouse next to his Tottenham quinine works.

In 1857, in recognition of his contribution to the study of the genus, Howard was made an honorary fellow of the Linnaean Society. The following year he purchased the original manuscripts of the Spanish botanist Pavon, together with the collection of cinchona specimens made during his ill-fated trip to Peru and Chile, and began a microscopic study of the barks. These studies would eventually lead to the publication in 1862 of his *'Nueva Quinologia'* – the most complete classification of cinchona at that time.

It is not known what Markham and Howard discussed, but there was no better authority on cinchona and it is safe to assume that Markham questioned him closely on how to distinguish the species with the highest quinine content – namely the red bark of Ecuador and the *calisayas* of Peru and Bolivia.

Next Markham visited the Horticultural Society in Chiswick to consult Robert Fortune on the design of several sets of Wardian cases for conveying the cinchona plants to India. These would be brought out separately by expert gardeners sent from Kew to rendezvous with Spruce and Markham on the coasts of, respectively, Ecuador and Peru, once their collections were ready. Markham also lobbied for an Admiralty vessel to convey the cases speedily to India, or failing that one of the Indian government's own steamships. But no one would give him a firm commitment. In contrast to the Dutch, who had provided a frigate in an effort to ensure the success of Hasskarl's mission, the British attitude was almost cavalier. When Markham wrote to the British Consul in Lima requesting letters of introduction to the Peruvian bark companies, for instance, he was blithely informed, 'I do not see any particular difficulties you would have to face in the prosecution of your mission.' Markham was not nearly so confident. War between Peru and Bolivia was imminent. More- over, he knew the *cascarilleros* who worked the highland forests were notoriously protective of their livelihood. Even if he reached the Bolivian border and succeeded in finding the 'true' *calisaya* it was by no means certain that he would be allowed to return with the seeds and plants.

Spruce's mood was also darkening. In August, after a two-week trek during which he was alternately frozen, scorched and drenched, he had finally reached Lucma, a town deep in the bark forests of the western Andes, and seen the *cascarilla roja* for himself. His guide, Bermeo, had discovered a slender new shoot growing from an old felled tree. When Bermeo slit it with his cutlass, Spruce marvelled as the colourless sap turned bright red on contact with the air. 'The more rapidly this change is effected, and the deeper is the ultimate tinge assumed, the more precious is the bark presumed to be,' he wrote. Because of the civil unrest Bermeo was convinced that no one had been in the woods for months and that they would find better examples deeper into the forest. But Spruce did not think it was worth riding further and by October he was back in Ambato. Three months earlier he had been forced to hang out the Union Jack after government troops, their ranks swollen by black and mixed-race conscripts, had marched on the town following their victory over rebel forces. On that occasion the troops had 'respected' his property but, as he wrote to Hooker, the country was now in a 'very unsettled state.' All around men and livestock were being pressed into the rival armies. To avoid being torn apart, many families had fled to the highlands with all their possessions strapped to mules. 'The war, if it actually comes, will be something like what you have read in India, yet nobody knows what it is to be about,' wrote Spruce, referring to the Indian Mutiny. 'These Spanish republics are not unlikely to squabble among one another until – like the Kilkenny cats – there is nothing left of them but their tails, and then Jonathan will step in and make an easy prey of their mangled carcasses . . .'

Spruce may not have been thinking about cinchona when he wrote those words but they would prove prescient. From Britain's point of view the political instability in Peru and Ecuador presented her with the perfect opportunity to seize the seeds and plants from under the noses of the South American republics. And in this case, Spruce and Markham would be the Jonathans.

*Chapter Six*

# THE QUEST

The gods that mortal beauty chase,
Still in a tree did end their race;
Apollo hunted Daphne so
Only that she might laurel grow;
And Pan did after Syrinx speed
Not as a nymph, but for a reed.

Andrew Marvell, 'Thoughts in a Garden'

BY THE END OF 1859 the Dutch were beginning to despair. After arriving in Java, Hasskarl had planted his *Cinchona calisaya* seeds in a volcanic range to the south of the capital, Batavia. But the soil was thin and the site ill-suited to cinchona and the plants had become more and more sickly. However, instead of cutting their losses and propagating a more promising variety the Dutch simply moved the plantation to the Malawar mountains.

This was a pity as in 1856 Hasskarl's successor, Dr Franz Junghuhn, had arrived in Java with two *C. calisaya* plants raised from Dr Weddell's seed. Unlike Hasskarl, Weddell had personally collected the *calisayas* in Bolivia but because they were less hardy and more difficult to cultivate the Dutch put less effort into their propagation. The result was that three years later the Dutch had nearly a million *Cinchona pahudiana* growing in the Malawar mountains, and just seven thousand of Weddell's *calisayas*. It was only when the

Dutch began testing the bark for quinine, however, that they realized their mistake. Dr de Vrij, the plantation's chemist, was astonished to find that the *pahudiana* contained just 0.4 per cent of the alkaloid whereas Weddell's *calisayas* contained up to 5 per cent. Indeed so minuscule was the quinine in Hasskarl's plants that it was doubtful that they were true *calisayas* at all. Clemente Henriquez, the Bolivian he had hired to collect the seeds and plants, was emerging as a man of considerable complexity. Not only, as Ledger attested, had he poisoned the soil in Hasskarl's Wardian cases but it now looked as though he had performed a subtle sleight of hand with the seeds too.

Markham was determined not to make the same mistake. The British cinchona hunters would not rely on outside agents but would harvest the plants and seeds in person. In addition, Markham arranged for Kew to send two expert gardeners – Robert Cross and John Weir – to nurture the cuttings and watch over the Wardian cases during the return voyage to England. The idea was that Cross would rendezvous with Spruce at Guayaquil once his seeds were ready to be sent to the coast, while Weir would accompany Markham into the *calisaya* forests of Bolivia and Peru. In addition, Markham also arranged for a fifth collector, Mr Pritchett, to travel to Huánuco in Peru and gather specimens of the grey barks.

Markham's organizational skills cannot be faulted. However, his political strategy left a lot to be desired. Convinced of the urgent need to gather the cinchonas before the South American forests were exhausted he made little effort to conceal his aims. Instead he broadcast the purpose of his mission widely in the naive belief that the Andean republics shared his philanthropic aims and would abide by the rules of 'fair play'. The Old World had contributed to the New such priceless gifts as wheat, barley, rice, sheep, cattle and horses, Markham argued. It was only right that the New World should now grant the Old a product of life-and-death importance: the cure for malaria. Besides, demand for quinine would always exceed supply. The Indian plantations might lead to a small fall in the world price of quinine but the knowledge gleaned from the cultivation of cinchonas by expert European botanists could only benefit South America in the long run.

Hitherto they have destroyed the cinchona trees in a spirit of reckless short-sightedness, and thus done more injury to their own interests than could possibly have arisen from any commercial competition ... It will then be a pleasure to supply them with the information which will have been gained by the experience of cultivators in India, and thus to assist them in the establishment of plantations on the slopes of the eastern Andes.[1]

What Markham appeared to have forgotten is that cinchona was an essential part of Peru's national identity. When Peru gained independence from Spain in 1821 a cinchona tree was enshrined in the national coat of arms along with an alpaca and a horn of plenty filled with gold – images that were meant to underline the agricultural, animal and material wealth inherited from the Incas.[2] Not only that but the Condesa de Chinchón's cure had taken place in Lima. Regardless of whether or not the story was true, it was widely believed. Under the circumstances it was naive of Markham in the extreme to think that the Peruvians would relinquish such an essential part of their botanical heritage without a fight. Unfortunately, by the time he realized this it was too late: as in the days of the Inca when imperial runners, fuelled by coca, conveyed messages the length of the Andes with astonishing speed, so news of Markham's expedition preceded his passage over the cordillera.

Markham set sail on his quest on 17 December 1859 accompanied by his wife, Minna, and John Weir. His first stop was Guayaquil, where he planned to make the arrangements for the collection of Spruce's plants and seeds. But Ecuador was 'in a complete state of anarchy', and with the Peruvian fleet moored in the estuary Markham found himself negotiating directly with the President of Peru. Fortunately Walter Cope, the British Consul, had already obtained passports guaranteeing the safe passage of Spruce's mules to the bark forests. But the political situation was apt to change at any moment and Markham left strict instructions for Cross to load the seeds and plants onto the first steamer for Southampton as soon as he arrived in Ecuador.

Lima, in contrast, was an oasis of calm. Disembarking on 26 January 1860, Markham was greeted as a homecoming son. He was now an eminent Inca scholar and the friends he had made during his travels seven years previously were delighted to see him and his new wife. One writer, reviewing Markham's book *Cuzco and Lima*, could barely contain his enthusiasm. 'Mr Markham does not come alone this time,' he gushed. 'He is accompanied by a young and beautiful wife, who participates in his enthusiasm and love for the privileged land which they now come to explore; and she is herself gifted with brilliant intelligence, and the most amiable qualities.'[3]

Markham's reaction to the review was characteristically naive. 'This has, I think, thrown people off the scent as to my real object, although it must necessarily be known to several,' he confided in his diary. Indeed it was.

Markham spent a month in Lima organizing supplies and equipment and discussing the condition of the cinchona forests with landowners in the eastern cordillera. Their prognosis was not encouraging. Ten years earlier, they informed Markham, it would have been relatively easy to harvest the plants. But in Carabaya true *calisayas* were now so scarce that collectors had to cut deeper and deeper into the forest. Conversely, on the Bolivian side of the border the forests were still rich in *calisayas* but war with Peru was imminent and the *cascarilleros* were more suspicious than ever of foreigners.

The intelligence placed Markham in a quandary. Should he proceed to Bolivia and risk running foul of the *cascarilleros* or, worse, being trapped behind the border by the outbreak of war? Or should he play it safe and go to Carabaya where, like Hasskarl, he might find only inferior seed?

The whole success of the mission, not to mention Markham's place in history, depended on his making the right decision and he was understandably nervous.

The forests where the cinchonas grow are almost inaccessible, without roads or habitations. There is great risk of being disabled by fevers in the humid forests, by *sorochi* [altitude sickness] in crossing the Andes, and by dysentery and ague on the coast. The plants, after they are procured, will have to pass on mules' backs over the frozen planes of the Andes, and the hot arid deserts on the coast before reaching the Wardian cases ... Many of these obstacles may, of course, be overcome by energy and care, others are in the hands of Providence.

At this stage Markham was still hoping to reach La Paz. Today this is a relatively simple matter. From Islay on the coast of Peru there is a railway all the way to Puno on the shores of Lake Titicaca from where you can catch a hydrofoil and bus to Bolivia's capital. In 1860, however, there was no railway and no roads – just a mule track that led across Peru's coastal desert to Arequipa and then wound up the cordillera and over the paramos to Puno. Crossing Lake Titicaca, the highest lake in the world, was equally problem-atic. In Markham's time the only vessels that plied the freezing cold waters were *balsas*, light reed sailboats. Although they were suppos-edly unsinkable, progress was necessarily slow and the *balsas* were limited in the loads they could carry. Moreover, once the eastern side of the lake was reached the problems were by no means over. To reach the bark forests below Apolobamba, Markham faced an arduous expedition across a series of snow-swept plains and down precipitous mud tracks.

Nevertheless, in early March he loaded his mules and set off across the coastal desert accompanied by Minna and John Weir. But en route he suffered a severe bilious attack and by the time they reached Arequipa he was very weak. At this point he decided to part company with Minna, fearing that if he did cross into Bolivia her life might be in danger. 'I cannot fully decide until I reach Puno,' he wrote in his journal, 'but I am fully resolved never to leave the coast of Peru, without a supply of *Calisaya* plants. With God's blessing I *will* succeed!'

Although it pained him to leave his 'beloved wife', Minna pointed out that from Arequipa she could pass on his communications to the

other cinchona hunters and keep him informed of political develop-
ments. Thus it was that on 23 March Markham started for Puno
along the same road he had taken in 1853.

His route took him towards Cusco before veering east up the *alto
de los huesos*, a long, zigzag path to the cordillera. It was the worst
season of the year to be travelling and they were soon being pelted
with hail and icy rain. On reaching Apo at four thousand two
hundred metres the majority of the party, including the mule-drivers,
began complaining of *sorochi* – 'violent pressure on the head, accompanied by acute pain and aches in the back of the neck.' In the night
their symptoms intensified and by morning Markham hardly had the
strength to mount his mule.

He was now in the most desolate country since his voyage to the
Arctic in search of Sir John Franklin ten years previously. Only the
herds of vicuña roaming the mountainside and the sight of a
*coraquenque*, an Andean condor, reminded Markham he was in South
America. Then, no sooner had they reached the Alto de Toledo, at
four thousand seven hundred and fifty metres the highest part of their
route, than they were forced to cross a series of bogs. With each
tentative step the swampy mud threatened to swallow their mules.
Eventually, however, they reached the swollen banks of the Tortorani
River and were greeted with the dazzling view of Lake Titicaca and
the snow-capped peaks of the Bolivian Andes behind it. By the time
Markham reached Puno on 27 March he was exhausted. Almost
immediately he discovered that the Peruvians had stationed three
divisions near the Bolivian border and were anticipating war. Not
only that but the rains had been excessive, turning the roads on the
eastern side of Lake Titicaca into mud-chutes. Given the Bolivian
ban on the export of *calisaya*, Markham concluded that it would be
'next to impossible for a private person to preserve his mules from
seizure' and that it was altogether too risky to cross the border.
Caravaya, on the other hand, lay in Peru and was nearby. Contrary
to his earlier advice Markham now convinced himself that if he
penetrated far enough into the Peruvian forests he would still be able
to find young *calisaya* trees in fruit. Moreover, because very little bark

was harvested there he reasoned that his party would not arouse the jealousy or suspicion of the natives. In fact, this proved another example of his wishful thinking.

While Markham was pondering his next move Spruce had been doing his best to ignore the civil war raging in Ecuador. Through discussions with local traders he had discovered that the best red bark did not come from Alausí at all but from the cinchona forests in the western foothills of Chimborazo. Covering an area of five thousand square kilometres, the forests were the property of two men. One, Dr Francisco Neyra, was a local notary, but by a stroke of luck the second was General Flores. Flores had recently been recalled to Ecuador after an absence of fifteen years by the provisional government to help take back Guayaquil from the rebels and Spruce now contacted Dr Taylor, the general's former doctor, to talk about renting his land. At first Flores was reluctant but Spruce persevered. The trees were about to blossom and, he insisted, he had to be on the spot to gather the seeds when they began to form. Hurriedly, he sent word to the British consulate in Guayaquil that he needed money to clinch the deal. Cope duly forwarded the funds entrusted to him by the India Office and after lengthy negotiations Flores and Neyra agreed to let the forest to him for $400. The only condition was that he left the bark intact.

Neyra now became very cooperative, offering Spruce the use of his *cascarilleros* from Guanujo, a town just beneath Chimborazo. Through Neyra Spruce also learnt that the most highly valued bark of all came from Limon, a ridge at twelve hundred metres surrounded by cane farms. Although the largest trees had been cut down some years before, the *cascarilleros* had carefully nurtured the new shoots and Spruce was informed the young trees were now stout enough to bear flowers and fruit. Spruce also needed to collect specimens of *Cinchona officinalis* from Loja, but Loja was separated from Limon by a fifteen-day journey. Realizing he could not be in both places at once, he rode to Riobamba to persuade Taylor to collect the *C. officinalis* on his behalf. Taylor having agreed to this, Spruce then returned to Ambato to rest and await the arrival of the dry season.

Ecuador was now divided into two opposing armies, with the rebels controlling Guayaquil and the low country and the Provisional government Quito and the sierra. But the threat of being swept up into one or other of these warring factions was nothing compared to the challenge of crossing Chimborazo. The dry season coincided with the Andean winter when conditions on the 'glory of the Andes' were well below freezing. In order to reach Limon, Spruce would first have to ride to Mocha and then ascend the north-west shoulder of the volcano to as high as four thousand metres. Then he would have to work his way down a precipitous, muddy slope to eighteen hundred metres along tracks so narrow that even mules found it difficult to keep their footing. Of course Humboldt and Bonpland had managed it sixty years previously, climbing to 5,878 metres – the highest point then reached by man. But even for someone in peak physical condition the mountain was a formidable challenge. How would Spruce, always suffering from one ailment or another, cope with such an arduous ascent? The question must have been playing on Spruce's mind, or perhaps it was simply a case of bad luck, but he now suffered a mysterious and debilitating attack. His journal entry of 29 April is certainly melodramatic. Headed 'The Break Down' it reads: 'Woke up this morning paralysed in my back legs.' Some time later, it appears, he went over the entry in black ink, underlining the words 'Break Down' twice and adding in parentheses, 'From that day forth I was never more able to sit straight up, or to walk about, without great pain and discomfort, soon passing to mental exhaustion.'

Spruce later described his condition as 'a rheumatic and nervous affection, almost amounting to paralysis.' While he could still move about and make preparations for the journey he now considered it doubtful that he 'should be able to bear the arduous fatigues of travelling in the forest' and decided to delegate his commission to Dr Taylor. Was this an extreme 'case of the vapours' brought on by the pressure of the impending mission, or was Spruce genuinely ill? One suggestion is that he may have been suffering from Guillain-Barre syndrome, a rare allergic reaction of the peripheral nerves usually brought on by a severe respiratory or gastrointestinal infection. Certainly his condition mystified doctors for years. According to Wallace, in 1869 doctors diagnosed the cause of the paralysis as a 'stricture of the rectum' – what today we might call a bad case of piles. But that hardly seems sufficient to explain symptoms as extreme as 'paralysis'.[4]

On the face of it Markham was made of sterner stuff. While Spruce was convalescing in Ambato, he had reached Crucero, the capital of Caravaya, and begun descending the eastern cordillera to Sandia, the town where Hasskarl had arrived disguised as a German six years previously. Two days from Crucero he arrived at a hut at the foot of a long cliff and met a ruddy-faced man who gave his name as Don Manuel Martel. A former colonel in the Peruvian army, Martel had lost a large amount of money in the bark trade. Now aged fifty-two, he claimed to have met Hasskarl in 1854 when he was travelling under the assumed name of Muller. He said that Hasskarl had offered him $40 to collect cinchona seed to which he had replied, 'not for $500'. Martel then pointedly told Markham how Hasskarl had hired Henriquez and how he had vowed that if he or anyone else ever again attempted to take cinchona plants out of Peru he would stir up the people and cut their feet off. 'There was evidently some allusion to myself in these remarks,' writes Markham, 'and I suspected, what afterwards proved to be the case, that Martel had, by some means, got information respecting the objects of my journey, and was desirous of thwarting them.'

Markham's suspicions would be proved right at Sandia. Forgoing a muleteer, he had had a frustrating journey to Crucero and across the four thousand metre pass that lay above the town. His pack-mules had bolted at every opportunity but rather than invest in his own mule train he had opted to exchange the animals at post-houses en route. This kept his costs low but also guaranteed that he was lumbered with the meanest and most recalcitrant beasts. The journey down from the pass had been particularly nerve-racking, as he had had to descend two thousand one hundred metres in just fifty kilometres. However, it was worth it for the sight that greeted him on arrival. Surrounded on all sides by mountains, Sandia is nestled in a steep ravine over which pour a series of spectacular waterfalls. The stepped hillsides produce some of the finest coffee and coca in all Peru. Moreover it was in the valley of Sandia that Dr Weddell first encountered the diminutive cinchona shrub he named *Cinchona josephiana* in honour of de Jussieu.

Markham's original plan was to make a leisurely survey of the cinchona forests, locate the most promising stands and then bide his time until August when the trees would be ripe and he could gather the seeds. After only two days in Sandia, however, he discovered that Martel had written to local elected officials, warning them of his intentions, and urging them to stop him. As if that were not bad enough, Martel had also begun stirring up other villages deeper into the cinchona forest. Markham's mission was fast becoming 'the talk of the whole country'. Unless he moved quickly he might not reach the coast alive.

Markham calculated that once he left Sandia there would be no possibility of finding fresh food and provisions, so he loaded up supplies that he hoped would last a month. In those days, explorers did not have the luxury of high-calorie powdered dinners or sophisticated water-purification systems. The food was simple – bread, cheese, chocolate and concentrated beef tea – and you used river water. In addition, Markham brought candles, ponchos, powder and shot, a tent, an airbed and a change of clothes. There would be seven in his party – himself, Weir, a young mestizo boy, Pablo Sevallos, and four Indians to carry the leather bags packed with supplies. No sooner had he left Sandia on the afternoon of 24 April, however, than one of the Indians deserted, leaving just three men to carry the provisions.

The trail led down a ravine along a series of ledges overhanging a fast-flowing river. It was narrow and dangerous, but the scenery was magnificent and the vegetation became richer and more tropical with each kilometre of the descent. Markham was encouraged by the fact that the few scattered huts they passed possessed no doors – testimony to the honesty of people in the region. To keep up with his Indian porters Markham had adopted the native habit of chewing coca. Like many an explorer since, he found it produced an 'agreeable soothing feeling' and meant he could abstain from eating food for long periods. More importantly, it enabled him to climb steep mountainsides 'with a feeling of lightness and elasticity' – a quality that he thought ought to recommend it to 'members of the Alpine Club'.

No doubt the coca added to Markham's appreciation of the dramatic scenery. Tier upon tier of coca terraces rose up one side of the ravine, their delicate green leaves contrasting with the deeper hues of the coffee plants, while on the other side the walls plunged dramatically down to the river. It was here that Markham encoun-tered the first wild cinchonas since his journey to the Madre de Dios with Father de Revello eight years before – *Cinchona josephiana*s with 'exquisite roseate flowers and rich green leaves with crimson veins.' Unfortunately, there were too few to be worth collecting. Neverthe-less, Markham noted down the best-looking specimens so that he would have no difficulty finding them, if necessary, on the return journey.

Next, he decided to leave the ravine he had been following since Sandia and descend to the Huari-huari. After camping by the river for the night, he then climbed up a steep ridge and crossed to the next valley along. Behind him now lay a series of spectacular ridges framed by distant snowy peaks. At last he was within touching distance of his goal – the cinchona forests hugging the Tambopata River. The last European to visit this area had been Dr Weddell in 1846. Markham's success now rested on his equalling the achievement of this great botanical explorer. It was a pivotal moment and one that seemed to bring to the fore all his fears and most deeply seated anxieties.

I am about to penetrate where no European has been before, and no human being for thirteen years, where there is no road, a dense matted forest, to suffer excessive fatigue, hunger, exposure, torments from insects, dangers from the nature of the country, from snakes and other animals, from savage Indians, and from the risk of accidents without the possibility of help: with the certainty of being vilified by those who sit at home and talk, if unsuccessful, and of having my services depreciated if successful. The feeling of having performed my duty manfully and well supports me through all this, and I know that my dear love will look on me with loving pride when I return, and that all true friends will do me justice.

One cannot read this soliloquy without feeling some sympathy for Markham. He knew he was not a botanist and was honest enough to recognize that his previous excursion to the Madre de Dios River hardly qualified him to lead such an important expedition. He was also intelligent enough to realize that from the India Office's point of view he was highly expendable. After all, what was one tax clerk more or less to the great British Empire?

But if his upper lip lacked the requisite Victorian stiffness he certainly did not show it in public. Instead he put on a brave face for his colleagues. To lessen everyone's anxieties he decided to turn the expedition into a game, naming his mule Joe after the *josephiana* and issuing the members of his party with pretend military ranks. Thus Savallos was promoted from aide de camp to lieutenant while he was to be referred to as Commander-in-Chief. The exercise must have triggered the military historian in him for he soon found himself musing on another British seaman-turned-adventurer, Sir Walter Raleigh. 'Our characters were, I think, cast in a similar mould. The same aspirations, the same love of enterprise, some of the same faults. Yet it is strange that Raleigh should have spent so much on the search for El Dorado . . . while I am now in perhaps the richest gold region in the world, and scarcely giving it a thought.'

Markham's first port of call was a hut on the Tambopata that Weddell had stopped at in 1846. Used as a rendezvous point by the local *cascarilleros*, it was owned by a local farmer, Don Juan de la

Cruz Gironda, and ideally situated for forays into the forest. Markham's supplies were already much reduced but fortunately Gironda agreed to supply him with enough food to get him back to Sandia. He also introduced Markham to an experienced local bark cutter, Mariano Martinez, who had guided Weddell. On 1 May they set off into the dense, tangled forest. Once again the party had swelled to seven. Martinez led the way, cutting a path through the jungle with his machete, with the others following behind in single file. The ground was choked with creepers, fallen bamboos and long tendrils that twisted round their ankles and tripped them at almost every step, and in many places they had to scramble along the verge of giddy precipices while the Tambopata surged beneath them. By the end of the first day Markham was exhausted. 'In some places we were half an hour forcing and cutting our way through a space of ten yards; and all the time, besides the torments of insects, I had a head ache and pain in the stomach. Looking back it seems like days, instead of hours that we have been forcing our way through the forest, and we have really only gone fifteen miles.'

For three days they continued like this, hacking their way through the jungle and scrambling up the riverbank whenever Martinez spotted a stand of cinchonas. The trees generally grew at a hundred and thirty to two hundred metres above the riverbank and gathering them was tiring. In some places, they had to cling to sheer precipices with only the half-rotten branches of trees as footholds, while in others they had to hack through foliage thick with thorns and hornets. Most evenings, Markham wrote, he would collapse by the campfire, 'sodden and wet to the skin, covered with moss and fungus, bitten all over by mosquitoes, my hands sliced in pieces by sharp grass'. Adding to their frustration was the scarcity of good trees. Relatively worthless cinchonas like *Cinchona ovata* were everywhere while the *calisayas* were generally found only on the most inaccessible ridges. Not surprisingly, after four days in the forest the Indian porters threatened to mutiny, saying they had been away from home long enough; besides, they had run out of maize and coca. Markham hurriedly sent one of the Indians back to Gironda to replenish their supplies and begged the others –

in Quechua — to stay. Luckily, the appeal worked. 'If they had deserted,' he admitted in his journal, 'all our plans would have been entirely frustrated.'

The Indian who had been to see Gironda soon returned with fresh food but the supplies could not sustain them indefinitely. Markham held out until 7 May, but when he saw that the provisions were once again running dangerously low he had to face reality: the time had come to turn round. They had managed to collect two hundred cinchona plants. It was a good amount to be getting on with and after laying them between layers of moss and Russian matting to keep them moist they set off for Gironda's clearing.

On the way back it began to rain heavily, making their earlier worries about the plants drying out seem ridiculous. Soon they were so wet that their hands were wrinkled 'like washerwomen's' and the damp had penetrated their gunpowder. On reaching a sheer precipice, Weir managed to scramble up the side and collect twenty-one more *calisayas*. The following day they were even more fortunate, finding a further hundred and nine of a variety known as *calisaya morada*, and by the time they reached Gironda's clearing they had more than five hundred plants, more than enough to fill the Wardian cases that were awaiting their return to Islay. All they had to do was pack them in moss and make their way back to Sandia and over the Andes. Then, on 11 May, just as they were about to leave, Gironda received an ominous letter from the *alcalde municipale* of Quiaca, ordering him to seize the plants and arrest Markham and Martinez immediately. The letter had been hand delivered by the son of Don Manuel Martel, the red-faced colonel Markham had met on the road to Sandia. Markham cursed his indiscretion. During their conversation he had made a passing reference to Martinez. Clearly Martel had guessed that, like Weddell, he intended to hire Martinez to guide him to the cinchonas and was using the fact to create difficulties for Gironda in the hope of getting his hands on his property.

Not surprisingly, the letter filled Gironda with alarm and he immediately proposed disposing of the plants, leaving Markham with just a few, which he could smuggle out without his involvement. But

Markham had come too far and been through too much to give up so easily. Arguing that the *alcalde* had no authority to order his arrest and that he had no intention of harming Peru's national interest, he told Gironda he was leaving immediately and, if necessary, would defend the plants with force. The threat worked and after sitting up with the cinchonas all night Markham set off at dawn the following morning. But he was by no means out of danger.

No sooner had he climbed out of the forest than he saw Martel's son and a party of *mestizos* waiting for him on the *pajonal*. As they drew nearer Martel began cursing the Indians in Quechua, demanding to know how they dared steal Peru's national property and warning them they would be arrested as soon as they reached Sandia. The situation was poised on a knife-edge. Markham drew his revolver. Martel hesitated. The powder was damp but Martel wasn't to know that. Slowly he measured Markham with his eyes; then he stepped back and allowed him to pass. Markham's nerve had held. Now he just had to get to the coast.

Unknown to Markham, however, Martel had been busy rallying the newly formed municipal *juntas* in the towns that lay along his escape route and by the time he reached Sandia three days later an alliance had been formed to prevent the cinchonas leaving Peru. The Sandians refused to sell him fresh mules and said he would have to go to Crucero, where Martel was waiting for him, to buy them instead. Markham knew full well that that would spell the end of his mission. Fortunately for him, one of Sandia's councillors was sympathetic to his plight and in return for his gun agreed to supply him with the mules he needed, as well as an Indian guide. In the hope of throwing Martel off the scent, Markham despatched Weir to Crucero and, avoiding the main road to Arequipa, set a direct compass course over the cordillera to Vilque instead.

It was a hazardous route but the difficulties were tempered by Markham's knowledge that his test was almost at an end. 'Tomorrow, I bid farewell to the montana of Caravaya, that lovely golden land, where I have worked harder and with more anxious care, and done better service than I ever did in my life before. The time has been one of intense anxiety and enjoyment – an earnest desire to do the work well, and a feeling of joy at having so great a work entrusted to me, and a chance of performing a really important service to mankind.' On the morning of 17 May he saddled his trusty mule Joe, and driving before him two others laden with the plants, set off accompanied by Angelino Paco, his Indian guide. Markham assumed that Paco knew the country but as they left the valley of Sandia behind it became clear that he had never taken this route before. Markham had no choice but to rely on his compass. Then, with night coming on and no moon, Markham pitched his tent behind a range of black cliffs and opened his pack. *Disaster*. His food and matches had been stolen in Sandia. All they had to sustain them was Paco's small store of parched maize.

They spent a hungry night huddled together for warmth and left early the next morning. Their route now led up the summit of the Cordillera of Caravaya and across a desolate, frosty plain populated only by vicuñas and wild geese. Eventually, after eleven hours in the saddle, they reached an abandoned shepherd's hut and spent another freezing night with the thermometer dipping as low as 20 degrees Fahrenheit. They awoke to discover the mules had bolted and spent three hours chasing them down. Despite their fatigue they then rode for another day, going to bed without supper. All the while Markham had to keep a close eye on the mules to prevent them from rolling and crushing the plants. At night, to protect the cinchonas from the frost, he curled up with them under his poncho. Never mind that he was starving and bitterly cold himself. All that mattered was that the plants were safe.

Finally on the fourth day out from Sandia they reached a small estancia where in exchange for the remainder of his coca an Indian family provided Markham with milk and cheese. The next day he reached a huge unmarked lake populated by immense flocks of flamingos, as well as ibises, ducks and cranes. As the flamingos whirled up in a long spiral column, their crimson wings and rose-coloured necks silhouetted against the azure Andean sky, Markham allowed himself a brief moment of reflection. 'It was,' he wrote, 'one of the most beautiful sights' he had ever seen.

On the 22nd they reached Vilque but Markham could not risk stopping and, after gathering fresh supplies, he left promptly the following afternoon. Ignoring a series of gales and icy squalls, he marched rapidly across the cordillera, reaching Arequipa on the 27th. Here he was reunited with Minna and, two days later, with Weir who, as he had anticipated, had found Martel lying in wait for him at Crucero. The sub-prefect had detained Weir but finding no plants on him he was forced to let him go. With no one to rally local opinion against him, Markham left Arequipa almost immediately, and the plants were safely deposited in the Wardian cases at Islay on 1 June. Of the 529 plants he had brought out of Caravaya just 73 had perished on the cordillera. His problems were by no means over, however. At Islay the superintendent of the Customs House refused to allow the plants to leave the port without an express order from the Minister of Finance. This was potentially an even bigger threat than Martel. The President of Peru had already issued a decree prohibiting cinchona from being exported and Markham calculated that it was only a matter of time before it was forwarded to the authorities in the interior and customs officers on the coast. However, Markham guessed that because of the ramshackle state of the country a copy of the decree would not yet exist in the office of the Minister of Finance and that if he rode to Lima he might be able to browbeat officials into giving him the necessary papers. 'Besides,' he wrote, 'all clerks in public offices are changed in every revolution, and there are no officials with more than two or three years' experience. My only hope was in their ignorance, for I well knew that their jealousy of foreigners would induce them to seize upon any plausible excuse for prohibiting the embarkation of the plants.'

Leaving Weir in charge of the Wardian cases, Markham rode directly to Lima, where he demanded an audience with the Minister of Finance, José Salcedo. It turned out that Salcedo had formerly been a Colonel of the Horse and had been appointed by the President – an 'illiterate but shrewd Indian' – to show his contempt for the other branches of public service. As Markham had predicted, he knew nothing about the order. Nevertheless, he had to use a combination of

cajolery and threats to persuade Salcedo to give the necessary permission and it was only after warning of dire diplomatic consequences
and several re-draftings of the letter that he obtained the correct form
of words.

The cinchonas meanwhile had begun to throw out buds and
young leaves – proof that they had recovered from the journey across
the cordillera – and on returning to Islay on the 23rd Markham
immediately had them hoisted on board a launch ready for transfer to
the steamer *Valparaiso*. But incredibly the plants were still not out of
danger. In the middle of the night an attempt was made to bribe the
boatmen to bore holes in the Wardian cases and pour boiling water
on them. Then, no sooner were the plants at sea, than one of the
panes of glass on the cases was smashed. Markham suspected a group
of Peruvians he had overhead grumbling about foreigners 'robbing the
country' and threatened to throw them overboard if he caught them
tampering with the cases again. The threat did the trick and the plants
arrived intact at Lima on 26 June, crossing the Isthmus of Panama
soon after. As Markham watched the American coast disappear
beneath the horizon he could barely contain his sense of achievement.

> It could not but be satisfactory to look back upon the extraordi-
> nary difficulties we had overcome, the hardships and dangers of
> the forests, the scarcity of the plants, the bewildering puzzle to
> find them amidst the dense Underwood, the endeavour to stop
> my journey . . . and then to see the great majority of the plants
> budding and looking healthy in the Wardian cases. So far as
> our work in South America was concerned, it had been
> performed with complete success.

Whatever the Cassandras at home might say, Markham could
return to Britain with his head held high. The quest was over. His
only regret was that he had been unable to persuade the British
government to take the cases straight across the Pacific to India on
HMS *Vixen*, which had been lying idle at Callao. Unfortunately for
Markham, that penny-pinching would later prove costly.

Chapter Seven

# SPRUCE'S RIDGE

The sounding cataract,
Haunted me like a passion; the tall rock,
The mountain, and the deep and gloomy wood,
Their colours and their forms, were then to me
An appetite, a feeling, and a love.

William Wordsworth

IT IS JUST FIFTY KILOMETRES as the condor flies from the summit of Chimborazo to the cinchona forests in the western foothills of the Quintanian Andes, but the descents are among the most dramatic in all the Americas. From the rim of the glacier at five thousand eight hundred metres you plunge through freezing clouds and a series of treacherous bogs to emerge on a bleak, wind-chafed *arenal*. On the *arenal* the ground is flat and the going easier, but it doesn't last. Soon you arrive at the Ensillada, 'the saddleback' – a craggy ridge on the western shoulder of the extinct volcano. From here you plunge down again, into a verdant bowl-shaped valley and up the other side to another ridge. Now you are poised above the cloudforest at three thousand metres looking towards the Pacific Ocean. Enjoy the view. From here on in the descents are almost vertical. To reach the zone where the cinchonas grow you must drop straight down and up and over another ridge, and another, and another, slipping and sliding along trails that are little more than mud-chutes. If your pack animals survive and your legs do not give out you will be exhausted and exhilarated. You will also have descended eighteen hundred metres in just twenty-five kilometres.

Even for someone in peak physical condition the trail is gruelling, but for Spruce it should have been next to impossible. While Markham was fighting his way out of the Tambopata valley, Spruce was still recovering from the mysterious rheumatic and nervous condition that had afflicted him in April. By early June he had been confined to his bed for two months. Unfortunately, we do not know what treatment he received or what thoughts went through his mind during this period as his journal from Ecuador is missing, but his sudden disability must have been mortifying. The India Office had entrusted him with the most important botanical commission of his career. To fail would have been forgivable but to not even try to gather the cinchonas was unthinkable. Somehow Spruce had to muster the same strength and determination that had seen him recover from malaria and other threats to his life on the Orinoco and Amazon and cross Chimborazo.

Spruce had always done what had been asked of him before but on this occasion it took Dr Taylor's intervention to effect a cure. On hearing of his friend's illness, Taylor had rushed to his bedside in Ambato and prescribed various remedies. We do not know what they were but they cannot have been very effective, as he was soon resorting to psychology, telling Spruce that if he could only get over the sierra he might find the drier, Pacific air on the western side of the mountain reviving. Incredibly, the pep talk worked and on 11 June Spruce hauled himself from his sickbed and set off with Taylor on horseback for Mocha, a small village to the east of Chimborazo, with a view to traversing the southern shoulder of the volcano and descending to Limon – the ridge where the *cascarilla roja* grew. If Spruce's report on the expedition is to be believed it was the most demanding he had ever undertaken. 'Not to interrupt the rest of my narrative with the continual groanings of an invalid,' he writes, 'I may say here, once for all, that . . . I was but too often in that state of prostration when to lie down quietly and die would have seemed a relief.'

His illness had left him so debilitated that on the first day out he needed two long rests, and by nightfall he and Taylor were still picking their way over the *paramo* of Sanancajas, a grassy area on Chimborazo's southern flank. Thick cloud had obscured their view of the mountain during the ride from Ambato but at sunset the cloud lifted, leaving, Spruce writes, 'a slender meniscus, assuming exactly the form of the cope of the mountain', clinging to the summit. At length this too dissipated, exposing the monarch of the Andes in all its 'glory' and allowing them to pick their way by the moonlight reflected off the glacier. Although the sight revived his spirits, by the time they reached Chuquipogyo, a small run-down settlement at four thousand metres, Spruce was so exhausted he found sleep impossible and the following morning was unable to mount his horse. Spruce does not record whether he had a headache and nausea – the most common signs of altitude sickness – but he was now at an altitude where stronger men had succumbed and took the whole of the next day and night to recuperate. The next morning, however, was fine with only a few drops of rain and sleet, and Spruce felt sufficiently strong to resume the journey.

Skirting round the edge of the glacier, he and Taylor soon found themselves on the *arenal*. Here the road became flat and smooth, like a 'gravel-walk in England'. They had now crossed the watershed between the Oriente and Pacific weather systems, and while on the eastern side of Chimborazo it had been rainy and overcast, on the western side of the mountain the sky was clear and a fierce wind buffeted their horses. They were still above three thousand six hundred metres and the only vegetation was small hassocks of *Stipa* and *Festuca*, but as they descended to the Ensillada they began to see bright-yellow calceolarias, red gentians, violas and other pretty Andean flowers. Then, at six hundred metres below the *arenal*, Spruce came upon the first trees – the birch-coloured *Polylepis*, with its peculiar flaking bark, *Podarcapus*, and *Araliacea*, known as tiger's paw because of its hairy palm-like leaves.

Ecuador was still embroiled in civil war and at the Ensillada they saw that several low straw huts had been erected to provide shelter for government soldiers preparing to march on the Peruvian-backed rebels at Guayaquil. As they approached, four raw-looking youths armed with lances rushed out and demanded their passports. Spruce considered unholstering his revolver and firing a shot in the air, but then he remembered he had a far better weapon — a bottle of aguardiente. The fiery brandy melted the soldiers' opposition and Spruce continued on down, crossing the 'saddleback' and dropping into the next valley. By nightfall they had reached Guaranda, a lively market town perched like Rome on seven hillsides. Here Spruce was detained for several days, buying fresh provisions and pack animals for the forthcoming descent to Limon. So far Spruce and Taylor had relied on mules but the trails on the western slopes of the Quintanian Andes are so steep, narrow and slippery that their provisions now had to be carried in single file by *cabrestillos* — tough Andean bulls. Before leaving Ambato, Spruce had made a deal with Dr Neyra, the owner of the bark forests, that he would hire eleven of his *cascarilleros* to guide him to the best trees and help him collect the plants and seeds. But at Guaranda he learnt the *cascarilleros* had been pressed into military service and were forbidden to leave.

Dr Neyra secured the services of four Indians instead, but Spruce soon discovered they knew little about cinchonas or their cultivation. Fortunately, by now Robert Cross — the Kew gardener whose job it was to nurse the cinchonas and convey them to India — had arrived at Guayaquil and Spruce sent him a message, via the British Consul, instructing him to rendezvous with him at Ventanas, a village just below Limon.

On 17 June Spruce and Taylor were finally ready to leave. They loaded their provisions of potatoes, peas and barley meal, taking care to make sure the sacks did not protrude too far from the bulls' backs, and set off for Guanujo, where a trail led up the opposite side of the valley to the next ridge and the pass of Llullundengo, a small V-shaped cutting that guards the entrance to the Pacific cloudforests. From here there was only one direction to go — straight down.

According to Spruce, the descent from Llullundengo at three thousand metres was 'the most precipitous and dangerous' he had ever negotiated. The trail was not so much a track as a near-vertical mud ladder rutted with camel-humps from the constant passage of animals' hooves. In places the humps were so slick with grease that it was all he could do to guide his horse from one to another without it losing its footing. One false step and Spruce risked tumbling headlong into the clouds.

His goal was a ridge some eighteen hundred metres below the pass, overlooking the River Limon. Even today the descent is both arduous and spectacular. For the first five hundred metres you feel like Jack scrambling down the beanstalk. Then the clouds disappear and the hillside is a riot of colour: yellow *Calceolariae*, blood-red *Melasto-maceae*, the violet of spreading *Pleroma*, and every now and then a bromeliad camped in the branches of a tree, its fiery tentacles reaching for the sky.

It took Spruce all day to reach his first campsite, some twelve hundred metres below the pass, beside the Río de las Tablas. But that valley was only the first in a series of troughs. From there he had to climb up and over another ridge and another, the trail becoming narrower and more treacherous with every descent. At one place, Spruce writes, the track was so deep and straight he had to throw his legs onto his horse's back to save them from being crushed, and at another, the path was so pitted with stones that there was 'a risk of both horse and rider turning a summerset'.

Gradually, as Spruce neared the cinchona region, the air became warmer and more humid. As he entered the rainforest, ferns and giant palms formed a canopy over his head. Then at just below twelve hundred metres, Spruce writes, 'we came out on the first chacras at Limon, where I almost immediately noted, and with no small satisfaction, a group of three red bark trees, each consisting of from two to four stems of 30 feet high, springing from old stools, and bearing a small quantity of fruit.'

From here he had just three more kilometres of gentle descent before arriving at the cane mill that was to be his home and collecting station for the next three months.

'*Cinchona succirubra* is a very handsome tree,' writes Spruce, 'and in looking out over the forest I could never see any other tree at all comparable to it for beauty. Across the narrow glen below our hut . . . there was a large old stool from which sprang several shoots, only one of which rose to a tree . . . This tree was 50 feet high . . . It had never flowered, but was so densely leafy that not a branch could be seen; and the large, broadly oval, deep green and shining leaves, mixed with decaying ones of a blood-red colour, gave the tree a most striking appearance.'

There are no trees the same size on Spruce's ridge today – they were all stripped of their bark and felled years ago – but the ruins of the cane mill are still there, and when the mist lifts the view is spectacular. The ridge runs east–west, falling gradually on the northern side to the Limon River, and very steeply on the southern side to a tributary of the Chausan. The top of the ridge has been given over to a banana plantation but the slopes are still littered with young *Cinchona succirubra* – descendants perhaps of the same trees described by Spruce a hunded and forty years ago.

Spruce and Taylor found their accommodation rudimentary. The cane mill was merely a long, low shed with rough, ill-fitting planks that let in the chilly mist and Spruce soon found that his clothes had turned mouldy and his cough had returned. From questioning one of the first settlers at Limon, Spruce learned that the forests above the ridge used to be full of bark trees, as well as bears and pumas. At first the settlers had used the trees for firewood, but soon dealers came from Guayaquil offering them money for the bark and, as they could still keep the firewood, they began felling trees throughout the forest. In no time every ridge and valley had been stripped bare, with the result that by the time the landowners excluded the bark-dealers with a view to preserving the trees, the damage had been done.

Incredibly, the settlers had no idea of the bark's true worth. According to Spruce the prevalent opinion was that the Europeans used it to make a chocolate-coloured dye. When he tried to explain that the bark was the source of the 'precious quinine which was of such vast use in medicine', Spruce reports they scoffed with disbelief, saying to one another, 'It's all very fine for him to stuff us with such a tale; of course, he won't tell us how the dye is made, or we should use it ourselves for our ponchos and our bayetas.'

Like Humboldt, Spruce observed that the *cascarilleros* also refused to take the bark for malaria, believing that its heat would only exacerbate the fever and that the correct treatment was *frescos* – cooling drinks. The same prejudice even extended to quinine, as Spruce discovered when he tried to offer some to a young mill-hand who had fallen ill on the way back from the low country around Ventanas. 'I offered to give them quinine, but they had evidently a great horror of it, and had I given it to the lad in the remissions of the fever, they would have mixed nostrums of their own, so that, had the case gone wrong, the blame would have been laid on us.'[1]

Spruce could not let such prejudices influence his own work and no sooner had he set up home in the mill than he began scouring the ridge for viable seeds to ship to India. It did not take him long to find thirty cinchonas in full flower, but when he collected specimens and dried them he discovered the seeds were not yet ripe. The reason was the damp climate. For most of the day the ridge was draped in a cool, impenetrable mist. It was only in the late morning that the sun broke the clouds, ripening the seeds, but by early afternoon the mist had rolled in again and the sunlight was gone. At Guaranda the *cascarilleros* had assured Spruce that he would find plenty of seedlings, but he now discovered that they were simply shoots from old stools and that the only young plants that were viable were the suckers of *Cinchona magnifolia* – worthless because the species contains hardly any quinine.

Spruce could scout the virgin forest for older *Cinchona succirubra* trees in the hope of finding young seedlings growing nearby, but most of the larger trees had already been stripped to their root balls and, without the aid of the *cascarilleros*, the chances of finding untouched stands was low. To succeed in his mission Spruce needed the help of an expert and sent Dr Taylor to Ventanas to look for Cross. But ten days later Spruce received word from the Spanish Minister that Cross had been taken ill at Guayaquil and had yet to set out.

' Spruce decided to press on with the work anyway. He recalled Taylor and together they began scouting the ridge, noting down the locations of the best trees. The bark forest stretched for about six and a half kilometres, and as there was a fair amount of sun at the end of June, Spruce had high hopes of the seeds ripening rapidly. But July was cool and foggy again with the result that most of the capsules scarcely increased in size while others were attacked by maggots and mould. The climate filled Spruce with despair. 'I began to fear we should get no ripe seeds this year, and as the seeds had been especially recommended to me in my instructions from England, it may be imagined how severe was my feeling of disappointment.'

Now, to add to his worries, the locals decided that he should buy seeds direct from them and one morning, while he was out making his rounds, he discovered that two of the trees had been stripped of their panicles. Concerned that the remaining trees would be ruined in the same way, Spruce toured the local *chacras* offering a gratuity to the owners to prevent anyone but him approaching the trees and telling them the seeds would be useless unless he collected them himself. 'This had the desired effect,' writes Spruce, 'and I do not think a single capsule was molested afterwards.'

However, his problems were far from over. About the same time that Taylor left Ventanas, the government troops garrisoned on Chimborazo began marching down from the sierra to attack the revolutionary forces that held Guayaquil and the low country. Contrary to all expectation they selected the route via Limon and Ventanas. 'For six weeks we were kept in continual alarm by the passage of troops, and it required all our vigilance to prevent our horses and other goods being stolen ... Indeed if I had had no companion who was independent of the political feuds of the country, I do not see how I could have got on at all.'

It was now impossible for Spruce to send Taylor to Loja to collect specimens of C. *officinalis* as he needed him to ride to Guaranda each month to replenish their precious stocks of barley and pease-meal that, due to the moist climate, rotted rapidly. Spruce could not send his Indian servants for fear of their being press-ganged into the army and without Taylor, he writes, 'I might literally have perished of hunger.'

Meanwhile, Spruce still had no idea what had become of Cross – he might have died or he might have left Guayaquil and be on his way to Limon. Spruce could not afford to wait and began noting down the location of healthy trees that had failed to flower that year with a view to striking his own cuttings. He was just about to start out for the trees with Taylor and two Indian guides when he heard that an Englishman had been spotted at Ventanas with a cargo of peculiar boxes. Spruce immediately sent Taylor to Ventanas to investigate. There he discovered that the Englishman was none other than Cross and that the peculiar boxes were the fifteen Wardian cases that Markham had deposited at Guayaquil the previous December. Cross had had all sorts of obstacles thrown in his way by the troops who held the river. He had scarcely been able to find enough men to paddle his canoes and the journey from Guayaquil had taken him nearly two weeks. Nevertheless, despite being pale and thin from his recent illness he was keen to start work and after resting for one day he began setting up an experimental nursery. Cross had been forced to leave the Wardian cases at Aguacatal, a village near Ventanas, for safekeeping, so to keep the cuttings shaded and free of fungus he built frames and an adjustable roof out of palm-fronds. By the beginning of August he had planted more than a thousand cuttings and within three weeks a number had begun to take root. At first the weather continued foggy, but by mid-August the days were scorching hot and the only way to keep the sun from drying out the plants was to ferry water to the nursery in bamboo buckets. Then, just as the cuttings were beginning to thrive, they were attacked by caterpillars. Cross dealt with these too but, Spruce writes, it was only thanks to his 'unremitting watchfulness' that the plants survived.

Meanwhile the sun had begun to ripen the capsules on the cinchona trees in the forest and on 13 August Spruce noticed they were beginning to burst at the base. He quickly ordered his Indian porters to climb the branches and begin breaking off the panicles one by one while he spread a sheet on the ground so that none of the seeds would be lost. In this way, within two weeks all the seeds had been harvested and by early September they were dry.

The pains he had taken to collect the seeds paid off. Cross sowed eight of the seeds on 16 August and by the first week of September all were producing healthy plants. By now his rooted cuttings were also thriving and he had more than enough to fill the Wardian cases. But Spruce wanted to be sure he had obtained all the best seeds and now rode south across the valley to San Antonio, where Pavon had originally collected the red bark, to take an inventory of the trees.

At San Antonio the cinchona forests extend to a lower elevation than at Limon, reaching almost to the Guayaquilian plain. In consequence the trees are more exposed to the sun and wind and the town is unhealthier, with fevers a common complaint. Not wishing to linger, Spruce collected five hundred capsules and hurried back to Limon. He now had a total of two and a half thousand capsules. As each capsule contained an average of forty seeds Spruce calculated that he had at least a hundred thousand – more than enough to satisfy the needs of empire.

Now, at last, he learnt that the provisional government troops under the command of General Flores had taken Guayaquil and that, consequently, communications with the interior had been reopened. Spruce decided to ride to Bodegas immediately and from there catch a steamboat direct to Guayaquil from where he could despatch a portion of the seeds to Kew while awaiting the arrival of Cross with the plants. He reached Bodegas (now Babahoyo) without difficulty but once there discovered that the only available steamer had been commandeered by the government. He had no choice but to wait eight days, finally arriving at Guayaquil on 7 October. Seven days later Spruce despatched two packets of seeds on a Panamanian-bound

steamer: one to Kew and Sir William Hooker; the second to the
Botanic Gardens in Jamaica.

Spruce had successfully completed the first part of his mission, but
concluding the second part would prove far harder than either he or
Cross could have imagined. Spruce had left Limon without knowing
when the plants would be sturdy enough to bring down to Ventanas.
As it was all but impossible to get a message to Cross he simply had
to sit it out in Guayaquil and await news from his colleague. This
was easier said than done. Revolution was still in the air and hardly a
day went by without a fire or some other commotion in the busy
coastal port. In addition, Guayaquil lies on a fault line and was now
hit by a series of violent earthquakes. Fortunately, the wooden house
Spruce had rented for himself and his botanical specimens was well
built and survived the shocks. Nevertheless, it was a relief when in
November he received word from Cross that the plants would be
ready by the end of the month.

On 24 November Spruce returned to Bodegas and proceeded
upriver to Aguacatal – the village where Cross had deposited the
Wardian cases the previous July. Spruce spent the next two days
carefully hammering the cases together. Then he cast about for a raft
big enough to accommodate the cases and allow space for cooking
and sleeping. He eventually found one a little further upriver. It
belonged to an elderly black man and was constructed from twelve
huge trunks, twenty metres long and thirty centimetres in diameter,
the largest that could safely navigate the river. The old man agreed to
rent the raft to Spruce for $90 and together they brought it down
to Aguacatal where Spruce loaded the Wardian cases ready to receive
the plants from Cross.

He did not arrive until 13 December. It had taken Cross longer
than he expected to construct bamboo baskets for transporting the
plants. He had not dared to entrust such a delicate operation to anyone
but himself and insisted on carefully wrapping each plant in wet

moss. The result was that only a few were lost in the descent from Limon – a consequence of the bulls running through the bush – and by the time he transferred them to the Wardian cases he had 637 ready for transport to India. Rather than run the risk of the glass in the cases breaking on the river, he left the windows off, stretching moistened strips of calico around the cases instead to protect the plants from the elements.

By now the rains had begun and the level of the river was rising rapidly. The only means of steering the raft was with long bamboo oars, two in the prow and one in the stern. On 24 December they set off, five in all: Spruce, Cross, two oarsmen at the front and the elderly black at the stern. According to Spruce the river 'ran like a sluice'. There were so many twists and turns it was difficult to keep the raft in midstream and out of the way of the branches and twiners that hung over the river. After several hours of steering the raft around these perils the craft suddenly went 'dead on' through a mass of overhanging branches. 'The effect,' writes Spruce, 'was tremendous: the heavy cases were hoisted up and dashed against each other; the roof of our cabin smashed in; and the old pilot was for some moments so completely involved in the branches and the wreck of the roof, that I expected nothing but that he had been carried away.'

Luckily, he managed to hang on but the deck now presented 'a lamentable sight'. Branches and sticks were strewn all over the raft and the roof was caved in. After running into the bushes twice more they finally found an area of the bank that was clear of foliage and hove to to make repairs. Miraculously, there were only a few slight cracks in the cases and none of them had turned over. Spruce spent a fitful night awake with one eye on the level of the river lest it suddenly fall and the raft be swamped by a landslide from the bank. Then, at daybreak, they continued downriver, Cross this time helping the old man to handle the oar at the stern.

At Caracoal the river widened and the banks were less overhung with branches so that the going became smoother. At noon they passed Bodegas and by nightfall they had reached the tidal part of the river. It was now simply a matter of riding the ebb and flow until they washed up at Guayaquil. But the going was so slow that on Christmas Day they were still stuck on the river.

Finally on 27 December they drifted into the estuary and were able to bring the raft into port. Spruce immediately leapt ashore to fetch a carpenter to assist Cross in repairing the cases. Next they transferred the cases to a launch and had them brought alongside the dock ready to be loaded onto the next available ship.

Three days later a goods steamer arrived from Lima. The ship was not due to sail again until 2 January and then only to Paita in northern Peru. From there, however, Cross could catch another steamer passing from Lima to Panama. Satisfied that the plants were safely on board and that he had done everything in his power to ensure the success of the mission, Spruce now took his leave of Cross confident that the plants were 'likely to go on prosperously'.

Like Markham, Spruce believed that in doing his patriotic duty he was also benefiting mankind. But in fulfilling his commission Spruce incurred the wrath of the Ecuadorian government and in his subsequent report to the India Office he felt obliged to justify his actions.

> I have seen enough of collecting the products of the forest to convince me, that *whatever vegetable substance is needful to man, he must ultimately cultivate the plant producing it* [Spruce's italics]. Whilst the demand for such precious substances as Peruvian bark, sarsaparilla, caoutchouc [rubber] etc must necessarily go on increasing, the supply yielded by the forest will decrease, and ultimately fail. My operations in the Red Bark woods have only partially opened the eyes of the Ecuatoreans to this fact, but have in a high degree excited their jealousy at the prospect of another nation participating in the possession of a treasure which they have not known how to preserve from deterioration and proxi-mate destruction, but which, with a little foresight, might have been an endless source of wealth to their country.

Spruce was right about the destruction. By the time he arrived in Limon the trade in bark was already much reduced. In 1859 the *cascarilleros* had only collected 2.2 tonnes of red bark and in 1860 none at all had been got out from Limon. The reason for the decline, of course, was the *cascarilleros*' ruthless felling of trees. In the valleys of the Chausan and Limon Spruce had seen only two hundred mature trees left standing. Of these only a few had attained their full grandeur of twenty-five metres, the rest being fifteen metres or under. Nearly all the trees were growths from old stools. He was unable to find a single plant that had seeded from a flowering tree in the forest, and in the meadows any seedlings that could have taken root were trodden upon by grazing cattle.

On the other hand, in 1859 a quintal – 100lb, or 45kg – of bark had fetched US $43. Within thirty years, thanks to the success of the Indian plantations, the price had dropped to $10 a quintal – barely enough to pay for the labour of getting it out of the forest. Markham's defence of the missions reiterated how much the Andean republics would benefit from the British example in India and adopt better cultivation methods. But, as we shall see, this never happened. Instead, the success of the Indian and Dutch plantations effectively killed the Andean bark industry. In this respect at least, Spruce's argument that it was impossible to stop men propagating economically valuable plants was more realistic than Markham's.

The Ecuadorians, however, were not nearly as forgiving of Spruce as the Peruvians had been of Markham. Although Spruce had not broken any law, within four months Ecuador had passed a decree forbidding foreigners from exporting plants, cuttings or seeds, and compelling the *cascarilleros* to plant around each felled tree six more plants or shoots of the same variety. The decree also forbade further exportation of the bark, requiring that in future quinine be manufac-tured on the spot, and inviting Bolivia and Colombia (Peru, under-standably given the recent animosities, was not included) to follow suit.

It was hopelessly unrealistic, of course. Spruce scoffed that the whole thing was framed 'on the dog in the manger principle' and that 'sticking six branches in the ground' was hardly a scientific way of seeking to restock the bark forests. Nevertheless, in extracting the red bark from Limon, Spruce – like Markham in Peru – had taken advantage of the confused political climate. Had the civil war finished a few months earlier it is unlikely he would have been allowed to export the plants.

Robert Cross had no such excuses. As soon as the *Cinchona succirubra* seeds and plants were safely delivered to India, he returned to South America to collect specimens of *Cinchona officinalis* from Loja. By now it was autumn 1861 and the Ecuadorian decree prohibiting the export of cinchona was in full force. Spruce had originally intended to send Taylor to Loja but had been forced to change his plans at the last moment because of the civil war. Markham, however, was determined to collect specimens of *all* the commercially significant barks and it was on his instructions that on 17 September Cross left Guayaquil in an open rowing boat and landed at Santa Rosa, the port for the province of Loja. From there he crossed a series of swamps and steep ridges, reaching Loja ten days later. On 1 October he began ascending Cajanuma – the mountain visited by La Condamine and Humboldt. Setting up camp in a hut belonging to a *cascarillero* near the summit, he began exploring the woods for *C. officinalis* stands. After several days of fruitless searching he suddenly spotted a number of fine young trees in a steep ravine. The trees were in flower and on closer examination he discovered some of the seeds were ripe. Thereafter, he continued searching all the ravines from sunrise to sunset, often abseiling to the bottom by means of overhanging vines. By the time he returned to Guayaquil in December he had amassed nearly a hundred thousand seeds.

Eighteen months later Markham called on Cross again – despatching him this time to Colombia to collect specimens of *C. pitayensis* and the so-called 'Santa Fe' and 'Cartagena barks' – respectively *C. lancifolia* and *C. cordifolia*. Leaving his home on the western slopes of Chimborazo, Cross proceeded direct to Popayán, which lies just across the Ecuadorian border in southern Colombia. From there he headed east to Syliva, the headquarters of the bark collectors near the volcano Purace. At Pitayo, on the forested slopes and ravines beneath the volcano, he collected four hundred and fifty ripened capsules of *C. pitayensis*, returning with them to Guayaquil in November.

By now, Markham writes, Cross was 'prostrated by ague' but it was not the end of his exertions. In 1868 Markham sent him back to Pitayo to collect specimens he had missed on his first trip. Then, in 1877, he called on him a fifth time, sending him to Caqueta and the Magdalena valley to collect the Santa Fe and Cartagena barks. Cross was once again attacked by 'swamp fever' and was only able to keep up with his Indian porters by the continual consumption of coca. But in March 1868 after innumerable sufferings and hardships he limped back to England triumphant.

In 1860 Markham had also succeeded in gathering specimens of the so-called grey barks from Huánuco, northern Peru. The result was that by 1864 he had collected cinchonas from four of the five regions he considered the most important – Pitayo, Limon, Loja, and Huánuco. He had also collected *calisaya* trees from Carabaya in southern Peru, of course, but without the so-called *calisaya vera* of northern Bolivia the set was incomplete. Unknown to Markham, however, Charles Ledger had been following his activities closely and now began to hatch his own plans.

On arriving in Australia in 1853, Ledger had gone straight to New South Wales where he presented his proposal for the import of alpaca to the government. According to him, officials gave him a verbal undertaking that if he succeeded in landing a hundred of the animals his expenses would be reimbursed and he would be granted ten thousand acres on which to graze them. Convinced that the 'dry' air of New South Wales was similar to that of the Peruvian highlands, Ledger hurried back to South America to be reunited with his flock, landing at Valparaiso in July 1853. By now Peru and Bolivia were at war and Ledger realized he could take advantage of the political confusion to move his flock, which was now in southern Bolivia, across the border to Argentina. From there he could drive them along the cordillera to Laguna Blanca, across the Chilean border and down to Puerto Caldera on the coast, from where they could be shipped to Australia.

It took him nearly five years. Accompanied by Manuel and his son, Santiago, Ledger rejoined his flock at San Cristóbal in November and began driving them to the Argentinian border. Of the four hundred and fifty alpaca that had set off from Ledger's estate in Chulluncayani, Peru, the previous year there were now just three hundred and twelve. Conditions were atrocious. It was mid-winter and in crossing the cordillera they found themselves mired in deep snow and ice. As the weather worsened, many of the animals perished in snowstorms, forcing Ledger to stop and purchase fresh alpaca from Indians along the way. To add to his worries, Ledger had run out of money and at one point had to ride sixteen hundred kilometres back to Valparaiso to raise fresh funds from his backers. Next he learnt that the Bolivians, angered by his crossing of the Peruvian border without a proper licence, had issued a warrant for his arrest. He hurried across the border to Argentina, giving a soldier who had been sent from Potosí to arrest him the slip.

By spring 1856 Ledger had reached Salta but just as he was contemplating a summer crossing of the Andes to Chile his flock suffered a massive infestation of leeches. Within days two hundred animals had died and he was back to square one. Returning to Bolivia to replenish the alpaca was out of the question. Instead, Ledger decided to buy llamas and wild vicuñas and crossbreed them with the alpaca until he had reconstituted the herd. The effort took him the better part of a year. In May 1857 he wintered the herd at Laguna Blanca, a freezing lake in a valley in the high tablelands west of Tucumán. Walled corals were built to contain the animals and the long days were taken up with nursing the crossbreeds and ice-skating. The surreal scene was well captured by Mamani's son who, signing himself 'Santiago Savage', depicted the activities in a series of vivid watercolours.

By May 1858 Ledger had a herd of six hundred and nineteen alpaca, llamas, vicuñas and cross-breeds and he was ready to drive the animals to the Chilean coast. It was a journey he would remember for the rest of his life. It took him eight days to cross the Andes into Chile, climbing through a series of passes as high as five thousand five hundred metres and sleeping at night on sheets of ice. Then he had to lead the herd down the western cordillera and across the parched Atacama Desert. By the time he reached Copiapo near the Chilean coast a month later he had lost a further hundred and seventy-nine animals and the herd numbered four hundred and twenty-one. Nevertheless, it was a Herculean feat. The townspeople of Copiapo had never seen alpaca before and for several days the city was deserted as they flocked to view the herd.

When Ledger finally reached Australia in November 1858, the *Sydney Morning Herald* praised his 'unparalleled daring', opining that he had accomplished a feat that had 'hitherto been considered altogether impracticable.' Unfortunately, his attempts to put the alpaca on a commercial footing were doomed. First, the New South Wales government reneged on its verbal promise, refusing to reimburse his expenses and forcing him to sell the flock to the state legislature to pay off his creditors. Then, no sooner had the legislature 're-hired' him to tend to the herd than it began pressuring him to sell the animals off in lots. The problem was competition from the Australian merino sheep, a far more profitable and practical animal than the alpaca and one that was perfectly adapted to the dry Australian climate. Nevertheless, Ledger persevered with his scheme and in 1862 his alpaca were exhibited at the International Exhibition in London, winning the gold medal. Ledger had to remain in Australia to lobby the bureaucrats, so his brother George collected the award on his behalf. Unfortunately Ledger's efforts came to nothing and the following year the flock was auctioned off, ending for good his dreams of an Australian alpaca industry.

Ledger was now broke. He had invested £7,000 of his own money in the alpaca venture and had lost it all. In addition, the New South Wales government was refusing to pay him three months' back salary. There was nothing for it but to return to South America, but to what purpose?

Three years previously, while negotiating with Australian officials, Ledger had learned of Markham's expedition to collect cinchonas. Keen to aid the missions, he had written Markham a long letter, advising him how to equip himself, how he should distrust everybody – even seemingly friendly priests – and where he should go in Bolivia to find *calisayas* of the same quality he and Mamani had seen during their expedition across the Peruvian border in 1851. Ledger had sent the letter to friends in Tacna with instructions for them to hand it to Markham when he next passed through. But by the time Ledger's letter arrived Markham had already left for Tambopata and, as he did not return to Tacna but proceeded direct to the Peruvian coast with the cinchonas, he never received it.[2]

Stuck in Australia, embroiled in the alpaca affair, however, Ledger did not know whether or not Markham had seen the letter. It was not until 1861 that he had his next news of Markham's mission. Ledger was in Sydney making preparations for Santiago's return to South America when he read in the *Home News* of the arrival in India of the cinchona seeds and plants collected by Markham in Peru. The article revealed that during his search for cinchona Markham had failed to enter Bolivia. Ledger quickly realized that in that case Markham could not have obtained *calisayas* of very good quality – certainly not trees equal to the ones he and Mamani had seen – and thus that his mission was, at best, only a partial success.

Ledger now began hatching a scheme to revive his fortunes. As Santiago was returning to Peru, Ledger would give him a letter to deliver to his father. Recalling all the details of their expedition ten years previously – the route they had taken through Apolobamba, the trail they had cut through the cloudforest with their machetes and, finally, the spot where they had stumbled on the fifty huge *calisaya* trees – Ledger instructed Mamani to return to Bolivia and collect as many seeds as possible. Once this was done he was to return to Tacna, by which time Ledger hoped to have arrived in Peru, and deliver the seeds to him in person.

Ledger's request smacked of desperation.[3] Retracing their steps through the *calisaya* forests was no small undertaking, especially for one man travelling alone. But Ledger was confident that if anyone could do it, it was his faithful Indian servant. The morning Santiago's boat was due to set sail he handed him the letter together with two hundred Spanish dollars (£40) – the last of his money. Mamani should treat it as a down payment, he told Santiago. When he returned to Tacna with the seeds, Ledger or his brother-in-law would be waiting with a further £500.

A few hours later Santiago set sail for Peru together with two other Indians who had accompanied Ledger on his epic journey with the alpaca and who had stuck by him throughout his troubles in Australia. For Ledger it was a last, desperate throw of the dice.

## Chapter Eight

# THE SHADOW IN THE FOREST

Old Manuel waited patiently, year after year, cutting bark
with his sons and looking for an opportunity of fulfilling
Mr Ledger's commission.

Clements Markham, *Peruvian Bark, A Popular Account*

BURIED DEEP IN the archives of the Pharmaceutical Society of Great
Britain is a faded photograph of a South American Indian. The man
is in his late twenties or early thirties and is standing on a rough path.
He is wearing jeans, a sombrero and the striped poncho favoured by
the highland Indians of northern Bolivia. A starched shirt and cravat
are just visible above the poncho's 'V', suggesting he has dressed
especially for the occasion. Yet, either by accident or design, the
photographer has chosen to show him with his hands raised in front
of his chest clasping the strings of his *mochila*. Indeed, were it not for
the Labrador seated faithfully at his feet, you would think from his
stern expression that he was about to stride purposefully out of the
frame and out of the story for ever.

The date on the photograph is 1860 and it could be of either
Manuel Incra Mamani or his son, Santiago.[1] We know very little
about Mamani, other than that he was from Coroico in the Yungas
and that he was an Indian of either Aymara or Quechua descent.
Although Mamani served Ledger faithfully for more than twenty
years, Ledger does not give more details or, perhaps, does not care to.

This is a shame, for it is thanks to Mamani that Ledger obtained the species of cinchona with the highest quinine content of all. More than Ledger, Markham or any of Markham's 'fellow labourers', it is Mamani who deserves to be remembered for making quinine widely available to the world.

The paucity of information about Mamani's character and motivation has traditionally presented historians of cinchona with a dilemma. Should he be seen simply as Ledger's amanuensis — an Indian faithfully doing the bidding of his 'master' — or was he a self-actualizing and conscious actor in the quest? The Spanish historian Marie Louise de Alaya Duran-Reynals controversially took the latter view. In her book, *The Fever Bark Tree*, written in 1946, she argues that Mamani's is 'a narrative in the best Homeric traditions' and should be seen in the context of the centuries-long subjugation of the Aymara people by first the Inca and then the Spanish. According to Duran-Reynals it was because 'destiny had appointed [the Aymaras] as guardians of the *Cinchona calisaya*' that no white man could hope to wrest the tree from Bolivia without their cooperation. Mamani, however, was 'one of the rare Indians of highland Bolivia who had left the native soil and, rarer still, had become the servant of a foreigner'. His decision to harvest the *calisaya* for Ledger, she suggests, was a betrayal of his people — but one that he took consciously and willingly out of his 'love of the master who had been kind to him'.

At the other extreme is Sir Clements Markham. In his *Peruvian Bark*, a popular account of the introduction of cinchona to India, Markham prefers to portray Mamani as Ledger's 'true-hearted' and 'faithful Indian servant'. In his narrative Mamani's deeper motivations go unexplored. Instead he assumes that Mamani was simply obeying orders. At one point he even refers to him overly familiarly as 'old Manuel' before adding, somewhat patronizingly, that 'it is very pleasant to have to record these noble traits of character in the Indians, the descendants of men who formed and organised the glorious empire of the Incas.'

In fact, no one knows whether or not Mamani was a Quechua and there is certainly no evidence to suggest that he was a direct descendant of Atahualpa, Tupac Amaru or any other Inca king. More importantly, there is nothing in Ledger's writings to suggest that he was any nobler than the next man, nor whether his primary motivation was gratitude or money. The truth is, we know so little about Mamani that we can project onto him almost any cultural and historical stereotype we please. He is the shadow in the forest, a cut-out-and-keep acetate for whatever prejudices we care to bring to the story.

There is one theory, however, that neither Markham nor Duran-Reynals seemed to have considered and that is that Mamani was descended from the Kallawaya – the traditional Indian healers of Apolobamba, the highland region of northern Bolivia through which he and Ledger passed while scouting a route for alpaca in 1851. The poncho Mamani is wearing in the photograph, for instance, is identical to the ones still worn today by Kallawaya from mountain villages near Bolivia's northern border with Peru. More importantly, the Kallawaya are expert naturalists. Every winter, when the rains cease, they descend from their mountain retreats to gather medicinal herbs and plants – including cinchona – from the cloudforests below Apolobamba. Then, dressed in their black breeches, striped ponchos, and broad-brimmed sombreros, and with their wallets of herbs strung across their backs, they walk in a direct line from village to village, practising their healing arts. Indeed, to this day it is said that the varieties of coca and cinchona most prized by the Kallawaya come from Apolo, an isolated jungle town two hundred kilometres north-east of Charazani. There, cinchona is still known by its traditional Aymara name, *calisaya*, from *cali* meaning 'best' and *saya* meaning 'bark' – 'best bark'. And it was there that Mamani returned, at Ledger's request, for the seeds and plants that would prove the most valuable kind of all.

Reaching Apolo is no easier today than it was in the mid-nineteenth century. Bolivia's military airline, Transportes Aeros Militares, used to operate a regular weekly flight but cancelled it in 2000 due to the poor condition of Apolo's runway and the lack of commercial passengers. Instead, soldiers and civilians wishing to reach the jungle outpost now have to board a bus or truck at La Paz's Cemetario station and endure a gruelling forty-eight-hour journey over some of the worst roads in the world. The one that hugs Lake Titicaca, for instance, is little more than an unmetalled track strewn with rocks and pitted with craters. Then as you plunge from the altiplano the descents become steadily more precipitous and hair-raising. The only thing that makes the ordeal bearable is the views. First, as you rise up out of La Paz, comes Illimani, its peaks burning like phosphorus in the morning sun. Then, as you begin to cross the altiplano, come Huayana Potosí and the Condoriri group, followed in quick succession by Illampu, Ancohuma and, glinting on the horizon, the Lagunas Glaciar.

We do not know whether Ledger and Mamani ever travelled this way but the route must have been well known to them, and in all probability this is the route Ledger recommended to Markham in 1858. Unfortunately Ledger's letter to Markham is now missing but Ledger often copied his own writings for different occasions, repeating the same details and many of the same phrases. Thus it is that in a letter addressed to John Howard in 1877 we find Ledger almost certainly reproducing the same advice he had given Markham twenty years earlier.

'In the first place,' begins the letter, 'there are *no laws* prohibiting the collection of plants or seeds, nor against taking them out of the country. There exists however the greater prejudice from the highest to the lowest inhabitant against anyone doing it. Were anyone publicly and openly to state his intention his life would be in the greatest danger.'

Ledger then goes on to give Howard detailed instructions on how to avoid detection – instructions that would have been invaluable to Markham when he was contemplating a foray into the same forests nineteen years earlier. The collecting party should consist of two men who speak Spanish and who are prepared to 'rough it' where necessary. They should pretend to be collectors of bird skins, as when the cinchonas are in flower the trees are surrounded by brilliantly coloured hummingbirds, but they must be careful never to relax their guard as 'every Indian is [a] most observant and suspicious person [and is] very difficult to hoodwink or deceive.'

To smooth their passage to the bark forests, Ledger suggests they obtain letters of introduction to local merchants and, most important of all, to the padres at the Missions lying along the route. A good start would be to visit the prior at the Convent of San Francisco in La Paz and 'give $25 to $50 to the poor box.' Then, proceeding along the eastern shore of Lake Titicaca, they should pass through the towns of Acoraimes and Escoma before veering to the right from where they can go 'direct to Peluchuco, then to Apolo, following on Mission to Mission until arriving on the shore of the Beni'.

Ledger concludes: 'There is not [sic] necessity to encumber oneself with anything . . . Quinine against fevers, ammonia against bites from venomous spiders, snakes (almost all the Indians have special native antidotes) . . . With tact, perseverance and *above all* for no one (not even the Consul) to know one's real object, a man well knowing *when* to pick and how to preserve seed could not fail in his mission.'

'A man well knowing *when* to pick . . .' Ledger clearly means to suggest that to succeed a collector would need the sort of expertise that only someone who had spent many years exploring the bark forests could possess – a man, in other words, much like himself. Yet the person who knew most about the trees was not Ledger but Mamani. It was Mamani who could distinguish the different types of cinchona simply by the colours and forms of their leaves, and it was Mamani who had observed the relationship between the topography of the Andes and the distribution of the most valuable quinine-bearing species. Furthermore, as a native of the highlands, Mamani would not arouse suspicion in the same way as a European collector.

Yet even for Mamani such an undertaking was fraught with difficulty and danger. Ten years had passed since he had last seen the stand of fifty huge *roja* trees that had so astonished Ledger. But even if he succeeded in retracing their steps to the headwaters of the Beni River near Apolo there was no guarantee he would be able to locate the trees again or that they would be in flower when he got there. Furthermore, if he was lucky enough to arrive just as the seeds were ripening he would still have to spend several days carefully drying them before transporting them to Ledger in Peru — a process that would inevitably arouse the interest and suspicion of any *cascarillero* who happened to stumble upon him.

Nevertheless, it would seem that no sooner had Santiago delivered Ledger's request to his father than Mamani set off for Apolo determined to fulfil the commission. From what Ledger tells us of their relationship it would never have occurred to him to do otherwise. After all they had been through together he and Mamani were no longer master and servant but friends, and Mamani could hardly refuse a friend such an important request.

When Ledger returned to Peru in 1865 he had no idea whether or not Mamani had succeeded in locating the fifty huge *roja* trees. It had been a full four years since he had waved farewell to Santiago at Sydney harbour and in all that time he had not received a single communication from his former guide. Ledger's first priority on reaching Tacna was to visit his three daughters who, because of the alpaca business, he had not seen for twelve years. The reunion must have been difficult, not least because while Ledger had been camped at Laguna Blanca their mother had died in highly straitened circum-stances. Although his father-in-law, Major Ortiz, had taken care of his daughters during his long absence, Ledger now had a new wife — Charlotte Oliver — and was up to his ears in debt. His only hope was Mamani. Had there been any news of his expedition?

To his relief he discovered that Mamani had already been in touch with Major Ortiz for money three times and had received $200 on each occasion. He had also asked Ledger's father-in-law to give him a message: 'Tell the *patron* that I am only waiting for a good season so as to secure thoroughly ripe seed.'

In fact, as Ledger now discovered when, late on the night of 19 May 1865, Mamani suddenly appeared on his doorstep in Tacna, he had had a very long wait indeed. As soon as he had received Ledger's instructions he and Santiago had travelled to Caupolicán province, south-east of Apolo, and began looking for the spot where they had first seen the *roja* trees. They found them, or at least trees very similar to the ones they had seen in 1851, without great difficulty. Unfortunately, it was too late in the season – the Bolivian winter had already arrived and there were no seeds to be had. Mamani had no choice but to retrace his steps and return with his sons the following March when he would have a better chance of finding the *calisayas* in flower.

This they did for the next *three* years. In 1862 they camped by the trees, cutting bark for their subsistence, and marking the most promising trees when they began to flower. But in early spring there was a severe frost and all the best seeds were destroyed, leaving only inferior sorts to be collected. Incredibly, the same thing had happened in 1863, and again in 1864, so that it was not until April 1865 that Mamani had finally been able to collect good seeds.

Mamani described how he had watched the trees become covered in beautiful creamy-white flowers like the ones they had seen so many years before. This spectacle was enhanced by the fact that the oldest trees were now covered with a scarlet and silver moss. Then, just before the seeds were about to fall, the undersides of the leaves turned dark purple, completing the brilliant display.

At first he had kept seeds collected from different trees in separate bags as Ledger had instructed, but one day while drying the seeds on his poncho there was a sudden gust of wind and they became mixed up. Nevertheless, the seeds were all there and accounted for in the two bags he now presented to Ledger. He had walked all the way from Coroico on foot – some sixteen hundred kilometres – over the freezing cordillera, sustained only by a little food and coca, to deliver them to his *patron*. Was he not pleased?

Ledger embraced Mamani gratefully. After all his disappointments with the alpaca, the seeds must have seemed like the answer to his prayers. He carefully emptied them onto a sheet. There was 40lb in all – in theory, more than enough to turn a healthy profit and revive his fortunes. He let the seeds sit in the sun for two hours every day for a month to make sure they were dry. Then he wrapped half of them in chinchilla skins, placed them in a box covered with hide, and addressing the package to his brother George in London shipped them to Britain via Cartagena and Panama. Next he paid Mamani $500 and as an additional show of gratitude gave him two mules, four donkeys, and a gun with ammunition. Finally, he told him that if he could procure another 20lb of seeds he would pay him a further $600.

When Ledger sent the packet of seeds to George he had no idea of their true worth. All he knew was that the British, like the Dutch, had been willing to fund a series of expensive missions to South America in search of high-quality *calisayas*. As a subsequent letter to George makes clear, he was happy to put his trust in the British, confident that a grateful government would soon be beating a path to his door. 'You might very greatly contribute towards obtaining for me *a recompense adequate to the services rendered,*' he wrote to George in June 1865. 'Sir William Hooker might bring the matter properly before the proper authorities and I feel that my services in this direction will meet with better return than my Alpaca toils.'

Unfortunately for Ledger his faith in British competence was misplaced. Sir William had just died and when George arrived at the gates of Kew he discovered that his son, Joseph Dalton Hooker, who had succeeded him, was ill and could not see him. The only person available was a superintendent who, not realizing the value of the seeds, declined to accept them and instead gave George a patronizing lecture on the cultivation of cinchona. Unknown to George his arrival had coincided with the India Office's decision to end its relationship with Kew. By now Spruce and Markham's seeds had reached India and were being raised in the government gardens at Ootacamund in Mysore. Kew, which had acted as a repository and nursery for the seeds and plants until they were ready to be shipped to the colonies, suddenly found itself surplus to requirements. The only other person who could possibly have helped was Markham, but he had left for India.

Not knowing what to do, George began touting the seeds around London. His first stop was the Exotic Nursery in Chelsea where he made a present of some seeds to the director, a Mr Veitch (not realizing their value, Mr Veitch innocently reported back to George in November that the seeds were 'germinating nicely'). Next he wrote to the Under-Secretary for the Colonies, offering to place the seeds at the government's disposal in the hope that when botanists had proved their value his brother would receive a 'just, fair and adequate' recompense from the government. George never received a reply. Instead, the Under-Secretary copied the letter to Joseph Hooker at Kew asking him to take the matter up directly with Ledger.

In a panic George offered the seeds to Professor Bentley of the Pharmaceutical Society, but he did not want them either and forwarded them to the Royal Botanical Society. George also gave some as a present to the Society of Arts only for them to send them to a Lady Hanbury. Finally, on Bentley's advice, he took the seeds to John Howard.

By now Howard was one of the leading quinine manufacturers in Britain and a pre-eminent authority on cinchona. More importantly from Ledger's point of view, Howard was in regular contact with the Hookers at Kew and the Dutch, in particular with Dr Franz Junghuhn and Wilhelm Van Gorkum, respectively the chemist and superintendent in charge of the cinchona plantations in Buitenzorg in Java.

George began by explaining how he had approached Kew and the Under-Secretary for the Colonies, only to be passed from pillar to post. Howard agreed that it was pointless trying to offer the seeds around London when all the competent British authorities were abroad. But had he considered the Dutch?

On Howard's advice George approached the Dutch Consul General in London. The Consul did not know what to make of the seeds so he passed the enquiry on to Professor Miquel, a well-known

Dutch botanist who had recently returned from making a collection of cinchonas in Java. Miquel was intrigued by George's story and after confirming that the seeds came from Caupolicán – an area of Bolivia that Dutch collectors like Hasskarl had been unable to penetrate – he recommended that the Consul should offer to buy 1lb of the seeds. Given all the money and effort that Ledger and Mamani had gone to, the amount the Dutch offered was derisory – just 100 guilders (£20) – but at least it was a start.

George now had 14lb of seeds left to dispose of. Worried that they would soon spoil and be unsaleable he approached Howard again. Surely he must know someone else who was interested? Howard suggested he approach a Mr Money, the Anglo-Indian owner of extensive cinchona plantations in India who was then vacationing in London. Money was not an expert and, at first, was unimpressed by George's explanation of how the seeds were the best in Bolivia and had been taken from an area that no European had ever ventured into. But after consulting Howard, and being assured that the seeds were viable, he agreed to buy them.

His offer was £50 for the lot, with a promise of a further £50 should ten thousand of the seeds germinate, take it or leave it. George took the money. Thus it was that the bulk of the seeds finally found their way via the back door to India – the place Ledger had originally wanted them to be cultivated – but not before they had also fallen into the hands of Britain's more commercially minded Dutch rivals.

The British authorities' indifference to the seeds wounded Ledger deeply. He had risked his last savings on the venture and once again had nothing to show for it.

'I feel convinced in my own mind that no white man would or could succeed in getting such splendid seed as my faithful Manuel did,' he wrote to Howard years later. 'It is so clear that he got the true Calisaya Rojo. In fact, and as the good poor fellow repeatedly told me, he got seed from particularly fine old trees that we had together seen and sat under.'

Gradually the perceived slight would become a canker, eating away at his pride and fuelling Ledger's sense of injustice. Again and again in his letters to Howard he dwells on what he sees as his harsh treatment by the British. Yet as far as the British authorities were concerned he was just another South American businessman on the make. Like many an expatriate before and since, Ledger had made the classic mistake of believing that his devotion to the mother country would be reciprocated.

At this point a less stubborn man would have abandoned the cinchona scheme and concentrated on something that he knew was likely to turn a profit – such as trading alpaca hides again. Instead Ledger sent Mamani back to the *calisaya* trees a second time. In so doing he sealed his friend's fate.

Ledger provides few details of the tragedy that resulted. All we know is that in 1869 he forwarded £200 to Mamani as a down payment on the next delivery of seeds. By now Mamani had returned to his home in Coroico, a beautiful mountain village overlooking the Yungas – the continuation south of the same subtropical valleys where he had collected the first batch of seeds. We do not know whether on receiving the funds Mamani made a second expedition to Apolo or whether he chose this time to gather seeds from *calisayas* nearer his home. It seems likely, however, that it was the latter. As Ledger wrote in a long letter to Howard in 1877 from Argentina: 'Poor Manuel is dead also; he was put in prison by [the] Corregidor of Coroico; beat so as to make him confess who the seed found on him was for.'

According to Santiago, his father had been returning from the bark forests when he was arrested. Somehow Coroico's chief of police had got wind of the fact that Mamani was collecting seeds to smuggle across the border, thus threatening Bolivia's valuable monopoly. He immediately had Mamani thrown in prison where he beat him to try to get him to reveal who he was working for. But Mamani stubbornly refused to betray Ledger. The chief of police withheld food and water for two weeks and beat Mamani again, but still he refused to reveal Ledger's part in the scheme. Finally, after twenty days the police chief released Mamani – as Ledger puts it – 'beaten and half-starved'.

The Corregidor had taken everything Mamani owned – his donkeys, his blankets and, in all likelihood, his striped poncho and *mochila* too. According to Santiago his father was barely able to stand up, and although the family did everything they could to nurse him back to health, his wounds were too serious and within a matter of days he was dead.

Ledger does not say whether he felt any guilt on hearing the melancholy fate of his friend. Santiago had ridden especially to Tacna to tell him the news and to account for the monies Ledger had advanced. According to Santiago, his father had been approached many times by other foreigners anxious to obtain seeds but had always refused, so it is probable his activities were common knowledge. But Ledger had also been fully aware of the risks and the fact remained that had he not asked his friend to venture into the forests a second time he would not have died. Incredibly, in spite of everything, Santiago himself now offered to return to the *calisaya* forests. This time Ledger wisely refused.

'Seeing the dangers to which these poor fellows were exposed,' Ledger wrote Howard, 'having no direct application for any, feeling also that I had been miserably recompensed for what I had previously done, I told him to collect no more on my account or for any one else.'

It is typical of Ledger that in lamenting Mamani's death he also cannot help reminding Howard of his own losses. His self-pity oozes from every line. But the more interesting question is what possessed Mamani to take such risks in the first place? Why return to the *calisaya* patch three years in a row and then walk sixteen hundred kilometres over the freezing cordillera? Was it simply for the money or was it, as Ledger and Duran-Reynals would have us believe, his sense of duty and devotion to his master? Or did Mamani have other motivations we can only guess at?

Ledger once remarked on how whenever Mamani came upon a tree felled by a *cascarillero* he would drop to his knees and say a prayer for '*los buenos padres*'. According to Ledger, it was the Jesuit fathers who had impressed upon him the importance of always planting five trees in place of every one felled in order that the forests should not become denuded. Perhaps the tree, not Ledger, was the real source of his devotion. After all Mamani had seen with his own eyes how the *cascarilleros* were gradually destroying the *calisayas* to the point where supplies of Bolivian quinine would soon be exhausted. Could it be that, like Markham, he wanted to ensure that the valuable anti-malarial would not be lost to the world?

We will never know. Mamani is the point where the facts run out and the trail ends. Like the faded photograph from the Royal Pharmaceutical Society he seems destined to remain for ever slightly out of focus.

Whatever spin Ledger subsequently put on his role in the affair, however, it is clear he was motivated first and foremost not by philanthropy but by money. After selling the seeds to the Dutch and the British, he succeeded in placing the remaining 20lb, £100 worth, with the government of Queensland. But the funds were nowhere near enough to compensate him for his outlay. In all he had spent £800 on procuring the *calisaya* seeds and had received just £170 in return. Yet any profits from the cultivation of the seeds would not accrue to him but to the Dutch or the aptly named Mr Money.

In fact, Mamani's seeds would prove far more valuable than Ledger or anyone else could have imagined – and ironically it was the Dutch, not the English, who reaped the rewards.

*Chapter Nine*

# A TALE OF TWO SEEDS

He lurks among the reeds, beside the marsh,
Red oleanders twisted in his hair
His eyes are haggard and his lips are harsh
Upon his breast the bones show gaunt and bare

The green and stagnant waters lick his feet,
And from their filmy, iridescent scum
Clouds of mosquitoes, gauzy in the heat,
Rise with His gifts: Death and Delirium.

*Malaria*, a lyric of India

IN 1864 FLORENCE NIGHTINGALE gave a prescient talk to the National Association for the Promotion of Social Science in Edinburgh. The title of her address was 'How people may live and not die in India' and her theme was the urgent need for public health measures to combat the twin ravages of cholera and malaria then sweeping the Asian subcontinent. By the 1860s as many as two million people a year were dying of malaria in India but as Nightingale pointed out infections were probably running at 'fifty times' that rate. 'The drain upon human life and happiness of *fever* in India is literally untold,' she began, but 'the mortality from malaria in India is a mere trifle compared with the ravage fever commits in sapping the strength and vigour of the country, in making the young old, the healthy infirm for life, the industrious helpless invalids, the rich poor, the thriving country a waste.'[1]

The malarious state of the country was only partly the fault of the mosquito. Thanks to the collapse of India's cotton-spinning industry and the East India Company's punitive land-tax policies, millions of workers had been displaced from the cities to the countryside where they found themselves little better than serfs. Forced to pay up to half their crop to the tax collector, they sank deeper and deeper into debt and began to neglect essential public works – such as irrigation and canal-building. The result was a huge increase in water-borne diseases like cholera, dysentery and, of course, malaria.

Ever since the Indian Mutiny had exposed the appalling con-ditions of British troops in Bengal, Nightingale had been campaigning tirelessly for improved irrigation and sanitation. Moreover, she had quickly realized that in India – unlike in the Crimea – malaria and cholera were not simply problems confined to barracks. From the Punjab to Madras and Burma to the Western Ghats, malaria had laid waste to large swathes of countryside, and even where the fevers had not brought, in the words of the popular lyric, 'death and delirium', they had so weakened the rural labour force that drainage works had gone neglected. Nightingale concluded that the only way to protect the army was to institute sanitary measures throughout the country, but this would take years and the army had to plan for a revolt next month. One idea was to station British troops on high ground, well away from the unhealthy 'miasmas' associated with low-lying swamps and jungles. But many of the hill stations in India were also malarious and if another mutiny broke out they would be isolated. Now, thanks to Markham and his 'fellow labourers', another solution was at hand.

The story of quinine after Markham's departure from South America is essentially a tale of two seeds – Spruce's *Cinchona succirubra* and Mamani's *C. calisaya*. It is a story that pits Dutch nurserymen and chemists against British gardeners and bureaucrats or, to put it another way, hard-headed realists against well-meaning but muddled 'amateurs'. But it is also the story of how the liberal instincts of health reformers like Nightingale combined with the enlightened self-interest of the British ruling classes in India. And running through the story is a tension that bedevils the debate over the development of anti-malarials to this day: can new malaria treatments be secured through the pursuit of profit alone or do they necessarily entail an element of philanthropy?

Interestingly, when the British and the Dutch first set out to raise cinchona in their colonies they assumed that philanthropy would be enough. Just as Markham had announced that his aim was to make a cheap cinchona febrifuge available to 'every pansari's shop' in India so in 1854 Rochussen, the Governor-General of the Netherland Indies, declared that the Dutch effort was 'no common speculation'. 'The eyes of Europe are fixed upon this enterprise which interests it in the highest degree; for it is, so to speak, to procure for the sick, the means of life, and to procure it at a cost which will not exceed his means.'

In fact, neither Britain's nor Holland's policy was quite so clear cut. The priority of civil servants at the India Office was the health of the British Army in India and the well being of the East India Company's white employees. If the cinchona missions, by securing increased supplies of cheap quinine, also brought the drug within the reach of the brown masses then so much the better. Similarly, while in Java the Dutch government sponsored the initial experiments with cinchona — effectively underwriting the costs of developing a chemi-cally lucrative strain — the decision whether or not to farm the tree was in the hands of private planters. Unless they could be shown — or they could be given guarantees — that cinchona was more profitable than coffee or sugar, philanthropy alone was never going to induce them to grow it.

The problem was that transporting seeds and plants to the colonies and developing the plantations was a far more complex horticultural and pharmacological task than anyone had anticipated. Indeed, for Markham the difficulties began the moment he despatched his collec-tions from the coast of Peru.

Before setting off for South America he had taken every precaution to ensure that his plants would survive the voyage to India. Mindful of Hasskarl's disastrous experience in 1854 he visited the Horticultural

Society expressly to consult the Chinese tea-collector Robert Fortune about the best design of Wardian cases. As a result of those discussions Markham commissioned thirty state-of-the-art cases, complete with battens for keeping the soil compacted and the plants separated into neat rows, and putty to ensure the glass seals were as airtight as possible. On arriving in South America Markham deposited fifteen of the cases at Guayaquil ready to receive Spruce's collection and brought the remaining fifteen with him to Islay. In addition, at Lima, he had a further six cases built to receive Pritchett's grey barks from Huánuco.

The only thing Markham didn't do was fit the cases with a false bottom. This innovation, designed to improve air circulation and drainage around the roots, would come later. In Markham's case it would probably have made little difference.

On leaving Peru, Markham's Wardian cases had contained more than four hundred and fifty seedlings. The original plan had been to send them direct to India by Royal Navy frigate but the promised ship never arrived and instead Markham was forced to book passage on a commercial steamer via Panama. The result was that by the time he and John Weir docked at Southampton in August 1860 only two hundred and seventy of his plants were still alive. The sensible course of action would have been to nurse the remaining plants at Kew and send them on to India at the end of the summer. But for some reason Markham decided to proceed straight to Bombay and the Nilgiri Hills, the site in south-west India he had chosen for the first experimental plantation.

The result was disaster. In crossing Egypt the cases were knocked about and one of the most valuable lost, dropped in the Red Sea, according to Markham, by 'truculent Arabs'. Next the engines failed and for twenty-four hours his ship was stalled in the sweltering heat of the Arabian summer, with temperatures rising as high as 107 degrees on deck. Then, on reaching Bombay, he learned that the steamer he had been planning to connect with had already left for Calicut, forcing him to remain in the bay for several days where the plants were exposed to the 'very pernicious climate'. The result was that it was not until mid-October – three and a half months after leaving Peru – that the plants finally reached the government planta-tions at Ootacamund, a hundred kilometres south of Mysore. Mark-ham had selected the Nilgiri Hills because of their resemblance to Carabaya, the province in Peru where he had gathered the plants. At Ootacamund he could also call on the skill of an expert horticulturist, William McIvor, the superintendent of the government gardens. Unfortunately, by the time the plants reached McIvor it was already too late. He planted them out but the delays had been fatal and by December all of Markham's *calisayas* were dead.

After all he had been through – the gruelling descent to the Tambopata River, the flight across the freezing cordillera to Arequipa, and his outwitting of Peruvian customs – it must have been a bitter blow. But in his subsequent account of the introduction of cinchona to India Markham makes no comment on the loss. One possible reason is that by 1880, when he came to publish *Peruvian Bark*, it was already apparent that the most valuable trees were not his but Spruce's and Mamani's. Under the circumstances, he probably considered there was little point in harping on his misfortune.

There may have been another reason too. The year after he left South America Robert Cross had followed exactly the same route to India without any problems. Cross set sail from Guayaquil with Spruce's *Cinchona succirubra* in January 1861, landed at Southampton in February and then proceeded across the Red Sea, arriving at Ootacamund in April with 463 healthy plants. Markham later attributed Cross's success to the fact that he had crossed Egypt in winter when the climate was cooler. But it also drew attention to the fact that Markham was not a trained botanist and it was not long before aspersions were also being cast on the methods being used by Markham and McIvor to propagate cinchona in India.

Their principal critic was Thomas Anderson, a young botanist who had been despatched to India by Sir William Hooker in 1862 with *Cinchona succirubra* and *C. calisaya* seeds carefully raised in Kew's nurseries. When Anderson, who had also visited Java, saw how Markham and McIvor were running the government plantations he was not impressed. In a report to the India Office he implied that Markham had played down the failure of his first batch of plants and had capitalized on the success that should have been due to Spruce and Cross. He also argued that the method of cultivation in the Nilgiri Hills was defective.

Ironically, what saved Markham and McIvor from ridicule was Spruce's *Cinchona succirubra*. The tree did so well at Nilgiri it was as if God had designed it with India in mind. In accordance with Spruce's instructions McIvor planted the saplings on an exposed site at Nedivattam, in the lower Nilgiri Hills, where they were guaranteed plenty of rain and sun. Meanwhile, at another site higher up the same mountain range, he began raising plants and seeds of *Cinchona officinalis* brought by Cross from Loja. The result was that by 1866 he had more than two hundred and forty-four thousand trees planted out. To Markham the transformation seemed 'miraculous'.

'The old jungle had disappeared,' he wrote, 'and in its place were the rows of Peruvian bark trees with their graceful and beautiful foliage.'

In describing the success of the *Cinchona succirubra* trees, however, Markham glossed over the fact that by now the *C. calisaya* seeds he had collected in Peru had also arrived in India. Owing to the lack of rainfall and differences in the soil and elevation, however, they did not fare nearly as well. In fact, the rootstock was soon attacked by parasites and McIvor had great difficulty getting any to grow at all. Under the circumstances, he had little choice but to concentrate on Spruce and Cross's species. The result was that by 1878 there were some three hundred and five thousand *Cinchona officinalis* trees, two hundred and sixty-one thousand *C. succirubra* and just five hundred and fifty-two of Markham's *C. calisayas* growing in the government plantations. As far as the India Office was concerned, Markham was on the right track and would soon be in a position to manufacture sulphate of quinine at a greatly reduced cost.

However, the faith of Markham's paymasters in London was misplaced: he would never be in a position to manufacture quinine cheaply – at least not as cheaply as the Dutch – for the simple reason

that Mamani's seeds were far more productive than Spruce's. Fortunately for Markham, however, the red bark was rich in other alkaloids
that he now proved were just as effective at clearing the malaria
parasites and that would make his dream of a cheap febrifuge a reality.

It is interesting to note how close the Dutch plantations were to
collapse when the 1lb bag of seeds that George Ledger had sold
to the Dutch Consul in London in 1865 reached Java. For more
than ten years Dutch botanists and chemists had been struggling to
develop a high-quinine-bearing strain at the government nurseries at
Tjinjiroean. Thanks to Hasskarl, however, the experiment had got
off to a disastrous start. Not only had he chosen the wrong mountain
range but also the species he brought back from Peru — *Cinchona
pahudiana* — contained hardly any quinine at all. Under the direction
of Hasskarl's successor, Dr Franz Junghuhn, the Dutch decided to
concentrate instead on plants raised from the original *C. calisaya* seeds
collected by the French botanist, Hugues Weddell, in Bolivia in 1850.
Then, in 1862, they began supplementing Weddell's *C. calisayas* with
*C. succirubra* and *C. officinalis* trees that in a spirit of cooperation
McIvor and Markham had forwarded from the British nurseries in
India.

Interestingly, it was the Dutch who first established that *C.
succirubra* was rich chiefly in cinchonidine, cinchonine and quinidine.
Indeed, in one assay the Dutch chemist, Dr de Vrij, found that
Spruce's bark contained as much as 8 per cent of the febrifugal
alkaloids. But since Java's principal aim was quinine production the
results were of little interest to the Dutch planters. Soon they were
mocking the government cinchona estates as 'the Governor's expensive
hobby', and by the time Mamani's seeds arrived many were on the
point of abandoning cinchona cultivation altogether.

At first there was little indication that Mamani's seeds would be
any different from all the other 'expensive' failures. When the new
superintendent of the gardens, Karel Wessel van Gorkum, opened the
small package from the Consul in London it gave off a strong smell

of ammonia and he feared the seeds had spoiled. Nevertheless, he managed to get twenty thousand to germinate and within a year he had twelve thousand healthy young seedlings. However, at this stage van Gorkum writes that he had 'no reason to suppose that we had come into possession of an especially valuable description of cinchona; on the contrary, we thought we were dealing with the identical *calisaya* we already possessed.'

Looking back, the Dutch could easily have compromised their own experiment. From a geneticist's point of view, Java was one of the worst places for Mamani's seedlings. By 1865 the Dutch colony was full of flowering cinchona trees of dubious commercial and genetic value. Because of cinchona's propensity to hybridization, once Mamani's trees flowered any one of the other species in Java could have cross-pollinated with them, contaminating the strain and diluting its genetic purity before the bark could be tested for quinine. As Mamani's C. *calisayas* had never been cultivated before and van Gorkum had no way of knowing when they might flower, this was no slight risk.

Fortunately for the Dutch, a brilliant young chemist had just arrived on the scene. J. C. Bernelot Moens had been sent to Java with express instructions to determine the alkaloid content of the trees in the government plantations. Unlike the British — who had to send their barks all the way to John Howard in Tottenham for analysis — Moens had all the equipment he needed installed on site. Beginning in 1872, he very carefully took strips of bark from the trees for testing. He had no great expectations. He had already tested a number of other cinchonas on the island, broadly confirming de Vrij's findings that they contained disappointingly small amounts of quinine. Imagine his surprise then when the results of his first tests on Mamani's C. *calisayas* came back. The young trees contained 8 per cent quinine — far more than any other species of similar age. Two years later the quinine content in the maturing trees had risen to 11 per cent and by 1876 it had reached 13 per cent.

It was an unheard of amount. In contrast, Moens found that the

*C. calisayas* raised from Weddell's seed contained a maximum of only 2 per cent quinine, while the variety that had survived from Hasskarl's ill-fated expedition contained even less. Indeed, the only species that bore comparison was Cross's *C. officinalis*. In 1873 de Vrij had visited Ootacamund and discovered that some of the offspring of Cross's Loja collection contained up to 9 per cent quinine. But later tests in Java confirmed that the alkaloid content of the barks varied widely depending on the age and variety, and that in the case of some trees it was as low as 1 per cent.

It was rapidly becoming clear to van Gorkum that the 1lb bag they had purchased from George Ledger contained a very unusual variety of *C. calisaya* indeed. But it was only when he sent 260kg to be auctioned at Amsterdam in 1877 that he realized just how unusual: the bark fetched 17.5 florins a kilo, double its reserve price; in contrast a kilo of *C. succirubra* bark fetched only 3.4 florins. 'The reputation of this description of cinchona was thus assured,' writes van Gorkum, 'and has since splendidly maintained itself at each auction.'

In retrospect it is surprising that the news did not spark an orgy of speculation on a par with the tulip craze of 1630. Then riots had threatened to break out in Amsterdam after a single bulb sold for $10,000. Mamani's bark had not fetched quite so spectacular a sum but in view of quinine's medicinal importance – after more than three hundred years it was still the only drug that cured malaria – it represented a far better long-term investment. The problem was, and this is the reason the Dutch reaction was more sober than in 1630, the investment *had to be* long term. It takes at least fifteen years for a *C. calisaya* tree to mature to the point where its quinine content is at a peak and its bark can be harvested. To ensure a constant supply of quinine, the Dutch planters would have to plant new seedlings every year so that they would always have new trees to replace ones that had been stripped the previous season. That entailed not only sufficient land to run several plantations in parallel, but investors with deep enough pockets to fund the plantations for fifteen years before they saw a return on their money. The problem was particularly acute in Java as the island was already overcrowded and the Dutch had to retain the older, less economically viable species of cinchona until Mamani's trees came on stream.

Perhaps the Dutch had learned the lesson of the tulip craze, or perhaps after so many disappointments with cinchona in the past they were more hard-headed. Whatever, van Gorkum now drew up a strict plan that contrasted sharply with the haphazard cultivation methods being pursued by McIvor in the Indian plantations. In future Java would concentrate on just three species: Mamani's *C. calisaya* and Cross's *C. officinalis* for quinine, and Spruce's *C. succirubra* for the other alkaloids. To ensure there was no contamination while inferior species were being phased out, van Gorkum cleared a small area of virgin forest for Mamani's *C. calisayas* away from the other trees and, as an additional precaution, had thousands of worthless varieties surrounding the plantation deflowered every year. It is no exaggeration to say that these few simple precautions saved the entire Dutch cinchona effort. In 1879, when the first trees were ready for harvest, most quinine bark still came from South America. However, by the 1930s Java was providing 97 per cent of the world's supply.

The question is why the British didn't achieve similar success. After all, through the Indian plantation owner, Mr Money, they had acquired far more of Mamani's seeds than the Dutch. Moreover, whereas in 1865 the Dutch government was under fire for squandering money, the Indian government had spent hardly anything, and Markham and McIvor – after weathering the initial criticism – enjoyed pretty much a free reign.

The short answer is that Markham's primary motivation was philanthropic, and as far as he and McIvor were concerned they had already found a tree perfectly adapted to India's needs – Spruce's *C. succirubra.*

By 1872 cinchona cultivation had spread to every corner of India. Following on from the success of the government plantations in Nilgiri, private plantations had sprung up in the coffee-growing districts of the Coorg, Travancore and Tinnevelly, as well as in Darjeeling in British Sikkim, Burma and Ceylon. All told, India now had more than four million cinchona trees and there was little doubt about the planters' favourite. Cross's *C. officinalis* might be the choice at higher elevations, but on the lower slopes *C. succirubra* was indubitably king. In Ceylon alone there were nearly one million red bark trees, prompting one visitor from the Pharmaceutical Society to comment:

> *Succirubra* is the variety in favour, the variety in demand, and the variety that thrives. It may be found growing luxuriantly every- where, in the mountain provinces, on fertile estates, and on the poorest patena soils ... So familiar indeed has it become to the eye of both colonist and native, that it is looked upon as indigenous; the latter having now the fullest confidence in it as a remedy, and not hesitating to help himself to a strip of bark from the nearest tree when occasion necessitates it.

But the preponderance of *C. succirubra* was not dictated simply by horticultural considerations: it was also the result of policy choices forced on the plantations early on by Markham and McIvor. By making his aim a cheap febrifuge for the masses, Markham had set out his stall. Unlike the Dutch he did not have the luxury of waiting for the government nurseries to produce a strain that was so rich in quinine its commercial advantages would be apparent to all. Hence his memorandum to the Revenue and Judicial Committee in 1865 starkly posing the question: 'Did the Government undertake Cin- chona cultivation in order that the use of quinine, in some form or another, might be extended to the people of India, now entirely debarred from its use, or did they undertake it as a mere speculation?' If the latter then the bark should be sent back to England and sold for the manufacture of quinine. But this would mean that the Indian masses would effectively be deprived of the use of the febrifuge. 'The object of the undertaking will be frustrated, and the Government will have entered upon a speculation which will no doubt pay well, but which is entirely foreign to its functions.'

Clearly Markham was worried about confusion within the Council of India about the purpose of the missions. By 1865 he was back
in London serving as a clerk to the Special Department and was well
placed to observe the council's innermost thoughts. Reading between
the lines of his memos he may also have been seeking a reason to
return to India. Interestingly it was about this time that he began
arguing for the preparation of a cheap febrifuge from all the alkaloids
which could be supplied 'from thousands of village dispensaries and
[which] would be within the reach of every *ryot* [peasant] in the
land.' What better excuse to return to India than the need to oversee
experimentation on the bark?

   The other factor was McIvor. He had already decided there was
little point in trying to cultivate quinine-rich *C. calisayas* in India
because of the problems they had acclimatizing. Instead, he was concentrating all his efforts on *C. succirubra* and *C. officinalis*. Unlike in
Java, where the Dutch had gone to pains to keep varieties of the same
species separate, McIvor was freely allowing hybridization in the hope
that a cross between *C. succirubra* and *C. officinalis* or *C. calisaya* would
spontaneously produce a hybrid higher in quinine than either. He also
experimented with 'mossing' and coppicing techniques to boost the
alkaloid content of the bark. John Eliot Howard, who was intimately
acquainted with both the Indian and Javanese plantations, viewed
McIvor's approach with scorn. 'In Java they are wisely thinning out
the inferior trees and allowing the best to develop themselves. In
British India, on the contrary, they are acting in a way that is as
consistent with common sense as to believe that by fusing together a
half-crown and a penny, one could produce a sovereign.'

   As far as Howard was concerned the sovereigns were Mamani's
seeds, which he had dubbed *Calisaya ledgeriana* in recognition of the
role Ledger had played in forwarding them to Europe. Indeed
Howard was so impressed with the Dutch results that in his
monolithic *Quinology of the East Indian Plantations* he described *Calisaya
ledgeriana* as the 'legitimate descendant of the finest sort of the Bolivian
forests' and 'the best, by far, of all.'

   As the world's leading authority on cinchona and the pharmacology of the bark, Howard's opinion ought to have counted for something. But in the case of India, it seems, Markham and McIvor were a law to themselves.

Mr Money had been reluctant to buy the seeds from George so it is not surprising to discover that soon after returning to India he had swapped them for a like amount of *C. succirubra*. But when the seeds reached McIvor all his attention was concentrated on *succirubra* and *officinalis*. Although he germinated the *ledgeriana*, planting some in Ootacamund and sending the rest to Sikkim where he believed the climate would be more suitable, either through uninterest or neglect the trees did not do well and were soon forgotten.[2]

Under any other circumstances this neglect would have been criminal. Not only did India have one of the highest incidences of malaria in the world but also in 1872 a series of deadly epidemics had swept through Bengal underlining the need for a plentiful and cheap supply of quinine. Fortunately, Markham had by now established that the other alkaloids in *succirubra* were almost as good at clearing fevers and that one of them − quinidine − was quinine's equal.

Every since Louis XIV had revealed Robert Talbor's secret formula for the 'English remedy' to the world it had been known that a rough decoction of powdered bark was usually sufficient to clear malarial fevers. But, following the initial studies on quinine, no one had thought to re-examine the other alkaloids in the bark to see if they might be equally efficacious. Beginning in 1865, however, Markham began lobbying for just such tests, arguing that local circumstances in India might favour a compromise febrifuge. In 1866 Viscount Cranbourne (later the Marquess of Salisbury), Secretary of State for India, agreed, ordering the establishment of Cinchona Commissions in Calcutta, Madras and Bombay staffed by medical officers tasked with conducting the experiments.

By today's standards the experiments were very rough and ready. Scientists had yet to identify the malaria plasmodium so instead of microscopic examination of blood smears the medics had to rely on their readings of patients' symptoms to determine whether or not the alkaloids had cleared the disease. There were also no controls. Instead, each of the alkaloids was administered to a different set of patients and the results tabulated. Nevertheless, taken at face value the results were astonishing. In the case of the Madras Commission, 846 patients were treated with quinine, 664 with quinidine, 559 with cinchonine and 403 with cinchonidine. In each case the alkaloids separately cleared the vast majority of fevers. Cinchonine fared the worse with thirteen failures, while quinine came second with six and cinchonidine and quinidine tied with four. However, the quinine and quinidine failure rates had to be set against the fact they had been administered to much larger numbers of patients.

The Commission's conclusion was that quinidine and quinine possessed 'equal febrifugal power', while cinchonidine was 'only slightly less efficacious'. Even cinchonine 'though considerably inferior to the other alkaloids [was] notwithstanding a valuable remedial agent in fever.'[3]

Not surprisingly Markham seized on the results, arguing that the government's aim should now be a 'mixture of all the alkaloids which would combine cheapness and efficacy in the highest degree.' If any-thing Howard was even more enthusiastic, arguing that all ordinary Indians needed to do was prepare a decoction from the bark – a process so simple 'it may be carried on by every family that has a few trees planted at its door.'

However, it was Markham's proposal that received approval. He was aided by the fact that although private planters were still pressing for a species of cinchona that could compete with C. ledgeriana in the international market, the India Office was rapidly losing patience with their demands.

In 1866, for instance, the Madras government had recruited an eminent chemist, John Broughton, to investigate the manufacture of a cheap febrifuge that would retail at no more than one rupee an ounce. Broughton succeeded, establishing a factory in Nedivattam producing a febrifuge he called 'amorphous quinine' at cost price. But the experiment was scuttled by government accountants who wanted to see a greater return on the sale of the bark from the Madras plantations.

Markham was furious, blaming the accountants for Broughton's subsequent resignation and arguing that their only object was 'to obtain harvests of bark to sell at profit in the London market.' Markham soon won the backing of Mr Hume, a secretary in the Indian government's agriculture department, who had seen at first hand how malaria had undermined the health of the rural labour force. The result was that when the Sikkim government appointed another chemist, C. H. Wood, to organize the manufacture of a cheap febrifuge, his argument that the government would not want to sell their alkaloids so cheaply so as to undermine private planters in 'the bazaars' met with an immediate and furious response. 'The question for Wood to consider,' fumed Cranbourne, 'is not what kind of bark fetches the highest price in the London market . . . but to grow the bark yielding the largest percentage of the febrifuge alkaloids generally . . . It should be understood that the object of Cinchona cultivation . . . is not a commercial speculation.'

Whether or not he realized it Cranbourne's sentiments exactly echoed those of the Governor-General of the Netherland Indies twenty years before. Wood got the message and began experimenting with quinetum — an extract of the alkaloids produced by dissolving the bark in hydrochloric acid and then repeatedly filtering and washing the resulting powder, invented by Dr De Vrij in 1872. Although the process was unsophisticated it had the advantage of being cheap and the result was that quinetum retailed for one rupee an ounce without loss to the Sikkim government.

By 1880, Markham could justifiably look back on cinchona cultivation in India with pride. India was now self-sufficient in bark. Not only that but the barks from the Nilgiri plantations were fetching higher prices in the London market than those from South America. Moreover, although the Indian plantations would never be as lucrative as the Javanese the whole cost of introducing and cultivating the tree in India had been repaid with profit. He could not resist pointing out that even as a 'mere commercial speculation' his enterprise had been a success. The Dutch had not been idle either. Thanks to their careful nurturing of *Cinchona ledgeriana* they were also about to bring quinine within reach of the masses and, ironically, they would do it by utilizing Spruce's trees in a way that had yet to occur to the British.

—

Although Moens had established that *C. ledgeriana* was the species richest in quinine, not all the offspring of Mamani's seeds contained equal levels of the alkaloid. Indeed some of the trees contained as little as 4 per cent, suggesting that they had not all been taken from the same area of Caupolicán or that the strain was itself a hybrid of others. Moens had already taken steps to ensure that *C. ledgeriana* did not hybridize with other species of cinchona in Java. Now he began refining the selection process. First, two trees with a high percentage of quinine were chosen. Next, the best seeds were selected and carefully nurtured to maturity. Then, once the trees had flowered, the descend-ants possessing the highest percentage of quinine were reselected. The result was a second-generation strain with 25 per cent more quinine than the first.

There was just one problem: the new quinine-rich strains of *C. ledgeriana* were even more difficult to grow than their predecessors. The rootstock was prone to attack by fungus and only thrived in virgin soils, which were in short supply in Java. By contrast *C. succirubra* had proved exceptionally robust and, as long as it was not overly shaded, flourished everywhere. The solution was obvious: in future shoots of young *C. ledgeriana* would be grafted onto *C. succirubra*. Not only would this give them a greater chance of survival but the grafting would ensure that the bark quality of the original selected tree was perpetuated from one generation to the next – something that could not be guaranteed with propagation by seeds alone.

The results were spectacular. In 1873, when Moens began his experiment, there were just ten thousand *C. ledgeriana* in Java. By 1880 there were nearly half a million, plus more than six hundred thousand *C. officinalis* and *C. succirubra*.

The Dutch success had a dramatic effect on world quinine prices. In 1880 the vast majority of the bark traded on the London market still came from South America and though the price had begun to slide quinine sulphate traded at nearly 500 French gold francs a kilo. By 1890, as the Javanese bark started to come on stream, the price had fallen to 60 francs a kilo, and seven years later it was down to about 30 francs.

The collapse in the price of quinine was excellent news for the millions of poor infected with malaria each year but a disaster for private planters and the native South American bark industry. One after another cinchona plantations in Darjeeling, Madras and Ceylon had to be dismantled and sold off for the 'more successful culture of tea'. Belatedly, the Indian planters had tried to follow the Dutch example, replacing Spruce's red bark with grafts of *C. ledgeriana* grown from the original seeds purchased by Mr Money. But they failed to produce the same quinine-rich strain, probably because the trees had already hybridized as a result of earlier neglect.

However, it was in South America – and Mamani's native Bolivia in particular – that the collapse in the price of quinine was felt most keenly. In 1851 the *calisaya* forests of Caupolicán and the Yungas were producing three million pounds of bark annually. Thanks to the Bolivian government's monopoly the trade brought $142,000 a year into the public treasury, accounting for 15 per cent of the republic's total tax revenues. The money from quinine not only funded essential public works, such as roads, it financed the construc-tion of La Paz Cathedral, one of the city's finest buildings. By 1880, however, Bolivia, Peru and Ecuador were exporting just one million pounds of bark combined. The effects of the quinine crash were felt most brutally in Sorata, a spectacular mountain retreat nestled below the summits of Illampu and Anchohuma north-east of La Paz. In 1875 a group of German plantation owners had begun building a spectacular trail from Sorata down to Mapiri, a steamy jungle town on the banks of the Mapiri River. The idea was to halve the time it took to bring cinchona bark up the mountain to Sorata, from where it could be sent direct to La Paz by road and over the cordillera to the coast of Peru. The ascents were brutal but worst of all was the *cuesta de amarga*, the 'slope of bitterness'. It was aptly named. By the time the Mapiri trail was opened in 1879 the price of quinine had already begun to fall and by the turn of the century the plantation owners had been forced to uproot most of the cinchona trees and replace them with rubber.

Nevertheless the success of the British and Dutch plantations should have been a source of great satisfaction to the two men who had made them possible. Both Spruce and Ledger had seen how the reckless stripping of the bark forests in South America had threatened to make the best species of cinchona extinct and to a greater or lesser degree both shared the conviction that only by exporting the seeds and plants to the colonies could the survival of this 'needful vegetable substance', as Spruce had put it, be secured for humanity. Ironically, however, no sooner were the cinchona plantations thriving than they too came to view them with bitterness. The focus of Spruce's resentment was Markham and the India Office, while Ledger's was primarily the Dutch. But in both cases their dissatisfaction came down to the same thing: money and what they regarded as inadequate public recognition for their achievements.

After sending his collection to India, Spruce's health had deteriorated rapidly. Whether it was a return of the mysterious paralysis that had visited him in Ambato, malaria or some other tropical disease contracted during his exertions in the bark forests and the descent to Guayaquil is unclear. With Spruce's luck it could have been all three. Whatever, he soon became feverish again and was in such pain that he could barely sit upright to complete his report to the India Office. For five months – from May to September 1861 – Spruce lay in his hammock, writing a little each day and stretching his legs when his paralysis abated sufficiently to allow him to walk around. Then in October there was another blow. After waving goodbye to Robert Cross, he had deposited his entire life savings – £700, including the £360 he had received from the India Office – in a bank, Gutierrez

& Co., in Guayaquil. But Gutierrez & Co. had just been declared bankrupt and now all his savings were gone. In desperation he appealed to the Foreign Office for some kind of consular position in South America that would pay him a small income and allow him to continue botanizing. But no offer was forthcoming and he became more and more despondent as he envisioned himself dying of fever and poverty in the marshes of Guayaquil never able to return to England and the company of his scientific colleagues. In a letter to Daniel Hanbury in October 1861, he complained: 'Had I worked as long in the East as I have done in the West, I might have reasonably calculated on a small pension when I was disabled from working; but I do not suppose there is any hope of such a thing in my case.'

Had Spruce's condition improved, as it had on previous occasions, his spirits might have lifted. But this time his paralysis worsened. He was only able to make two further short expeditions, one to the plain of Guayaquil, the other to the coast, and by the end of 1862 he was so disabled that further collecting was out of the question. Writing again to Hanbury he gave full vent to his bitterness:

> I had never calculated on losing the use of my limbs, and yet nothing was more likely to happen, if the sort of life I led be considered. When after loss of health came wreck of fortune, simple though my wants be and modest as were my aspirations, I felt for a time completely prostrated. The fact is I have been far too constant to botany – several times in the course of my travels I might have taken to some occupation far more lucrative – and I have met many men, who beginning without a cent have made far more money in 2 or 3 years than I in 13, and that without being exposed to thunderstorms, and pelting rain – sitting in a canoe up to the knees in water – eating of bad and scant food once a day – getting no sleep at night from the attacks of venomous insects – to say nothing of the certainty of having every now and then to look death in the face, as I have done.

In his next breath Spruce asks Hanbury to 'excuse these personal details' but clearly his sense of injustice was mounting. 'Too late I have found that there is no sympathy for me where most I might have expected it,' he declares.

In 1863 Spruce travelled to Paita, in northern Peru, in the hope that the drier desert climate would prove more conducive to his health. While there he succeeded in making excursions to Piura and Chira and drew up a report, at Markham's request, on the Peruvian system of cotton cultivation. But the miraculous recovery he had been hoping for never came and by 1864 he had run out of options. His health broken by his adventures in the Amazon and Andes, and with no funds to speak of, he now faced the prospect he had been fearing all along – a penurious return to England. Six years earlier he had written to Bentham: 'Poverty is such a positive crime in England that to be there without money or lucrative employment is a contingency not to be reflected on with dread.' Now, as he bid goodbye to South America – his home for the last fifteen years – the dreaded prospect was staring him in the face. After all his exertions in the cause of botany the least he could have expected was a small welcoming committee. In the course of his travels he had collected seven thousand flowering plants and ferns, as well as numerous maps and Indian vocabularies. According to Bentham his researches were the most important 'since the days of Humboldt'. Yet when he disembarked at Southampton on 28 May 1864 there was no one to meet him. Instead, he went straight to Kew where, between spasms of pain, he threw himself into work, sorting out his massive collection. His labours would eventually result in the publication, in 1885, of his six-hundred-page *Hepaticae of the Amazon and of the Andes of Peru and Ecuador*, describing seven hundred species and varieties of plants, four hundred of which were new to botany.

It was a monumental effort, the more so because – although he was now back among friends – his health continued to deteriorate. Shortly before Christmas 1864 he had suddenly developed a fever and started to shiver. A doctor was called to his bedside at Kew and immediately diagnosed ague. Oddly, in view of the fact that this was clearly not Spruce's first experience of malaria, he wrote to Hanbury that in all his time in South America he had never suffered an 'intermittent fever' although 'I have had my full share of *remittent* and *continued* fever' (his italics). Interestingly he included in the latter categories the fever that had nearly killed him on the Orinoco, suggesting that he only considered intermittent fevers to be true malaria. But as before he took quinine – ample supplies of which he had brought back with him from Peru – and was cured.

His paralysis, however, continued to defy treatment. On Hanbury's advice he consulted a number of prominent specialists in London but the symptoms continued, so much so that according to Alfred Wallace, 'for months or even years together, he was unable to sit up at a table to write or to use a microscope, and could never do so for more than a few minutes at a time with intervals of rest on a couch.'

It was a country doctor – a Dr Hartley of Malton – who eventually identified the cause as a 'stricture of the rectum'. Spruce had signalled the area as the 'seat' of his disease for years but said that the specialists had preferred to prescribe his symptoms to hypochondria and never so much as thought of 'passing a bougie[4] into the rectum'. Now, following treatment with enemas and gentle opiates, the pain subsided and Spruce was once again able to work at his microscope and take short walks. But his condition had become chronic and the discomfort remained with him until the end of his life.

By now Spruce's influential friends had rallied to his cause and had set him up in a small cottage at Welburn, near Castle Howard, not far from the village where he had been born. Thanks to the intervention of George Howard, the Earl of Carlisle, his plight had also been brought to the attention of Lord Palmerston, the former prime minister, and in 1865 the government agreed to award him a small pension of £50 a year. In view of the large revenues beginning to be generated by the Indian plantations it was a miserly sum, and hardly enough to live on. Markham was appalled and immediately wrote to the Revenue Department calling on the government to top up his pension to £100. The India Office refused, granting him a one-off payment of £200 instead. Incensed, Markham wrote again, pointing out that Spruce was still owed £97 for his work in Ecuador and that more than any other collector he merited special recognition for his 'great and valuable service' to India in gathering *Cinchona succirubra*. The India Office sanctioned the £97 payment, but it was not until 1877 that it reluctantly acceded to Markham's demand to grant Spruce a further £50 annual pension.

According to Markham, Spruce's modesty and 'high sense of honour' prevented him making representations on his own behalf. But in a letter to Howard in 1869 Spruce privately gave expression to his anger and, interestingly, he appears to have blamed Markham. Howard had written to ask Spruce where he could obtain information about his role in introducing *C. succirubra* to India. Spruce replied that the information should have been included in the 'Blue Book' – the parliamentary record of the correspondence relating to Markham's missions – but for some reason had been left out. Spruce pointed out that he had first proposed gathering cinchona in Ecuador in 1858 – two years before Markham – but that his proposal had been held in abeyance by the Foreign Office until the Indian Mutiny had been 'definitely quelled'. Then, without mentioning Markham by name, Spruce continued:

> Afterwards, as you know, the direction of the enterprise was put into other hands and this is perhaps the reason why the whole of the above-mentioned correspondence was omitted from the report; thus robbing one of the merit (very slight, possibly) of having been the first person who, already practically acquainted with the country and the plants, proposed to procure seeds etc of the Peruvian Bark for forming plantations in the East Indies and other of our colonies, and showed how it could be done.

In fact, Spruce had not been the first to make such a proposal. That distinction belonged to Forbes Royle. However, it was certainly true that Spruce had been the first British botanist to actually arrive in the Andes and make his services available, and as Markham's own notebooks from the period make clear, he was fully aware of Spruce's proposal to the Foreign Office. Given that it was Markham who arranged for the Blue Books to be published in the first place it is curious therefore that he did not see fit to include Spruce's letters in the parliamentary record. Perhaps there is an innocent explanation, perhaps not. The fact that Markham went to such lengths to petition for a pension for Spruce – and without his instigation – may be suggestive of a guilty conscience. On the other hand, he repeatedly drew attention to Spruce's pivotal role in introducing the red bark to India – hardly the actions, you would have thought, of someone who wanted to claim all the glory for himself.

Spruce was not the only one concerned about the historical record. From South America Ledger had also been monitoring the progress of the cinchona plantations, and while he was proud that Mamani's seeds had turned out to be so productive he was also beginning to resent the fact that he had not been afforded sufficient recognition for his role in the enterprise. Interestingly, Ledger also selected Howard as his confidant but, unlike Spruce, he was not nearly so shy about pressing his claims.

Ledger's extraordinary correspondence with Howard begins in 1874 and continues for almost nine years. His letters are by turns supplicating and boastful and, despite his attempts to disguise his motives, his resentment is frequently all too apparent. But when he isn't complaining to Howard about his 'ill-treatment' by the British and Dutch, or soliciting his support for compensation, his letters are full of wonderfully vivid details of his adventures in the Andes and poignant anecdotes about Mamani.

All the strengths and weaknesses of Ledger's character are displayed in the first letter, written three years after Mamani's death. He had now abandoned Peru and moved to the province of Salta, in Argentina, where he had reverted to his former occupation as a general trader. As he struggled to make a living dealing in alpaca ponchos and chinchilla hides, Howard – by now the owner of the most important quinine works in England and an esteemed member of the Linnaean and Pharmaceutical societies – became the sole conduit for his hopes and dreams.

'It is, as you may imagine, a source of great pleasure to me to see that the Cinchona seed forwarded by my aforementioned brother in

1865 has turned out so satisfactorily,' he begins. 'I am quite ignorant of botany. I have for many years taken and still take the liveliest interest in the successful cultivation of this most valuable tree in the dominions of Great Britain, rendering my native land independent for supplies from Bolivia or any other country . . . Had it not been for my kind brother, George Ledger, exerting himself, neglecting very likely his own business, carrying on a long correspondence: after all, this valuable seed in other hands would most likely have been lost.'

The false modesty of these opening sentences is typical. In the next few paragraphs Ledger outlines the history of his expeditions in the bark forests of Peru and Bolivia, making it clear that, though the insights into the location of the best *calisayas* were Mamani's, he was the first to propose putting the knowledge to good use. In 1845, he reminded Howard, he had written via his father to the British government, urging them to raise *calisayas* in Jamaica, India and Ceylon so as to be independent of Bolivia in the production of quinine but had 'never heard in what spirit my ideas were received'. Next he had written to Markham explaining where to go to in Bolivia to collect the best *calisayas* and what precautions to take 'so as not to excite suspicion as to his *real* object', but his letter had arrived too late to be of use. Ledger reminded Howard that Markham had never made it to Bolivia, yet in 1862 he had put up the money for Mamani to travel to Apolo and collect the *calisaya* seeds. Having painted a moving portrait of Mamani's loyalty and devotion to the cause, Ledger concludes:

> After having witnessed the great precautions taken by different parties to 'pack' the seed of the Cinchona for transmission to Europe, failing in almost every case to arrive in a 'live' state, it is wonderful indeed how the '*seed*' sent by me in 1865 produces such splendid results . . . I cannot but feel that I have met with most inadequate acknowledgement after all my exertions, outlays and dedication of so many years. Surely, after the success attending the seed sent by me, the Govt of India and the Govt of the Netherlands should award me a sum of money commen-surate with the importance and value of the service rendered.

There was some merit in Ledger's demands. The Dutch had paid him 100 guilders for the seeds and an additional 500 guilders when they germinated – a total of just 600 guilders (£120). Yet their plantations were now poised to reap huge profits. Similarly, although Ledger was not to know that the British would eventually squander his gift, Markham had to acknowledge that Ledger's expenditure in gathering the seeds had 'far exceeded' the £50 he had received from Mr Money for their sale. Further fuelling Ledger's resentment was the knowledge that the Dutch had spent thousands on Hasskarl's expedition and showered him with honours when his seeds had turned out to be worthless.

At first Howard was more than happy to help Ledger petition the Netherland Indies government for compensation. In part this was because he recognized the force of Ledger's argument but also because by now he could see that the *Cinchona ledgeriana* obtained by the British had been allowed to hybridize and he wanted him to obtain more seed for the Indian plantations. Unfortunately, Ledger's demands proved unrealistic – he wanted £2,000 to return to the *calisaya* forests – and Howard had to drop the proposal. Nevertheless, in the meantime, in an attempt to appease Ledger, Markham had also agreed to petition the British government for a £200 honorarium on his behalf.

Not everyone shared Howard's view of Ledger's contribution. Moens, the Dutch chemist, argued that Ledger's part in the success of the plantations was 'very slight'.

> The seeds have been gathered by an old servant of his, whilst he was on his travel back from Australia to Peru . . . If cinchona growers would make a statue for the clever cascarillero Manuel Incra Mamani, some reason could be found for that. But Ledger has indeed only a very small part in the history, and procured the seed without danger and without trouble, and without knowing indeed that he had got hold of such a precious kind of seeds.

Later Moens was even harsher, claiming that Ledger had built up his role in the enterprise only after he 'knew how valuable a kind of cinchona he had been the means of procuring.'

Moens went too far. Ledger may not have risked his own life to collect the seeds, but he certainly risked his money and there is little doubt that he knew their potential. Moreover, in 1879 he discovered that the Dutch had offered to pay one of his former clerks £400 for 25 lb of seeds of equal quality to those his brother had sold the Consul in London in 1865. It was with some justification then that Ledger concluded he had not been treated 'in good faith or honesty'.

As the exchanges became more heated Howard desperately tried to find a middle way. Judiciously he argued that while botanists owed their knowledge of the best kind of *calisaya* bark to 'the experience and practical sagacity of an Indian' it was to Ledger that belonged 'the whole credit of the enterprise of obtaining the precious seed to which the hope of future success attaches in Java and perhaps in other parts of the East Indies.'

However, it was Moens who won the initial skirmish. Rejecting his petition for further compensation, in 1880 the Dutch agreed to award Ledger a premium of 1,200 guilders (£242). The British were even more peremptory, rejecting Markham's appeal for a £200 honorarium for Ledger out of hand.

Ledger tried to disguise his disappointment. Waiving his claim for compensation against the British, he wrote to Howard, 'I am delighted to hear that fine Ledgeriana are at last! thriving in India and Ceylon. Hurrah! Three times three!' However in almost the same breath Ledger made it clear that it was Mamani who had got 'the true calisaya' and that he was determined to continuing petitioning the Dutch.

Eventually his nagging paid off, although not in quite the way he expected. Howard had already begun referring to the seeds as *Calisaya ledgeriana*. Now in 1881 Moens, perhaps in response to Howard's representations and anxious to find some way of placating Ledger, formally christened the species *Cinchona ledgeriana*.

In botanical terms at least it was the ultimate accolade. At long last Ledger had received the public recognition he craved, and in writing to Howard in 1881 he seems cheerfully resigned to his place in history. 'I am indeed glad, very glad, to see Cinchonas being so successfully cultivated in so many parts of the world and to see my humble name handed down to posterity as one of the helpers in the great work.'

If Howard thought he had heard the last of Ledger's demands, however, he was very much mistaken. For, of all Ledger's talents, his greatest was his capacity to bear a grudge. Had his other schemes for making money ever borne fruit he might have forgotten the matter. But Ledger's tragedy was that he never found a product as valuable as Mamani's seeds. And when, like Spruce, he too lost everything in a banking disaster, he had nothing else to exploit.

The British had never entirely given up hope of matching the output of the Dutch plantations. Although the seeds that George had sold to Mr Money had been allowed to hybridize in India, he had also given some to Howard. These he had carefully nurtured, first at his greenhouse in Tottenham and later in the nurseries at Kew Gardens. Beginning in 1875 Kew began sending cuttings raised from these original seeds to Ceylon and Jamaica. But the soil and altitude there must have been inferior to Java, or else the Dutch management of their plantations was more scientific. Either way the Javanese plantations continued to produce twice as much quinine per acre as the British and gradually the India Office realized there was no point trying to compete. In future the Nilgiri and Sikkim plantations would cultivate bark solely for the production of quinetum, thus meeting the domestic needs of British subjects in India. Meanwhile, British demand for quinine outside of India would be met either by leasing plantations from the Dutch in Java or by purchasing quinine on the open market.

From both a political and commercial point of view the compromise made perfect sense. Malaria was such a widespread problem and the challenge of cultivating cinchona so difficult that from the beginning both countries had been happy to exchange seeds and scientific know-how in search of a lucrative strain. Now that the Dutch had succeeded and the price of quinine was beginning to fall there seemed little to be gained from holding out for more. Quinetum was now available at any post office in Bengal for half a farthing a dose. The truth was that even at this highly subsidized price it was still beyond the means of most Indians. Contract coolies, and their wives and families, in high-risk areas could afford it. But for the self-employed or indigent, half a farthing was too high a proportion of their income. The conclusion was clear. There was a limit to philanthropy and in India the British had reached it. If any profits were to be made from the bark in future, it would come from selling quinine to those who could afford it – in other words 'rich' Europeans and Americans.

If Ledger had not been living in isolation in Argentina he might have seen the logic of these arguments for himself and saved himself a lot of grief. Instead, displaying the same misjudgement that had plagued the alpaca venture, he invested the money the Dutch had awarded him in buying the latest quinine preparations from Howard. It was, of course, a disaster: in 1880 the price of quinine began to slide precipitously and by 1881 the margins Ledger had been hoping to trade on had evaporated.

There was now little to keep Ledger and his wife in South America. In letters from friends and family in Peru and Bolivia he learnt that animosity to him in those countries was growing. Because of the success of the Dutch plantations, made possible by the seeds he had 'stolen' from Bolivia, Ledger was now being accused of having 'destroyed a trade employing 20,000 persons' and 'depriving many of fortune'.

From Ledger's point of view of course he had not gained any-thing. Although he had cleared his debts, his only assets were the few alpaca he had brought with him from Bolivia. He and Charlotte now decided that there was little point in remaining in Argentina and that they should return to Australia, where they still had family and the prospect of making a living. When in 1883 Ledger's father died and it became clear that George's health was not good either he made up his mind. He would catch a steamer to London for the funeral reception and then, after a last visit to the Stockwell family home, emigrate to Australia.

Ledger must have had mixed emotions as he embarked at Buenos Aires. He was now sixty-five and had not set foot in Britain for forty-seven years. In 1836, when he set sail for Peru on the *Swallow*, he had been full of youthful enthusiasm. Now, as he crossed the equator once again, he had plenty of time to reflect on what could have been if only he had possessed the 'right' connections. More than anyone else, Markham had been the key. If only he had known about his mission sooner or his letter had not missed him at Tacna, the British might now be enjoying the fruits of his quinine-bearing seeds and he would be a rich man.

It would be interesting to know if Ledger expressed any of these regrets when he reached London and was finally introduced to Markham at Howard's office in Tottenham. Howard had also invited Moens but he declined. He did not like Ledger – that much is clear.

There is no record of the meeting, but in all probability Ledger kept his thoughts to himself. Markham had been unstinting in his support and there would have been little point in antagonizing him. In his book on cinchona cultivation, Markham had written that although Ledger had not 'served under' him, as soon as he heard about the mission he had 'set to work, actively and zealously, to co-operate in the good cause.'

Markham could afford to be generous. Unlike Ledger, cinchona had made his name. In 1868, on the strength of his success in Peru and India, Markham had been appointed official geographer to Robert Napier's expedition to Abyssinia. Other honours soon followed: he was made a Fellow of the Royal Society and Honorary Secretary of the Royal Geographical Society. In 1872, with the help of Kew, he had despatched collectors to the Amazon to seize another valuable botanical product of South America – *Hevea* rubber, an assignment that Henry Wickham succeeded in realizing four years later when he managed to smuggle seventy thousand *Hevea* seeds onto an English steamer at Belem. Next Markham began promoting polar exploration, joining an expedition to Greenland in 1875. Since then he had dedicated himself to historical writing and was now encouraging expeditions to the South Pole.

We know from Ledger's subsequent letters to Howard that they mainly went over old ground, discussing how the British had made a hash of cinchona cultivation and had ignored all competent advice. Previously Ledger had told Howard how much he appreciated Markham's support for those who had 'served under him' and in all probability he repeated similar sentiments in his presence. Secretly, however, Ledger could not forget that he had been to Bolivia whereas Markham had not.

But there was little point dwelling on that now. The meeting had convinced Ledger there was nothing further for him in Britain and that he should leave for Australia immediately. Two days before embarking he wrote to Howard one more time to thank him for his 'kindness and support'. The letter concludes: 'Something may "turn up" and indeed it would be most welcome ... As before repeatedly stated I'm no "Botanist" – the little I know has been acquired practically and from what I heard from my faithful old servant and friend Manuel and other most intelligent Bolivian Indians.'

It was the end of their correspondence. Shortly after Ledger's departure Howard died. From now on only Markham could help him.

*Chapter Ten*

# THE GREAT WHITE HOPE

Without exaggeration and without excessive optimism we must continue to get quinine used as much as possible.

Angelo Celli

ONE OF THE MOST REMARKABLE aspects of the story of cinchona is that for two hundred and fifty years everyone knew that the bark cured malaria but no one had the faintest idea why. Despite spending fifteen years in the Amazon and Andes, for instance, Spruce never once seems to have questioned the medical orthodoxy that malaria was the result of 'poisonous exhalations' from the land. Nor does he seem to have asked himself why cinchona, rather than any other plant, should block the fever cycle. Like Wallace, Darwin and other eminent nineteenth-century naturalists, Spruce simply had no concept of the 'germ theory' of disease. Nor did he have much interest in plant pharmacology or chemotherapy. As far as Spruce was concerned malaria was simply an intractable fact of life – the cost, if you like, of working in the tropics – and quinine another of nature's imponderables.

While Spruce, Ledger and Markham were hunting for cinchona, however, another group of malaria pioneers were following a parallel trail. Like the naturalists, they would need determination, tenacity and a fair degree of luck. The difference is they could do it all from the comfort of a laboratory bench.

The life cycle of the malaria parasite is complicated and involved but for present purposes the only bit that needs concern us is the merozoite or so-called 'ring' stage. This is when the young parasites emerge from the liver and suddenly begin feeding on red blood cells from the inside. Thanks to powerful electron microscopes we now know that the merozoite burrows through the wall of the corpuscle and begins avidly devouring the cell's protein – the haemoglobin. In the process, however, it also releases the iron-bearing haem, which is toxic. In order to stop itself being poisoned, the merozoite locks the haem away as malaria pigment. Quinine interrupts this process by binding to the haem in a manner that is still not fully understood, and preventing the production of the malaria pigment. In other words, it causes the young parasites to choke on the products of their own digestion.

The point is, if you know what you are doing, this process is easily seen through a microscope. The malaria pigment appears as a black dot or dark granule within the circular bodies of the merozoites. If quinine is not introduced, and the merozoites are left to follow their natural course of development, some of them grow so big as to fill, or almost fill, the entire red blood cell. Next they divide, emerge from the blood cells and invade fresh red corpuscles, sparking the fever attack. Eventually, after several such cycles, some merozoites cease dividing and develop instead into sexual-stage gametocytes. Viewed through a microscope the gametocytes appear as crescents in the case of falcipa-rum malaria, and spheres in the case of other types of malaria.

At first these gametocytes just hang about in the blood waiting for another female *Anopheles* to bite. But once reingested by the mosquito, the males undergo a further spectacular transformation – sprouting flagella, or filaments. These are the sperm, the male gametes that will fertilize the female gametes inside the mosquito's stomach, nearly completing the life cycle of the parasite.

Microscopes have been around since the end of the seventeenth century – in other words, at least as long as physicians have known about cinchona. However, it was only when Louis Pasteur's and Robert Koch's groundbreaking work on bacterial infections renewed interest in microscopy that scientists began taking a closer look at the blood of malaria patients. Once they did it was simply a matter of time before someone stumbled on the truth. The dark, iron-bearing malaria pigments are like droppings along a trail. If you follow their path, quite soon you will discover the characteristic forms of the parasite. And if you happen to be looking at fresh blood from someone with a malaria infection you might even see them moving.

The first person to notice the pigments was a German psychiatrist, Heinrich Meckel. In 1847 he was examining the blood of a lunatic with an enlarged spleen when he recorded a series of 'black irregular rounded granules united ... to globular, egg-shaped or fusiform bodies.' Meckel did not mention whether or not the patient had intermittent fever but soon other researchers were taking note of the pigmentation and gradually doctors began to associate 'melanism', as the phenomenon became known, with malaria.

In 1858 the German pathologist Frerichs demonstrated that the black particles resulted from the destruction of human red blood cells. Then in the 1870s Achilles Kelsch, a French army pathologist at the Val-de-Grâce military hospital in Paris, noted that the pigments were formed at precisely the time the fever came on.

However, the real breakthrough came in 1880 when another French army doctor, Charles-Louis-Alfonse Laveran, in Algiers, decided to take a closer look at the pigments. Like Kelsch, Laveran only had a very basic microscope to work with but, unlike Kelsch, Laveran got lucky. On 5 November 1880 a twenty-four-year-old soldier of the 8th Squadron of Artillery presented himself to Laveran complaining that he was still suffering fever and chills despite having been treated with quinine three weeks earlier (he had probably been given an inadequate dose). Laveran had already found a large number of crescents – the gametocytes of falciparum – in the soldier's blood. Now, before dosing him with quinine again, he took another blood sample and placed it on a slide. This time Laveran not only saw the crescents but, astoundingly, a number of sphere-like bodies with moving filaments. It was the first time anyone had observed the malaria parasite – in this case, in its sexual stage. 'I was astonished to observe that at the periphery of this body was a series of fine, transparent filaments that moved very actively and beyond question were alive,' Laveran later recalled.[1]

Incredibly, Laveran's discovery was ignored for four years. Despite clearly seeing the parasite, his observations were dismissed mainly because most leading scientists were convinced that malaria must be a bacillus like the ones discovered by Pasteur and Koch. Indeed, it was not until the invention of the oil-immersion lens microscope in 1884 and improved aniline stains brought the parasite into sharper focus that the Italians – the arbiters of malaria research – began to take Laveran's findings seriously. In autumn 1884 and throughout 1885 the Italian researchers Ettore Marchiafarva and Angelo Celli patiently examined hundreds of blood slides, assembling what was, in effect, a series of freeze-frames of the parasite's development. At the same time another Italian, Camillo Golgi, observed that the parasites seemed to be synchronized – they divided almost simultaneously and at regular intervals – and that their division coincided with the onset of fever. These observations would eventually lead in 1892 to the conclusion that the crescents and rings seen by Laveran twelve years earlier were all forms assumed by a single species of parasite, and in 1897 to the realization that the flagellating gametocyte was the same parasite in its sexual form.

As far as quinine's reputation was concerned, however, there was no need to await these further revelations. Although the scientific community was slow to accept Laveran's conclusion that malaria was a parasitic illness, his observations provided clear and dramatic proof that quinine stopped the pigmentation process in its tracks. Laveran was still a long way from explaining how quinine achieved this remarkable feat, but you only had to look at the blood of a malaria patient who had been treated with quinine to see that the black pigments disappeared. In the future quinine could no longer be viewed merely as a therapeutic, a drug for easing fever. To use the sort of military terminology that Laveran – who after all was an army doctor – might have appreciated, it was now a weapon, a magic bullet against the disease itself.

But while the microscope broadened quinine's horizons it also, for the first time, marked the drug's limitations. For, following Laveran, it soon became clear that quinine had no discernible effect on the crescents and spheres.[2] The gametocytes persisted no matter how much you dosed them. In other words, quinine killed the parasites in the blood cells but it had no effect on their sexual form and thus could not be considered a complete sterilizing treatment which could prevent transmission. 'Even when giving quinine every day by subcutaneous injection, and in large doses for a whole month,' wrote Celli in 1901, 'I have not often succeeded in destroying the crescent forms . . . upon these forms of the parasite, which are the most dangerous from the epidemic point of view, quinine has no influence . . . therefore a complete rational prophylaxis by means of disinfection . . . is not easy, nor is it always possible.'

However, in order for quinine's limitations to become apparent to Celli another army doctor, the British surgeon-captain Ronald Ross, first had to made the crucial link between the parasite and the mosquito. This Ross did in 1897, dissecting an *Anopheles* in Secunderabad and discovering the plasmodium (in its oocyst form) hidden in its stomach wall. But not only did Spruce, Ledger et al. not know about the plasmodium; they did not know about the mosquito either.

To be fair no one did, though there had been suspicions. The earliest plausible reference to the mosquito as a vector comes in an early Indian text known as the Susruta. Written by a Vedic scribe in the sixth century BC, it refers to five kinds of disease-carrying *masakah* (mosquitoes) whose bite is accompanied by, among other symptoms, 'fever, pain of limbs . . . shivering . . . burning sensation, intense cold.' The Babylonians portrayed their pestilence-causing god Nergal as a two-winged fly, while the Canaanites called him Beelzebub, 'prince of flies'.

Similarly, although the association between malaria and 'bad air' is an Italian idea, some classical Roman writers dropped tantalizing hints that there might be more to it than that. Varro in his *De Re Rustica* posited that invisible micro-organisms breeding in marshes and stagnant waters might be responsible for the disease and recommended that houses be built in high and well-ventilated places so that the small 'bestiolale' would be blown away. And writing at the end of the first century, Columella pointed out that marshes bred 'animals armed with mischievous stings, which fly upon us in exceeding thick swarms; and also send forth, from the mud and fermented dirt, envenomed pests of water snakes . . . whereby hidden diseases are often contracted.'

Unfortunately, so great was the Roman obsession with the foul air emanating from swamps that these tantalizing glimpses of the truth were ignored, not least by Hippocrates, who was convinced that the cause was stagnant water. The result was that by the seventeenth century – when malaria became widespread in Europe – the association between malaria and the insalubrity of marshes was well established. The French term for malaria, *le paludisme*, for instance, comes like the Spanish *el paludismo* from the Latin word *palus*, meaning swamp. Similarly, although the English term 'ague' refers to the characteristic swelling of the spleen in malaria patients – the so-called 'ague cake' – in *The Tempest* Shakespeare has Caliban call forth: 'All the infections that the sun sucks up/ From bogs, fens, flats on Prosper fall and make him/ By inch-meal a disease'.

Interestingly, the first person in the modern era to make explicit his suspicions about the mosquito's role in transmitting malaria was another French doctor, working like Laveran in the tropics. More intriguing still, this doctor was based in Caracas, Venezuela, less than eight hundred kilometres from the Orinoco, and published his theory just months before Spruce succumbed to fever on the river.

Born in Guadeloupe in 1803, Dr Louis Daniel Beauperthuy had a strong biological bent. Like Laveran, he enjoyed nothing better than looking at blood through a microscope and after studying medicine in Paris he had returned to his native Caribbean to be closer to the seat of such diseases as leprosy, yellow fever and malaria.

Whenever an epidemic broke out, Beauperthuy would study it on the spot and in 1854 his work as a health officer for the Venezuelan government brought him to Cumaná, then in the grip of a yellow fever outbreak. Beauperthuy was familiar with the miasma theory of malaria, but could not help noticing that though Cumaná was humid there were no swamps. There were, however, plenty of mosquitoes. Noting that the Roman historian Herodotus had referred to mosquitoes as 'winged snakes', Beauperthuy decided to take the idea a stage further. In May 1854, as Spruce was making his way downstream to Maipures, Beauperthuy wrote in the *Gaceta Official de Cumaná*:

> The mosquito plunges its proboscis into the skin ... and introduces a poison which has properties akin to snake venom ... Marshes do not communicate to the atmosphere anything more than humidity, and the small amount of hydrogen they give off does not cause in man the slightest indisposition in equatorial and inter-tropical regions renowned for their unhealthiness. Nor is it the putrescence of the water that makes it unhealthy, but the presence of mosquitoes.

Although Beauperthuy rather ruined his theory by conjecturing that the source of the 'poison' introduced by the mosquito was decomposing animal matter, it was a stunning leap and soon others were edging towards similar theories. By the middle of the nineteenth century malaria was rampant all along the watercourses from the Mississippi to the Potomac. However, a number of American doctors had begun to notice that malaria was also prevalent in the hill country, where marshes and stagnant water were absent. In 1848 Josiah Clark Nott, a doctor from Alabama, had tentatively raised the possibility that the culprit might be the mosquito because of its ability to 'take flight'. However, it was not until 1882 that another doctor was prepared to be more outspoken.

Albert Freeman Africanus King was an Englishman who went to America as a boy, became an obstetrician and practised for nearly fifty years in the nation's capital. Washington DC had been so malarious during the Civil War that General McLellan's Army of the Potomac had been unable to capture the city and had to withdraw to Malvern Hill where his men promptly came down with 'Chickahominy fever'. Twenty years later, it was no better. The United States Sanitary Commission had already commissioned a report on how to tackle Washington's 'miasmatic fevers'. Now, in a paper before the Philosophical Society, King listed nineteen reasons why he believed mosquitoes were the vectors of malaria and challenged the city's fathers to erect a massive wire screen as high as the Washington Monument around the capital to test his theory.

Unfortunately King's novel suggestion was dismissed. His distinguished medical colleagues still considered the mosquito theory too fantastic and King is best remembered today for attending to Lincoln on the night he was assassinated at the Ford's Theatre. The one thing that could have given King's musings credibility was Laveran's theory about the parasite. But though Laveran had published his findings three years earlier they had met with such indifference that few doctors in America, including King it seems, were aware of them.

It was the British who were destined to provide the crucial link between the mosquito and the parasite and they did it, not through an intuitive leap but by steady, laborious experimentation. The first step was taken by Dr Patrick Manson, a medical officer in the Chinese Imperial Customs Service. In 1876, while dissecting mosquitoes in Amoy that had fed on human volunteers infected with elephantiasis, a parasitical infection of the filarial worm, Manson discovered filariae in the mosquitoes' stomach walls. However, although he studied filariasis for several years he never followed the parasites to full maturity and thus never saw them proceed to the mosquito's head, enter its proboscis and, at the moment of biting, slide down the puncture into a new human host.

Manson's failure to take his studies to their logical conclusion led him into a cul-de-sac that could easily have prevented Ross, his disciple, from ever discovering the true transmission process. On his return to England Manson had reasoned that mosquitoes were simply nursemaids to the filariae and that the parasite only passed to humans when they drank from water infected with filariae-containing mosquito larvae. Nevertheless, Manson inspired Ross sufficiently to persuade him to invest in a microscope and begin examining mosquitoes for signs of the malaria parasite.

A reluctant medic, whose first love was poetry, Ross seems to

19. Postcards by the artist Albert Guillaume, issued by the French War Ministry during the First World War. The first card urges soldiers to take quinine every day. The captions on the second card read, 'he does not have a mosquito net' and 'he has slept well under his mosquito net'.

20. A 1927 poster from British India, spelling out the benefits of quinine, and the dangers of not taking it.

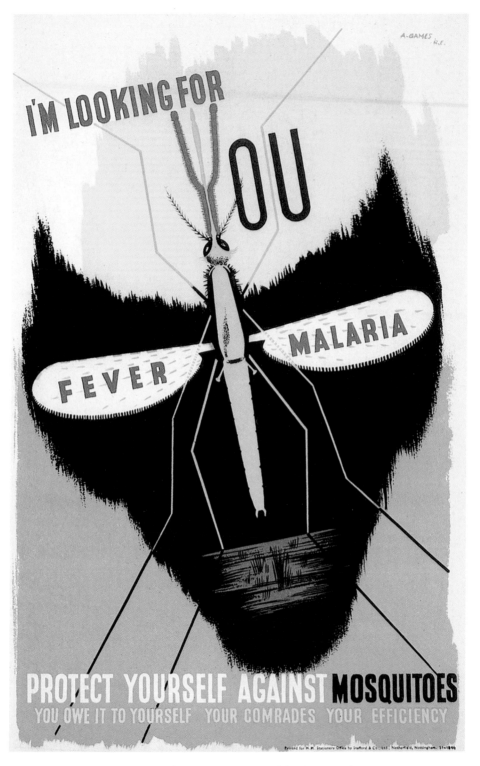

21. British public health poster, warning of the dangers of mosquitoes
and malaria.

The cold stage

The hot stage

22. RAF cartoon showing the three clinical stages of a malaria attack.

The sweating stage

23. An early nineteenth-century cartoon showing three members of the Roman Campagna Malaria Commission, carrying their gear.

24. An advertisement for Burroughs Wellcome, showing the various situations in which a 'tabloid' medicine chest would be helpful. The portable medical kits were a big hit with explorers like Henry Morton Stanley.

25. Pipe dream: a British malariologist poses in essential tropical headgear.

26. Cinchona bark being dried in the sun, circa 1950. Following the Second World War, quinine was supplanted by chloroquine and other synthetic drugs.

27. Cartoon celebrating Charles-Louis-Alfonse Laveran's discovery of the malaria parasite in the blood of a feverish French solider in Algiers in 1880. In the picture Laveran metaphorically lances the mosquito enemy from atop a camel . . .

28 . . . and Manuel Elkin Patarroyo, the Colombian immunologist who hopes to employ pipettes and hypodermics to similar effect by developing a malaria vaccine.

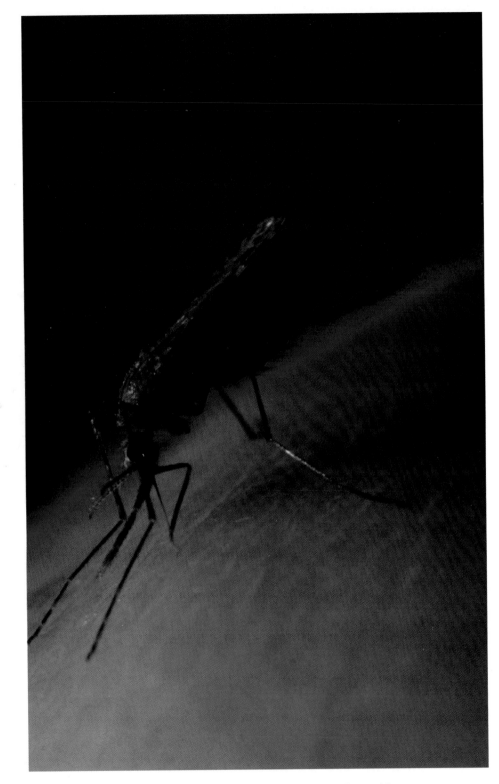

29. *Anopheles gambiae*, the deadliest insect in the world.

have had little understanding of parasitology or mosquito taxonomy. However, he was a dogged researcher and, stationed in a remote, malarious Indian outpost, found himself ideally placed and with plenty of time to pursue the insect vector. Interestingly, shortly before he made his breakthrough at Secunderabad, Ross had passed by the cinchona plantations at Ootacamund – or 'Ooty' as he liked to refer to the hill station. At the time Ross had been on his way to the highly malarious Sigur Ghat to trawl the pools and lagoons for mosquito larvae and in preparation had been dosing himself with five grains (325mg) of quinine daily. But quinine, as we know now, is a poor prophylactic and when he reached the ghat Ross suffered a 'severe go of fever'. To cure himself, he upped the dose but he later recalled that the experience left him 'weak and depressed for a long time'.

Indeed, it was only while straining his eyes one steamy summer evening back in Secunderabad that the young military physician's spirits finally lifted. Ross later referred to that day – 20 August 1897 – as 'Mosquito Day'. That was when he saw for the first time a spherical body (oocyst) on the stomach wall of an *Anopheles* that had previously fed on a malarious patient. He recognized that it contained pigment identical to that seen in the malaria parasite. Then, the following July, in Calcutta, while examining bird malaria transmitted by the culex mosquito, Ross saw the oocysts burst, invade the insect's thoracic cavity as 'threads' and migrate to the mosquito's salivary gland ready to be inoculated. As far as Ross was concerned the *culex* was all the proof that he needed. 'Hence I think I may now say QED and congratulate you on the mosquito theory indeed,' he wrote to Manson.

The congratulations were a little premature. Ross never seemed to have fully grasped the fact that it was only a certain type of mosquito that transmitted malaria in humans and never went on to examine whether anophelines – or 'dapple-winged' mosquitoes as he called them – also contained oocysts and threads. That proof was left to Giovanni Grassi, Professor of Anatomy at Rome University. But unfortunately for the Italians, Grassi's paper showing that human malarias were only transmitted by species of *Anopheles* was not published until four months after Ross had announced his discovery to the British Medical Association. The result was that it was the Englishman, not the Italian, who in 1902 was awarded the Nobel prize.

What Spruce would have made of Ross's breakthrough had he lived to see it is anyone's guess. Perhaps he would have found irony in the fact that while he had been struggling to sit up straight at his own microscope in order to put his collection of mosses and liverworts in order, Ross had been using the same instrument to such dramatic effect.

His doctor's belated diagnosis of a 'stricture of the rectum' had done little to ease his suffering. In 1869 he wrote to a friend from Welburn that 'sitting up to the microscope has brought on bleeding of the intestines to such an extent that I fear I must renounce the task altogether'. For the next eighteen months he was in too much pain to use his microscope at all, and it was only in the spring of 1871 that he 'plucked up the courage' to disinter it and resume work on his hepaticae.

In 1873 Spruce moved to a small cottage in Coneysthorpe, just outside the gates of Castle Howard. The sitting room was just three and a half metres square and the bedroom even smaller. Although he had a housekeeper and young girl to nurse him, and the Howard family looked in on him, his options were few. Too infirm and poor to contemplate further travel, all his efforts were now devoted to organizing his massive collection. It was meticulous, painstaking work but as Wallace would later recall Spruce was 'a man who, however depressing were his conditions or surroundings, made the best of his life' and by 1885 his six-hundred-page work on Amazonian hepaticae was complete.

Of all the areas he had visited, it was the Río Negro that had enthralled him most, and where he had discovered a great number of the species and genera new to science. But he had also been captivated by the Andean cloudforests not least because the same damp, clinging mists that were conducive to cinchona also favoured the growth of mosses, lichen and fungi. Indeed, plant pharmacologists believe today that the alkaloids in the bark probably evolved in response to this mossy environment, their bitterness helping to discourage fungi and other plant predators. But if such a thought ever occurred to Spruce he never recorded it. Although he liked to think of himself as a Darwinian, his response to plants was first and foremost aesthetic. 'I like to look on plants as sentient beings,' he once wrote in response to some deprecatory remarks about his beloved hepaticae.

> It is true that the Hepaticae have hardly as yet yielded any substance to man capable of stupefying him, or of forcing his stomach to empty its content, nor are they good for food; but if man cannot torture them to his uses or abuses, they are infinitely useful where God has placed them ... they are, at the least, useful to, and beautiful in, themselves — surely the primary motive for every individual existence.

Spruce too had been 'infinitely useful' in Ecuador, the place where fate had placed him. After all, it was thanks to Spruce that Ross, and thousands of other malaria sufferers in India, survived to lead productive lives. Moreover, the trail Spruce had followed had been fraught with real danger whereas the only pitfalls Ross had risked were professional ones. But there was no Nobel prize for Spruce, none of the acclaim that accompanied 'great' scientific achievement. Instead, in 1864 he received an honorary doctorate in philosophy from the Imperial German Academy in Berlin, and two years later an honorary fellowship from the Royal Geographical Society. Then, in 1893, he was elected an associate of the Linnaean Society.

It was too little, too late. Spruce was now seventy-six and so incapacitated that he could barely walk, let alone write. Four years previously he had suffered another paralytic attack, as a result of which he had been unable to leave his cottage for two months. Now, shortly after Christmas 1893, he contracted influenza and, after a severe attack, he died on 28 December.

Spruce was buried at Terrington, the parish in which he had

been born, beside his father and mother. The Countess of Carlisle sent a wreath from Castle Howard as a token of remembrance, but the only people present at the graveside were Matthew Slater, the executor of Spruce's estate, and a few close friends from Coneysthorpe.

After completing his book on Amazonian hepaticae, Spruce's last years had been spent working on British and European hepaticae, having no strength left to write a popular account of his travels. That task now fell to Wallace. Fortunately, Spruce was a conscientious and descriptive diarist, as well as a prodigious letter writer, and under Wallace's skilful editing – informed by his own experiences in the Amazon – an enduring testimonial emerged. Spruce may not have understood malaria or how quinine worked, but he was one of the last great naturalist-explorers. And from the botanical notes and journals he kept in South America emerges a vivid picture not only of the plant life and geography of the Amazon and Andes but of the customs and habits of the indigenous peoples among whom he spent the most arduous and, arguably, the best years of his life.

Given his reputation as a collector the only surprise is that Spruce never discovered a new species of cinchona. Instead his name is commemorated in two genera of moss and liverwort named, respectively, *Sprucea* and *Sprucella*, and two species of British liverwort, *Marsupella sprucei* and *Orthotrichum sprucei*.

Unlike Spruce, disease does not appear to have figured much in Ledger's life or his imagination. During his travels over the cordillera into Bolivia and Chile he suffered altitude sickness and no doubt he endured his fair share of dysentery. But in all his time in South America he never once refers to an intermittent fever or having to take quinine. And even in later life, after Ross's discoveries had been announced to the world, there is no record in Ledger's letters of so much as a passing interest in the pathology of malaria – the disease that his seeds had done so much to alleviate.

In 1891, however, like Spruce two years later, Ledger succumbed to influenza. The epidemic fell upon him and his wife in Goulburn, in New South Wales. He and Charlotte had bought a small farm there with money from his father's inheritance and the sale of the remaining alpaca in Argentina. The plan was to retire on their modest savings — some £1,500 in all, which Ledger had deposited in a local branch of the Australian Banking Company. But the flu was a severe one and Charlotte died. An obituary notice in the local paper mentioned that Ledger too was 'very low and not expected to live throughout the day.'

That notice would later lead to rumours in Britain that Ledger was also dead. In fact he survived, but in some ways it may have been better had he not. For the same day that Charlotte's obituary notice appeared another article in same paper announced that the Australian Banking Company had 'suspended payments'. The fall in the price of wool, coupled with the embezzlement of funds by a senior director, had eaten into all the bank's deposits. A year later, the bankruptcy was confirmed and Ledger — like Spruce thirty years earlier — found himself bereft of savings.

Now aged seventy-three, Ledger was broke and all alone. His only hope was Markham. Following the success of the Indian plantations and the Napier mission to Abyssinia in 1868, Markham had been showered with honours and in 1893 was elected President of the RGS. If anyone could secure him a pension from the British and Dutch, reasoned Ledger, it was Markham.

Once again Ledger put pen to paper and once again Markham renewed the appeals, writing a long letter to the *Chemist and Druggist* outlining Ledger's plight. To the eminent quinologists and chemists who subscribed to the specialist weekly, the news that Ledger was alive and broke in Australia came as a surprise. 'A lost cinchona-pioneer found,' announced the headline. A few weeks later the *Chemist and Druggist* went a stage further, writing a long editorial in support of Ledger's claim and calling on planters, importers and quinine manufacturers everywhere to contribute to a fund on his behalf.

Ledger had been 'very shabbily rewarded', opined the editorial. 'We doubt whether, as a matter of bare commercial principle, it would be possible for Mr Ledger to show any cause why either the Dutch or Indian Governments, to whom, for a hundred pounds or so, he supplied seed that has produced cinchona bark worth many thousands of times the sum paid for it, should do anything for him in his old age. Fortunately, however, for those in distress, sentiment counts for something in the governments of the world . . .'

It was the same argument Markham had put to the Secretary of State for India in 1880 and the unsentimental British were no more inclined to accept it now than they had been in the past. At first the Dutch were not moved either. At this point Ledger was only asking to be reimbursed for the monies he had spent procuring the ledgeriana seeds. But the Dutch rejected the request out of hand, saying he had already received 'repeated liberal payments' – a reference to the total of nearly £400 he had been paid since 1865. The phrase infuriated Ledger.

'Had I been born in Holland I should have been covered with medals and be a wealthy person now,' he fumed, adding that by refusing to compensate him the Dutch were condemning him 'to end my days in an asylum for the destitute.'

It was hyperbole, of course. By 1895 Ledger had mortgaged his cottage and was living on the interest from the money raised. But his income was only £3 a month and the *Handelsblad* of Amsterdam, one of the leading Dutch daily papers, was sufficiently appalled to take up his cause. Calling on the Dutch government to grant him a pension of £100 a year, the paper began a sustained campaign. Markham quickly pitched in, adding his weight as President of the RGS to write direct to the Dutch Minister for the Colonies.

At first the Netherlands Indies government resisted, but gradually under the weight of public pressure it was forced to give in and in 1896 the Dutch parliament voted Ledger a £100 pension 'for distinguished services rendered by him to the cinchona industry.' On 4 May 1897 – Ledger's seventy-ninth birthday – the Dutch Minister for the Colonies formally notified him of the annuity. After more than twenty years of canvassing and complaining Ledger's fight was finally over.

In the last photograph of him, taken shortly before his seventy-ninth birthday, Ledger is shown seated in a Victorian parlour, with one foot propped on a cushion and his top hat resting upside down on his writing desk. His left hand is still gloved, as though he has just come in from a brisk walk, while his lips are clamped tightly shut, giving him a stern and forbidding look. The portrait was probably meant to convey Victorian respectability but his eyes seem to burn with bitterness and it is hard not to see in his piercing gaze unrequited resentment for all his misfortunes.

Very little is known of Ledger's old age. He lived eight more years, finally dying in May 1905 at the age of eighty-seven of bronchitis brought on by senile decay. He was buried beside his Australian sister-in-law, Emma Garratt, in Rookwood Cemetery, a sprawling Methodist burial ground outside Sydney. At the time of his death he was so poor that his name did not appear on the tombstone.

By the turn of the century quinine was the Great White Hope. With abundant and cheap supplies of the drug flowing out of Java it seemed only a matter of time before malaria was eradicated from every corner of the globe. Interestingly, quinine's biggest supporter was Robert Koch, the German bacteriologist who had been one of the most vocal sceptics of Laveran's claims to have seen the parasite. In New Guinea Koch had seen for himself how efficiently quinine cleared the parasite from patients' blood and he now became the leading advocate of quinine prophylaxis, a method he believed 'could make every malarial place free or almost free of malaria' within nine months.

The Italians concurred. Some, like Celli, went even further. 'Without exaggeration, and without excessive optimism,' he wrote in 1901, 'we must continue to get quinine used as much as possible; we must administer it promptly, assiduously and in greater quantities than Koch prescribed.'

But quinine alone would never be the complete answer to malaria for several reasons. First, as Celli had already observed, it did not act on the gametocytes nor did it affect the growing liver stages of the parasite.[3] Second, if used for a prolonged period it had unpleasant side effects, including headaches, nausea, ringing in the ears and, in cases of extreme falciparum infection, blackwater fever – an auto-immune response in which blood haemoglobin suddenly breaks down, staining the urine a dark red or black. Third, and perhaps most importantly, quinine's 'affordability' could not last: sooner or later the economics of bark production in Java would force up the price.

However, by now the identification of the mosquito as the culprit had raised the possibility of complementary strategies – ones that, in tandem with quinine, could deliver man to the promised land of a malaria-free world. In 1900 Manson oversaw a series of experiments on the Roman Campagna in which he demonstrated that it was possible to block the transmission of the parasite from mosquito to man through the simple expedient of screens. In India, meanwhile, Ross had done complex calculations to show that if you filled in enough ditches and greased enough ponds and puddles with oil you could stop *Anopheles* from breeding. Then there was the Italian idea of extensive public sanitation works that drew inspiration from Rome's ancient *cloaca maxima*.

In 1901, at a conference on malaria in Eastbourne, Koch – just returned from New Guinea – outlined a four-point plan for eradicat-ing malaria. Pride of place still went to quinine – especially in the tropics – but nets, screens, blitzing mosquito breeding grounds and removing malarious patients were now almost as important. A year later the Italian government decided to follow 'Koch's Way', establish-ing a state quinine service to subsidize production and distribution of the drug. In the first year of operation alone, the government sold more than 2.2 tonnes, chiefly in sugar-coated tablets, and by 1907 sales exceeded 24 tonnes. At the same time it began a vigorous campaign of bonification – draining swamps and marshes and filling in unsanitary ditches. The result was that deaths from malaria in Italy fell from a high of fifteen thousand in 1900 to just over two thousand by 1914.

In India, 'Ross's Way' took precedence. At Mian Mir, a notoriously malarial plateau in Lahore, the British army cleared and oiled irrigation ditches, exported infectious patients and administered quinine in both preventive and curative doses. Unfortunately, the results were not encouraging. By 1909 two-thirds of local children were still being infected – as many as when the experiment had begun – and General Kitchener decided to stop the experiment. Meanwhile in India as a whole, malaria cases were still running at a hundred million a year. The difference was that, thanks to quinine and quinetum, by 1910 deaths were down to one million – half the level of fifty years previously when Markham began cinchona production in Mysore. However, it was in South America – the only place in the world to have previously been malaria-free and that, until now, had profited least from quinine's extraction – that, appropriately, the new control measures were about to enjoy their finest hour.

Ever since the Spanish conquistador Vasco Núñez de Balboa first laid eyes on the 'southern sea' from a hill on the Isthmus of Panama in 1513, men had dreamt of a canal linking the Atlantic with the Pacific. Initially, governments had thought it a simple matter of digging and dredging. But as Joseph de Jussieu could have told them, the Isthmus was a death trap: in 1735 the French botanist had almost succumbed to fever at Puerto Bello, reviving only after taking an infusion of cinchona bark. And La Condamine and the other Academicians had been so anxious to flee Puerto Bello's 'dangerous climate' that they had hurried on to Ecuador after only a few days.

The *Anopheles* was only one of the reasons the Isthmus was so feared. Panama also teemed with *Aedes aegypti* – the carriers of yellow fever – and in combination the twin vectors were deadly. If the 'yellow jack' didn't get you in the first week, malaria inevitably would.

The French learned the lesson the hard way. In 1879 Ferdinand de Lesseps, triumphant from engineering the Suez Canal, began laying a railway line across the Isthmus in preparation for gouging a

canal through the jungle. No one knows exactly how many Frenchmen died — twenty-two thousand was one estimate — or what
proportion of the fatalities were black labourers imported from the
West Indies. But it is said that for every sleeper laid a man lost his life
and in 1889 Lesseps was forced to abandon the project.

It took a man in the Rossian mould to realize the scale of the
problem and draw up an appropriate battle plan. That man was
William Crawford Gorgas, a colonel in the American medical corps
who had been raised in the malarious Confederate state of Virginia.
Gorgas was not an instant convert to Ross's theories. He came to
mosquito control reluctantly, through his experiences with yellow
fever, first at Fort Brown, Texas, where in 1882 he was stricken with
the disease and almost died, and later in Havana where he came
under the sway of the Cuban doctor Carlos Finlay and the US
Army surgeon Walter Reed, a brilliant medical researcher who had
previously studied the typhoid bacillus.

Since 1881 Finlay had been arguing that yellow fever was
transmitted by 'stegs' — the *Aedes* mosquito, also known as *Stegomyia*
— but it was only when Reed was sent to Havana in 1900 to
investigate the disease and allowed *Aedes* to feed on three of his
assistants that Finlay's suspicions were confirmed (they all died).
Although Gorgas remained 'unconvinced' by these experiments he
immediately instituted a strict quarantine regime and set about oiling
the cisterns and pools in Havana's backstreets where the mosquitoes
bred. The result was that by the summer of 1902 yellow fever had
been completely eradicated and deaths from malaria had been reduced
to seventy-seven. 'For the first time since the English occupation in
1762,' Gorgas wrote to Ross, 'we have an October free from yellow
fever, and malaria decreased more than one half.'

When in 1904 the United States began taking an active interest
in the problem of the canal route, Gorgas was the natural choice to
head the campaign against the mosquito. At first he encountered
stubborn opposition from Commission officials who considered the
mosquito-transmission theory 'balderdash', but the chief engineer,
John Stevens, had seen workers suffering at first hand and decided to

give him a chance. Getting rid of yellow fever was relatively straightforward. As in Cuba, Gorgas launched an all-out attack on the
*Aedes*, screening the water barrels where they bred and coating ponds,
cisterns and cesspools with oil once a week. At the same time, he
launched an extensive pyrethrum fumigation campaign and, as a final
precaution, screened in those who had already contracted the disease.
The result was that by 1906 yellow fever had been completely
eradicated.

Reducing malaria took a little longer and required four lines of
attack. First, Gorgas eliminated the *Anopheles*' breeding grounds by
draining and filling in swamps and spraying oil on lakes, streams and
ditches the length of the canal route. Second, he employed full-time
'swatters' to kill mosquitoes harboured in workers' quarters. Third, he
erected screens outside every veranda. Fourth and last, he deployed
quinine. Establishing a chain of more than twenty dispensaries
between Cristóbal and Balboa, he offered men a prophylactic dose of
150 mg twice a day. In one year alone, these makeshift health centres
dispensed 1.3 tonnes of quinine and to get round some men's aversion
to its bitter taste Gorgas even offered the drug diluted in 'extra-sweet
pink lemonade'.[4]

The result was that within three years Gorgas had cut the
incidence of malaria by more than half and thereafter there was a
steady decline in cases from eight hundred out of every thousand canal
workers in 1906 to seventy in every thousand by 1913. And by the
time the first ship passed through the canal in 1914 deaths from all
causes had fallen to just six per thousand. It would not be long,
Gorgas predicted, before 'life in the tropics for the Anglo-Saxon will
be more healthful than in the temperate zone.'

The construction of the Panama Canal was a remarkable achievement not least because it showed that disease need no longer be
considered a barrier to progress. The lessons were clear. If you were
determined enough and brought military organization to bear, the
tropics could be tamed. Well, almost. By 1916 Gorgas's measures had
succeeded in reducing malaria cases in Panama to sixteen in every
thousand but, unlike with yellow fever, he would never completely

eradicate the disease. The reason was that the workers continued to harbour the gametocytes in their blood, and until every last *Anopheles* in Panama was exterminated – a truly impossible undertaking – malaria could rebound at any time.

It is not known what Markham made of the canal. By the turn of the century all his energy and attention was focused on another geographical challenge – mapping the Antarctic. In 1901 he had despatched Robert Falcon Scott to the south pole on the *Discovery* and by 1910 he was fully occupied with fitting out Scott's second, tragic expedition. However, Markham had always been fascinated with the problem of the circumnavigation of the globe, and the linking of the seas must have struck him as a remarkable achievement, not least because during the cinchona mission he had had to cross the Isthmus twice – once on the way out from Southampton, the second time on his way back with the seeds. Through his histories of Columbus and the early Spanish colonists Markham was also well aware of the Isthmus's dreadful reputation for fevers. Now, thanks in part to his humanitarian efforts, quinine had helped make the Isthmus safe.

Unfortunately, the same was not true of India. The failure of the Mian Mir project coincided with a serious epidemic. In 1911 malaria raged throughout the country with a severity comparable to that of ten years earlier. The problem was not the lack of quinine but the authorities' failure to mount a consistent, military-style campaign against the *Anopheles*' breeding grounds. Irrigation and drainage works had been commenced but they had not gone nearly far enough. Florence Nightingale's prescription fifty years earlier that 'the salvation of the Indian Army must be brought about by sanitary measures everywhere' had been ignored. Regular malaria surveys were commissioned but they just confirmed what everyone already knew. As the Malaria Advisory Board put it, the war against malaria required 'continuity of policy and extreme thoroughness'. Without both, the parasite would never be defeated. Nevertheless, Markham could at least take comfort in the fact that the cinchona missions had brought the cure within the reach of ordinary Indians. Or could he?

In June 1911 Leeds University had presented him with a doctorate in science. Conferring the degree the university's chancellor, the Duke of Devonshire, had singled out his missions for unique praise: 'To have established in our Indian Empire ... the cultivation of a prophylactic for its desolating malarial disease, was a service to humanity such as few may hope to render by the undivided labours of a lifetime.'

But Markham's philanthropic vision was already in ruins. The problem was that despite the evidence that quinetum was as effective as quinine at curing malaria, the medical profession preferred the refined drug. The result was that by 1913 consumption of Markham's cheap cinchona febrifuge had fallen to just 725kg and India — in common with the rest of the world — was receiving most of its quinine from Java. In 1910 Markham had written to the Secretary of State for India 'deploring' the rundown state of the Indian cinchona planta-tions, but rather than encourage planters in Ceylon to switch to *Cinchona ledgeriana* production in order to compete with the Dutch the British simply leased their own plantations in Java. At first the arrangement worked well. After all it mattered little where the bark came from as long as the end product — quinine — was plentiful and cheap. Indeed rivalry between the planters in Java and the European manufacturers who controlled the production of quinine had generally exerted a downward pressure on quinine prices. In 1892, in an effort to keep bark prices low, for instance, the manufacturers had formed a syndicate under the direction of the German quinine producers to ensure that no one outbid the other. But the Dutch planters resented the European manufacturers' monopoly and in 1896 set up their own factory in Bandoeng, Java, with the aim of manufacturing quinine direct for the Amsterdam market. The result was that by 1898 the Bandoeng factory was producing some 100kg of quinine a day and began undercutting European quinine prices. But, paradoxically, the reduction of bark shipments to Europe brought about by the

Bandoeng factory led to a steady rise in the unit price of bark on the Amsterdam market. The result was that bark prices, having reached a low of just over 2 cents a unit at the end of 1896, began to rally again, rising 6 cents in the first eleven months of 1897 and peaking at 12.25 cents a unit in September 1900.[5]

By 1911, the European manufacturers had come to the realization that the only way to protect their profits was to invite the Dutch planters to join their accord. Two years later, in 1913, this is exactly what happened. Under an agreement known as the First Quinine Convention, the European manufacturers agreed to purchase the bark equivalent of 515 tonnes of quinine annually from the Javanese planters at the minimum price of 5 Dutch cents per unit. If quinine prices increased over a certain fixed amount, the manufacturers would share their excess profits with the planters by increasing the amount they paid for a unit of bark. To ensure no one cheated by, for instance, exporting excess bark to third parties or dumping quinine, a committee, consisting of three planters' and three manufacturers' representatives, was established in Amsterdam to enforce the agreement. Its name was the Kina Bureau.

The idea was that the bureau would regulate the agreement for five years, from July 1913 to July 1918. Clearly, it was a monopolistic arrangement. The only thing acting as a brake on prices was the excess supply of bark from the Java plantations. If, however, demand for quinine should suddenly go up or the plantations should suddenly contract, there would be nothing to prevent the bureau setting any price it liked. Fortunately, before the Kina Bureau had a chance to flex its muscles the First World War broke out and the British and French manufacturers were forced to sever ties with their German confrères. Within a year Allied troops were dug in all along the Eastern Front with only the drone of mosquitoes for company. It was to change everything.

*Chapter Eleven*

# THE MALARIA FIGHTERS

The history of malaria in war might almost be taken to be
the history of war itself.

C. H. Melville

JUST AT THE POINT where Washington DC runs into the state of
Virginia is a monument to the military's enduring fascination with
malaria. From the outside the joint US Army–Navy medical research
institute looks like any another recent addition to the American
suburbs. A fifty-thousand-square-metre glass and brick box, it rises
above the colonial-era houses that line the pretty backstreets of
Bethesda, Maryland, like some sinister and unwelcome corporate
invader. But once you step across the threshold of 'Building 503' –
as it is known to the military scientists who labour inside it – the
impression changes. Ten huge slate murals line the atrium, softening
the light pouring through the plate-glass windows and guiding the
visitor into the heart of a state-of-the-art medical research facility. The
murals are inset with portraits of famous army doctors, like Walter
Reed – the man who put the mosquito in Gorgas's ear, so to speak,
and helped eliminate yellow fever from Cuba. But it is not the images
of the moustachioed pioneers of military science that make the most
lasting impression, but the imprecations against malaria etched in the
slates. 'This will be a long war if for every division I have facing the
enemy, I must count on a second division in hospital with malaria
and a third division convalescing from this debilitating disease,' reads

one from General Douglas MacArthur in 1943. And from C. H.
Melville in 1895: 'The history of malaria in war might almost be
taken to be the history of war itself.'

Melville was exaggerating, but only slightly. Malaria has rarely
been the decisive factor in wars. But from the death of Alaric the
Goth from fever at the gates of Rome, to Cartagena, Walcheren and
the American Civil War, it – or at least the mosquito – has repeatedly
influenced the outcome of military engagements. Moreover, the
relationship is far from one way: just as malaria has affected warfare,
so the legacy of war has often been an increase in malaria. In 1923–6
there were ten million cases and sixty thousand deaths following the
devastation wrought by the civil war in Russia, and it was during
the Vietnam War that drug-resistant strains of malaria appeared for the
first time in south-east Asia. That is why army doctors have a special
responsibility for malaria and why the language of malaria control is
so often couched in military terms. From Ross's 'mosquito brigades'
to Gorgas's 'war on the mosquito' to the World Health Organisation's
benighted 'global eradication' campaign in the 1960s, we have
imagined that it is simply a matter of 'blitzing' the mosquito and the
scourge of malaria will disappear.

But, of course, it is not that simple. As the century has worn on,
the mosquito has proved far more resilient than Reed, Ross or Gorgas
could ever have suspected. The WHO no longer talks of eradicating
the mosquito battalions ranged across Africa and the Asian subcontinent with DDT, for instance, but of 'rolling them back' through a
series of continuous campaigns employing bed nets, malaria prophylaxis and new-generation pesticides. Nevertheless, the link remains
and nowhere more so than at the Walter Reed Army Institute for
Research (WRAIR) in Maryland.

As pharmaceutical companies have retreated from the front line of
malaria research, the heirs to Walter Reed have increasingly had to
step into the breach. The US Army invests about $4 million annually
in the hunt for new anti-malarials. It is pure self-interest, of course.
In nearly every engagement in the last hundred years, the US Army
and Navy have suffered more casualties to diseases than to enemy fire.

Nonetheless, without WRAIR's continuous drug development programme, there would be no new anti-malarials waiting in reserve and
thus nothing to stop the relentless march of drug-resistant parasites
across the face of the globe.

More than any other war in the last century, it was the First World
War that convinced Allied military planners that they would have to
take an active interest in malaria prophylaxis, and it was in Greece
that the lesson was driven home.

There are five species of *Anopheles* in Macedonia, each one
specialized in a different type of terrain, but if you are considering a
war in northern Greece there are only two you really need to worry
about. *A. maculipennis* is a 'sea-level' mosquito. It is found all over
Macedonia but it is most prevalent in the Struma and Vardar valleys
and the deltas of the Vardar and Galiko rivers west of Salonika. It
breeds in lakes, marshes, the holes left by horses' hooves and even in
discarded tin cans. Its cousin *A. superpictus* rules the hill country. It
breeds in brackish water and pools at nine to twelve hundred metres
above sea level, but it is also found lower down the valleys, near the
point where the streams break upon the plains. During December to
March it is so cold in Macedonia that neither species has much
opportunity for reproduction, but in May the temperatures, especially
in the valleys, begin to soar and by August Salonika is a sweltering
90 degrees Fahrenheit.

At first Britain and France hesitated to commit troops to the
Balkans, preferring to leave the Serbs to resist the Central Powers
alone. But when in September 1915 the Bulgarians threatened to join
the assault on the Serb line the Allies had no choice but to respond.
The Allied plan was to evacuate Serb fighters from Yugoslavia and
establish a new base with which to block the German advance in
northern Greece. The site that the British and French chose was
Salonika.

The Franco-British expeditionary force knew they would face a
problem with malaria, which is why they timed their arrival in the

delta for October – the end of the mosquito-breeding season. What they could not have known is that hundreds of thousands of Greek refugees infected with falciparum malaria had fled to Macedonia from Asia and the Caucasus just prior to the landings, greatly stoking the levels of infection.

The Allies' first mistake was to set up camps and field hospitals in the hill country above Lake Langaza, in the belief that they would be out of range of the *Anopheles* come the summer breeding season. Their second was to advance up the Struma and Vardar river valleys the following June, seemingly oblivious to the *A. maculipennis* multiplying in the marshes.

By July the British and French were strung out in a long line, running east–west from the mouth of the Struma River to Lake Dojran and over the hills to Vardar and the Monastir Road. The result was catastrophe. Hospital admissions for malaria rose steadily, from 4,500 in July to 7,500 in August and close to 9,000 in September 1916. The following summer was even worse, with 30,000 cases in September and October alone.

Ross, by now a lieutenant colonel, visited the Monastir road and suggested forming mosquito brigades to drain marshes, clear streams and kill larvae. In addition, bivouacs were improvised and special bell-shaped nets manufactured. But nothing seemed to work. By the end of 1917 a further 70,000 troops had come down with malaria and the field hospitals were so overwhelmed that medics were having to evacuate the most chronic cases to England at the rate of 1,000 a week.

The final figures make sober reading. By October 1918, out of a force of 160,000, there had been 162,000 hospital admissions, half of them for falciparum malaria. In other words some men contracted malaria more than once. Nor were the consequences confined to Greece. Men returning from the front brought the disease home, sparking mini-outbreaks in Kent, and long after the war was over many veterans continued to suffer recurring attacks.

Salonika underlined the importance in warfare not only of malaria but also of quinine. Every morning troops were expected to fall in in an orderly line and take their medication. Although officers complained that a quinine prophylaxis regimen was difficult to enforce – both because of the drug's unpleasant side effects and the old soldier's canard that it caused impotence – there was little doubting the drug's value. Despite the huge numbers of casualties at Salonika there were just 821 deaths from malaria during the whole campaign. Quinine may not have prevented soldiers contracting the disease but once they had been admitted to hospital it saved their lives. And it wasn't just in Macedonia that quinine was needed. In East Africa, malaria had decimated Indian troops specially selected for colonial duty in the mistaken belief that they would be immune to it. Similarly, when the British pursued the Turks into the malarious Jordan valley in the autumn of 1918 they were confronted by propaganda leaflets warning, 'The flies die in Jericho in July, and the men in August.' It was no idle threat: within weeks almost half the 40,000-strong British force had been hospitalized with malaria.

Soon the army medical department was clamouring for quinine, but because of the neglect of the Indian plantations there was now only one place to get it – Java. At the outbreak of hostilities the Quinine Convention had been torn up and both Britain and Germany had imposed export controls on the drug. The war was causing severe disruption to shipping lanes and it was feared that with supplies of bark from Java becoming increasingly erratic, quinine stocks would be rapidly exhausted. In 1917, in an effort to cut off quinine to the Central Powers, the British forced the Dutch to close the German-owned Chininefabriek factory in Amsterdam. However, Germany had taken the precaution of cultivating hybrids of *Cinchona ledgeriana* and *C. succirubra* in East Africa and by 1917 its Tanzanian plantations were producing 2.72 tonnes of top-quality bark a year. Fortunately in early 1918 the British quinine manufacturer Howard and Sons was able to reach an agreement with the six British-owned plantations in Java to buy up their entire annual output of bark. Then, in September, the Allies also agreed to buy the entire output of the Bandoeng factory, insisting on an immediate delivery of 0.5 tonnes of quinine and 406 tonnes of bark. The result was that by the end of the war Bandoeng accounted for more than three-quarters of the world's production and quinine had once again become a priceless commodity.

It was a sad end to Markham's philanthropic dream, but fortunately he was spared the anguish of seeing it. In 1905 he had stepped down from the Royal Geographical Society after twelve years' service as president – the longest of anyone before or since – and in 1912 he resigned from his other positions. Now aged eighty-two, his aim was to write one last history – a compendium of everything that was known about 'the Ends of the Earth', the polar regions to which he had devoted much of his life, both as an explorer to Greenland in 1875 and more recently as the sponsor of Scott's two voyages to the Antarctic. Then, in February 1913, came the news that Scott had reached the south pole the previous year only to perish in a blizzard on the return journey. Markham had loved Scott like a son and was deeply saddened by his death. Perhaps that explains why, when a deputation of old boys from Westminster asked him to sit for a portrait for his alma mater he chose to allude, not to the voyages of the *Discovery* or his own polar adventures, but to an earlier epic – the hunt for red cinchona. Markham was presented with the painting by the artist George Henry, showing him seated beside Pavon's *Cinchona uritusigna*, at a gathering of friends and well-wishers in Cambridge. The only reference to Markham's 'other' career as the father of polar exploration was a small silver sledge perched on the mantelpiece.

The following year, despite the war raging in western Europe, Markham travelled with Minna to Madeira for a holiday, dodging German submarines on their return via Portugal. By January 1916 he was very much preoccupied with the war, confiding in his diary that it was 'a very sad and portentous New Year ... [with] at home the enemies of efficient methods of resistance still clinging to office.' But although he recorded that Belgium, northern France, Poland and Serbia were 'all conquered' there was no mention of Salonika or of the mounting importance of quinine to the war effort. Instead, almost his last thoughts were connected with the death of Scott.

'Sturdy little Peter Scott came and walked with us in the Square garden,' reads the last entry but one in his diary. 'I often think of his dear father and the men he has trained to fight his country's battles.'

A few days later, on 29 January, he was reading in bed by candlelight at his home in Eccleston Square when the candle toppled and set light to his bedclothes. Although he screamed for help and the flames were quickly extinguished, it seems that the shock was too great for him and, after lying unconscious for twenty hours, he died. He was eighty-five.

Why he chose to read by candle when there was a perfectly good electric light in his room is not known. Perhaps it was a habit he had picked up in the navy and, despite having swapped his hammock for a bed, was unable to change. Whatever, it was a gruesome and – one is tempted to say – cursed end, almost as if Markham was driven to his grave by the same flames that had consumed Ruiz and Pavon's collections in Peru two centuries before.

By the end of the war the price of quinine had more doubled, and by 1920 it had reached a high of 52 florins a kilo. But peace gradu-ally brought a return to economic normality. Dutch planters could no longer count on the military to buy up all their excess bark. Furthermore, with the worldwide decrease in purchasing power that followed the war, neither could consumers be relied upon to maintain quinine's price. Some way had to be found of growing sufficient bark to fulfil the requirements of European quinine manufacturers but at a price that would ensure planters had an incentive to remain in business. The result was the Second Quinine Convention.

Under the new agreement, signed in 1918, manufacturers agreed to pay planters a minimum of six Dutch cents per unit for their bark – one cent more than the pre-war price – and guaranteed to buy 750 tonnes in the first year of the contract and 515 tonnes in each year thereafter. In addition, if the price of quinine exceeded the contract price then the manufacturers would split the difference with the planters by paying higher unit prices for their bark.

Overall it was a good deal for the manufacturers and an excellent one for planters. The problem from the consumers' point of view was that the only signatories were the Dutch – the European manufacturers having gone out of business during the war, leaving just the three Netherlands factories and the factory in Bandoeng. The result was that 80 per cent of the world's production of quinine was now regulated by the Kina Bureau in Amsterdam. In theory the bureau could set any price for quinine it wanted and the world would have to pay. Although by 1924 the price of quinine had fallen to 35 florins a kilo, the US government argued that it was still too high and that quinine could be produced far more cheaply from barks sold at cost price. As a statement of bald economic fact this was undeniably true. There was just one flaw in the argument: if you reduced the price of the bark too far no one could be persuaded to grow it.[1] The truth was that the limits of 'poor man's quinine', as one post-war writer put it, had already been reached in India where the British had pioneered a cheap febrifuge – quinetum – only to find that at cost price it was still too expensive for the vast majority of Indians. The result was that by 1921, only one-sixth of all malaria sufferers in India had access to quinine and deaths from the disease were running at 1.3 million annually. One commentator estimated that just to treat those attending hospital the government would have to import 57 tonnes of quinine a year, but that the true demand could be closer to 680 tonnes.[2]

In 1917, Herbert Hoover, then an up and coming food adminis- trator in the United States government, had been so alarmed by the prospect of a wartime quinine shortage that he had telegrammed US officials in the Philippines with just two words: 'Raise quinine'. Now, ten years later, the US Department of Justice decided to launch its own war, bringing an antitrust suit against the Kina bureau, accusing it of price-fixing. In 1928 Federal agents impounded five tons of Dutch-produced quinine at the port of New York. At the same time, the department of commerce, acting on Hoover's advice, began

encouraging US quinine manufacturers to invest in their own planta/
tions so as to be independent of Java for supplies of bark. Before the
plantations could get off the ground, however, the US reached an
accord with the Kina bureau under which it agreed to refrain from
further monopolistic practices.[3]

By now the limitations of quinine were apparent, not only to the
military but also to economists. What the generals wanted was a drug
that could be given to the troops before they entered a malarial area
which would ensure they never developed the disease. What the
economists and strategic planners wanted was an anti/malarial that
was cheap and that could be turned on and off at will without having
to worry about supplies falling into enemy hands. The problem with
quinine was that it was short/acting and toxic if maintained at the
levels needed for a prophylactic dosage. Common complaints included
nausea, blurred vision and ringing in the ears – all of which made a
medical regimen difficult to enforce. After nearly three hundred years
of continual use the miraculous 'fever bark' had run its course. In
future, the solution to malaria would no longer be sought in nature
but in synthetics, or so the military thought.

Ever since Pelletier and Caventou had isolated quinine from cinchona
bark in 1820 chemists had been searching for a way to synthesize the
drug. The first to attempt it was the German chemist Friedlieb Runge
in 1834. But though Runge succeeded in deriving quinoline, an
organic base, from coal tar, the synthesis of quinine defeated him.
Then in 1856 a young British chemist, William Perkin, was experi/
menting with quinine synthesis when he stumbled on Mauveine,
the first of the aniline dyes. Perkin quickly abandoned the hunt for
a quinine substitute and devoted himself instead to marketing his
lucrative new dyestuff.

Curiously, it was while experimenting with another synthetic dye
that a scientist made the first significant advance. In 1891 the German
immunologist Paul Ehrlich used methylene blue to treat two sailors
who had returned to Berlin with tertian malaria. Ehrlich had already

noted how methylene blue would stain — combine with — blood cells and certain microbes. Now, to his surprise, he saw that the dye also had a powerful inhibiting effect on the parasites in the sailors' blood.

However, because at the time there was no suitable model for comparing human and animal malarias Ehrlich did not pursue the research line further. Instead, he began experimenting with other dyes in his search for a 'magic bullet' for syphilis, synthesizing numerous compounds until, in 1909, on his six hundred and sixth attempt, he came up with arsphenamine (Salvarsan).

Indeed, it was only when scientists confirmed in the 1930s that the life cycle of the malaria parasite in birds was identical to falciparum infections in humans that it became possible to investigate synthetic therapies for malaria in a systematic way. Again, the Germans led the way and once again the First World War was the impetus.

Because of the Allied blockade on quinine from Java, German troops in East Africa had suffered even more than the British. Determined never to be a hostage to quinine again, the German government asked its scientists to renew the search for a substitute. The centre of operations was I.G. Farben, part of the Bayer Dye Works in Elberfeld. Beginning with methylene blue they started testing thousands of compounds until, in 1926, they hit on one that worked. Its name was Plasmochin (pamaquine) and it possessed one distinct advantage over quinine: it rendered the sexual stage of the parasite non-infectious. Unfortunately, it was also highly toxic and was soon abandoned. Then in 1932 the Farben scientists discovered Atabrine (mepacrine), a dye almost identical in its action to quinine. In fact, although it turned patients' skin yellow, in many ways it was superior, persisting in the blood for at least a week after the first dose and providing better long-term prophylaxis. Once again, however, it was toxic and difficult to tolerate.

The breakthrough came in 1934 with the synthesis of Resochin and, a few years later, Sontochin. These were a new type of synthetic — a class of compounds known as 4-amino quinolines. Like quinine they targeted the blood stage of the parasite but they were much faster acting. Both, however, had toxic side effects and Farben did not go on to explore the 4-quinoline group further, possibly, it is said, because Hermann Goering held the patent and would have been the only one to have profited from sales. This was a big mistake for, as US scientists at Farben's sister company, Winthrop Stearns, would discover ten years later, both compounds were closely related to chloroquine, possibly the best anti-malarial ever developed. Indeed, Resochin and chloroquine were subsequently found to be identical. Ironically, Farben had passed the formula for Resochin to the US company in the late 1930s but Winthrop simply shelved it. What persuaded them to take another look was the outbreak of the Second World War.

This time round it was the Allies who were deprived of quinine. With the German invasion of Holland, stocks at the Kina bureau's plants in Amsterdam and Maarsen became the property of the Nazis. Then, in 1942, the Japanese invaded Java, seizing the Dutch plantations and with them 90 per cent of the world's supply of bark. The War Production Board issued an emergency decree restricting the use of quinine to the military and launched a desperate campaign to pool chemists' dwindling stocks. To aid the effort, President Roosevelt even forwarded 45 kg of the drug that he had been given as a gift by the President of Peru. Next the Board of Economic Warfare began looking for alternative sources of bark. Deals were quickly struck with the Andean republics to buy up their annual output. But because of the success of the Java plantations very little bark was now under cultivation. Then there was the problem of quality control.

Like the seventeenth-century European apothecaries before them, American chemists now discovered that the quinine content of the wild South American barks were extremely variable. There was no alternative, decided the planners and military strategists, but to recruit a group of botanists prepared to risk their lives by returning to the bark forests to gather seeds and plants of the most valuable species. Beginning in 1942, this is exactly what happened: the Board of Economic Warfare organized a series of missions to Colombia, Ecuador and Peru manned by handpicked botanists and forestry experts seconded from the Department of Agriculture and leading

US universities. Their job was to follow in the footsteps of La Condamine, Mutis, Spruce and Markham, exploring some of the most inaccessible parts of the Andes in search of species with obscure names like *Cinchona pitayensis, officinalis, succirubra* and, of course, *calisaya*.

Travel in the Andes had changed little in a hundred years and the botanists faced many of the same risks as the nineteenth-century pioneers before them: precipitous slopes, recalcitrant mules, roaring mountain streams, and exhaustion from the dizzying altitude. As Froelich Rainey, the director of the Ecuadorian mission, later admitted: 'Scrambling up a narrow gorge where mud and water, belly deep, alternated with irregular boulders and rock slides, I learned that none of my former experience with mountain trails and riding animals applied in the Andes.' But at least Rainey survived. One of his colleagues, Arthur Featherstonehaugh, an ex-marine, was not so lucky. Gazing out over the Quintanian Andes at three thousand metres, Rainey was appalled to see 'Feather's' face turn a blotchy grey. 'He was panting with such force that he could scarcely speak. After a time he was ready to go on, but he looked desperately ill and we urged him to ride again and rest ... We were rigging a stretcher for Feather when I heard his low, terrified voice, "Frol, come here!" Those were his last words ...'

With the help of Ecuadorian botanists, Rainey eventually found Spruce's red bark growing in the foothills of the eastern Andes near El Topo. The result was extensive new Ecuadorian plantations, producing totaquinine. Similar plantations with local species were also begun in Peru and Colombia and by the end of the war South America was contributing 2,720 tonnes of bark a year to the Allied war effort. The only country that refused to cooperate was Bolivia. Instead, like the Dutch a hundred years before, the Board of Economic Warfare was forced to despatch agents to La Paz. Like Hasskarl they had little success and once again *calisaya* remained the most elusive bark of all.

However, there was one place the Americans knew they could obtain *calisaya* seeds – the south-west Pacific. When in 1917 Herbert

Hoover had ordered officials in the Philippines to 'raise quinine' no one had taken much notice. But four years later the Philippines had a governor-general with the medical background to realize the importance of Hoover's order. General Leonard Wood was a Harvard-educated doctor who had begun his army career in the medical corps. As Governor-General in Cuba in 1899 he had funded Walter Reed's yellow fever studies. When in 1921 he saw a young forest ranger in the Philippines die of malaria for lack of quinine, he decided to find the money to carry out Hoover's order too. Commandeering $4,000 from a special contingency fund, Wood sent the money to the US Consul in Java and received a bottle of *Cinchona ledgeriana* by return military post (the price had gone up somewhat since Ledger's time). Those seeds became the responsibility of Arthur Fischer, the Director of the Philippines Bureau of Forestry. Within six years Fischer was raising *C. ledgeriana* and *C. succirubra* plants at Baguio, on Luzon. Then, in 1927, he moved the plantations to Mindanao, the island at the southern end of the same chain, where the climate was more humid. In 1936 the first shipment of bark from Mindanao reached Manila and by 1941 Fischer had established a factory for the production of totaquinine in the Philippine capital. By the time the Japanese invaded Pearl Harbor it was producing 2.5 kg of the febrifuge a day.

The Philippines, along with Papua New Guinea and the Solomon islands, is one of the most malarious places on earth. Prior to the Second World War, it is estimated that as many as two million people were infected with the disease, with ten thousand dying each year. The only thing that kept the mortality rate from spiking even higher was quinine, but with the Japanese invasion in 1942 the American and Filipino troops garrisoned on the island suddenly found themselves cut off from their supply lines. As the Americans retreated to Bataan and Corregidor infections shot up, and by early spring 80 per cent of the troops had come down with malaria. Among them was one Arthur Fischer, now a colonel in the intelligence service. In March 1942, ill with fever, he persuaded his commanding officer to allow him to fly the gauntlet to Mindanao, where he hurriedly improvised a makeshift factory for the production of cinchona febrifuge. But before he had an opportunity to return, the weakened American forces in Bataan surrendered, leaving Fischer and just a small guerrilla force to fight a rearguard action against the Japanese in Mindanao. Armed with totaquinine, the guerrilla fighters maintained their resistance and, according to Father Haggerty, a Catholic priest who remained on Mindanao through the occupation, the bark was shipped all over the southern Philippines, saving 'tens of thousands of lives'.

Meanwhile, General MacArthur, the commander of the South Pacific forces who had ordered the hasty withdrawal to Bataan and who now had himself retreated to Australia, issued orders for the evacuation. Three Flying Fortresses were despatched to Mindanao with instructions to bring back important military personnel. The first two planes were shot down but a third, containing Colonel Fischer and a milk churn packed with the *C. ledgeriana* seed, got through. No sooner had he landed in Australia than Fischer and his churn was on the next plane to Washington where, still feverish, he delivered the seeds to the Department of Agriculture. Within days those seeds had germinated and *ledgeriana* plants were being raised in a government hothouse in Glenn Dale, Maryland, not far from where the joint forces medical research institute stands today. By the end of the war, the plants had been transplanted to Ecuador and were thriving on the higher slopes of the Quintanian Andes. Thus it was that by this curious and circuitous route Mamani's *calisayas* returned to the continent from which they had been torn.

Unfortunately, the *ledgeriana* plantations in Ecuador came too late to aid the war effort. Besides, by 1943 the US had found a better solution to the quinine shortage: Atabrine. Army researchers had first tested the compound on soldiers in Panama in 1938, but discarded it after troops reported unpleasant side effects such as vomiting, diarrhoea and yellow discoloration of the skin. Spurred on by the war, however, in 1942 the government brought army and civilian chemists together under the auspices of the National Research Council to test synthetic compounds, both old and new. At first it was feared that Atabrine might contain a toxic fraction not in the original German product, but Winthrop researchers soon confirmed this was not the case and in the autumn of 1942 began distributing the drug to troops in the south-west Pacific.

The most pressing need was in Buna, Papua New Guinea, and at Guadalcanal, in the Solomon Islands. In August 1942 US marines had made an unopposed landing on Guadalcanal following intelligence reports that the Japanese were planning an airfield there that could block sea lanes between the US and Australia. The Japanese quickly reinforced the island and brought in their navy, effectively isolating the marines in an area of high falciparum transmission. At first little attention was paid to malaria discipline. As one senior officer reportedly put it: 'We are here to kill Japs and to hell with mosquitoes.' But within months of the landing attitudes changed dramatically as the force was ravaged by the disease. By the end of the year, 80 per cent of the marines had contracted malaria and one infantry unit had had to be evacuated to New Zealand for rehabilitation.

On Buna, where American and Australian troops had launched a joint offensive in November, the situation was even worse. General Robert Eichelberger, who had been ordered by MacArthur 'to take Buna or not come back alive', found that the two-hundred-man rifle companies he had been sent to relieve were down to sixty-five men, all of them febrile. In total, in the fighting throughout Papua New Guinea, nearly 28,000 Australian and American troops were admitted to field hospitals with malaria. In comparison, casualties from the fighting were just 7,700. It was these sorts of statistics that forced MacArthur to take malaria seriously.

At first soldiers rebelled against the new Atabrine discipline. Army medics had yet to refine the dosage and the side effects were so unpleasant that many men threw the tablets into latrines or buried them under mattresses rather than take them. Further trials were conducted both in the US and Australia, and after establishing that the drug was better tolerated with a large primer dose followed by smaller maintenance doses, in the spring of 1943 the therapy was renewed, this time with success. In Papua New Guinea, in particular,

Australian medics showed that if a tablet of Atabrine was taken each day a soldier could operate for months in an endemic zone and that if the therapy was continued after leaving the area falciparum was completely eradicated from the blood. Not only that but, unlike quinine, Atabrine eliminated the sexual forms of the parasite, meaning that soldiers returning from the jungle would no longer be at risk of infecting colleagues a transport to the front line.[4]

However, Atabrine was still far from ideal. The 'ideal' anti-malarial would be chloroquine, but after screening fourteen thousand compounds neither Winthrop nor the finest scientific brains in the US Army had found it. Then came the fall of Tunis and, with it, the suggestion by French doctors that the Americans might like to experiment with Sontochin, the Farben compound that they had been using with some success in North Africa. It was Sontochin that led the Winthrop researchers to discover chloroquine and to the realization that it was identical to Resochin, the German compound that had been gathering dust on their shelves for nearly ten years.

The synthesis of chloroquine came too late to make any difference to the war in the Pacific or to the Allied landings in Sicily – another endemic front where, once more, diseases, including malaria, accounted for more casualties in the US Seventh and British Eighth armies than enemy fire. But following the Second World War chloroquine quickly became the drug of choice throughout the tropics. In Ehrlich's parlance, chloroquine was the 'magic bullet', a fast-acting, easy to administer prophylactic that afforded complete protection against all forms of malaria. Like quinine, chloroquine is what is known as a 'blood schizontocide', in other words it hits the parasite when it tries to invade red blood cells. But unlike quinine, it also takes out the parasites of the vivax, ovale and malariae strains in their sexual stage, blocking transmission. The only flaw in chloroquine's armour is that it has no effect on the gametocytes of falciparum. But that was of little consequence as the military now had reinforcements available in the form of pamaquine and primaquine, the new easy-to-tolerate variants of plasmochin, that did destroy falciparum's crescents and also prevented relapses from vivax malaria. When, in 1944 Imperial

Chemical Industries succeeded in synthesizing proguanil (Paludrine in the US), a new compound unrelated to the quinoline group that hit both the blood and liver forms of the falciparum parasite, the military's arsenal was complete. At long last it seemed quinine could be consigned to druggists' dustbins.

Chloroquine was not only a boon to the military, it heralded a new dawn for Indian coolies, Thai rice-farmers and millions of ordinary Africans too. At last, a malaria-free world seemed like a real possibility. In the 1930s Mussolini had launched an extensive bonification campaign of the Roman Campagna, ending malaria transmission in the Pontina by 1948. In Brazil, a military-style pyrethrum-spraying campaign had succeeded in exterminating *Anopheles gambiae*, the deadly African vector of malaria that had suddenly appeared uninvited in the Natal in 1930, sparking the worst malaria epidemic in South American history. Now, adopting the military vernacular, the World Health Organisation began trials aimed at nothing less than the 'global eradication' of malaria. Its weapons? Chloroquine and a promising new insecticide, DDT. The on-again, off-again debate over DDT is beyond the scope of this book. It cleared malaria from Italy in the immediate post-war period when the deliberate breaching of dykes by retreating German panzer divisions had threatened to undo all the bonification that had gone before; in the 1950s it virtually eradicated malaria from Cyprus, Greece, Venezuela, Sri Lanka and – for a time – large parts of India. But by the 1970s DDT-resistant strains of mosquitoes had begun to emerge and following a vociferous campaign by environmentalists concerned about DDT's affect on birds and other wildlife, in 1982 the US banned it.[5]

In contrast there has never been anything controversial about chloroquine. By the 1960s a bottle of chloroquine was as ubiquitous in colonial homes as bottles of quinine water had been in India a century earlier. Chloroquinized salt was being distributed by the ton to Brazil, Cambodia, the Philippines and New Guinea, and the US

Administration for International Development (USAID) bought millions of tablets to give away in Africa and India. Unfortunately, chloroquine's honeymoon was over almost as soon as it began. The reason was the evolution of the parasite. Army medics had long known that, if left untreated, falciparum could be as deadly as a concealed enemy sniper, but neither military nor non-military scientists had fully appreciated that the malaria parasite also possessed hidden biological cloaking devices and was skilled at taking evasive action.

Interestingly, the first hint of the emergence of drug-resistant strains of malaria came in South America. In 1910 German engineers returning by Amazonian steamer from north-west Brazil came down with falciparum malaria. The men, who had been labouring on a railway construction project near the frontier with Bolivia, dosed themselves with quinine but on their return to Hamburg doctors discovered they still had parasites swimming in their blood. The dosage was increased but it was only after repeated treatments that they were cured. In 1918 German doctors noticed similar resistance to quinine in troops with vivax malaria returning from the Macedonian front. Then, in 1960, in the Magdalena valley in Colombia, and just across the border in the Lake Maracaibo area of south-west Venezuela, doctors simultaneously reported the first cases of chloroquine resistance. These were the very areas where Spruce and Bonpland had come down with malignant tertian fevers more than a hundred years before. In the case of two seismographic explorers who had contracted falciparum in the Magdalena valley, not only did the infection not respond to chloroquine, it did not respond to quinine either. One possible reason for the emergence of cross-resistant strains in these areas, scientists theorized, was their proximity to the cinchona forests of Colombia and Ecuador — the places where quinine had been in use for the longest period and where the parasite would have had sufficient time to develop immunity. But when in 1962 scientists also began to see the emergence of chloroquine resistance in Malaya, Cambodia, Vietnam and Thailand this theory began to seem less probable. Perhaps resistance was simply the result of under-dosage and

over-dependence on the quinoline-based drugs? Whatever, drug resistance spread rapidly throughout south-east Asia and, once again, it
was the military that had to find ways of combating the problem.

At the beginning of the war in Indochina, the French had used
quinine and Atabrine as a prophylactic but by 1952 chloroquine had
become the drug of choice both because it was easy to administer –
you only had to take one 300 mg tablet a week – and had fewer side
effects.[6] Chloroquine prophylaxis led to a dramatic decline in infections in the French forces, but no sooner had the US entered the
conflict than the first signs of parasite resistance began to emerge.
At first Army medics persevered with the so-called 'CP' tablet – a
combination of chloroquine and primaquine that had been shown to
be effective against both falciparum and relapses from vivax malaria.
But by 1966 it was clear that the therapy was no longer working. In
December 1965 the overall rate of infections in the army was running
at ninety-eight per thousand and in the Ia Drang valley some units
were suffering infection rates as high as six hundred per thousand.
There was no choice but to resort to quinine again.

However, except where it was given intravenously, the relapse
rates remained high. The medics called up reinforcements – pyrimeth-
amine, a new synthetic that targeted the parasite's enzymes, and
dapsone, a slow-acting blood schizontocide – and the infections began
to fall. But by now it was apparent that no single drug – whether a
synthetic or a purified alkaloid like quinine – could hope to defeat
resistant strains of malaria. Whatever chemical you threw at the
parasite, sooner or later it would find a way to evade it. What was
more, there was now nothing left in reserve.

Gradually it was beginning to dawn on malariologists that the
only form of chemotherapy that could stand a chance of working in
the long term was one that combined several chemicals or alkaloids at
once. In other words, a combination not unlike the cheap cinchona
febrifuge pioneered by Markham in India. Once again, the US
government looked to the bark, restoring overgrown plantations in
Guatemala, Indonesia and Zaire and manufacturing totaquinine for
distribution to GIs. Thus it was that three hundred years after the

Jesuits brought the 'miraculous cure' to Europe it was still saving lives
– this time in Vietnam and Cambodia.

As the war in Vietnam was coming to an end, Wilbur Milhous, a
bright young field medic from South Carolina, was called in by his
commanding officer. Instead of going to the front how would he like
to go back to university and learn something about malaria? 'Well, I
didn't know the first thing about malaria,' recalls Milhous, 'but in the
army when an officer suggests you do something you do it.' Sitting in
his office in Building 503 today, surrounded by souvenirs from the
Amazon, Africa and other endemic malaria regions of the world,
Milhous has little doubt he made the right decision.

After getting his Ph.D., Milhous joined WRAIR in 1983,
quickly rising to the rank of colonel. He is now director of WRAIR's
division for experimental therapeutics with a budget of $4 million a
year to spend on new drugs and therapies for malaria. It is not as
much as he would like, but it is better than nothing and it puts him
in the front line of malaria research. Fansidar, halofantrine, mefloquine
– you name it, WRAIR has had a hand in nearly every new anti-
malaria drug to have emerged from Western laboratories in the last
thirty years. But so rapid is the spread of resistance that it is a constant
battle to stay ahead. Indeed, some experts believe that drug resistance
is so prevalent that the world is facing its severest crisis since the
discovery of quinine.

On the wall above his desk, Milhous has a flow chart tracing the
progress of drugs currently in the pipeline. Malarone – a new Glaxo-
SmithKline prophylactic against falciparum that combines proguanil,
an old army compound, with atovaquone – has already been licensed
for use in Kenya and is in the final phase III trial stage in the US.
Just behind it is tafenoquine, a new 'super prophylactic' that WRAIR
has also developed jointly with Glaxo. Then there are the derivatives
of a 'new' plant compound, artemisinin: artesunate, artemotil, and one
formulation Milhous believes could be particularly promising, artelinic
acid.

Milhous first heard about artemisinin in 1982 when he was a fellow at Burroughs Wellcome and received a report from the WHO malaria steering group in Geneva about a promising new Chinese plant called *qing-hao*. Rumours of a miraculous new Chinese cure for malaria had been circulating for years. The Chinese had first published their findings in the *Chinese Medical Journal* in 1979 but when the WHO approached Chinese scientists for samples of the plant so that they could conduct their own assay they were rebuffed. 'This was just after the Nixon era, remember. Mao Tse-tung was still in power and the Chinese were very sceptical about sharing information and news,' says Milhous.

It turned out that *qing-hao* had been known to Chinese herbalists for more than two thousand years. The first Western botanist to describe it was Linnaeus, who gave it the name *Artemisia annua*, but to the green-fingered it is better known by its colloquial name, sweet wormwood. Like cinchona and other members of the Compositae family to which it is related (sagebrush, tarragon, absinthe), sweet wormwood is noted for its aromatic bitterness. English herbalists had used it for years, but it was only when, at the height of the Cultural Revolution, Mao ordered his scientists to 'solve' the problem of malaria then sweeping China's southern provinces that *qing-hao* was 'rediscovered'. It first appeared in a Chinese recipe book in 168 BC as a treatment for haemorrhoids. Then in *The Handbook for Emergency Treatments*, a book written by Ge Hang in AD 340, it was recommended as a treatment for chills and fevers. Ge Hang instructed fever-sufferers to soak *qing-hao* in one *sheng* (about 1 litre) of tea, squeeze out the juice and drink the remaining liquid. Following Hang's recipe, Chinese scientists prepared a decoction and fed it to mice infected with *P. berghei*, a lethal rodent malaria parasite. Incredibly, they found that *qing-hao* was as good as choloroquine and quinine at clearing the parasite and also cured chloroquine-resistant strains of the rodent malaria. By 1972 Chinese pharmacists had succeeded in crystallizing the active principle – qinghaosu, or artemisinin – and Mao's scientists began testing it on humans. Seven years later they reported their findings. According to the Chinese, artemisinin cured falciparum malaria more rapidly and with less toxicity than either chloroquine or quinine. Moreover, it also worked against strains that were chloro-quine-resistant.

Artemisinin came as a bombshell to the US military. Just as the Galenists and English Puritans had been reluctant to accept the 'popish remedy' three hundred years before, so the heirs to Walter Reed cast doubts on the Chinese claims about artemisinin. How was it possible that a bunch of 'reds' had beaten Walter Reed's finest brains to such a significant discovery? The Chinese, they pointed out, had made similar claims in the past – most notably when they said they could cure malaria with acupuncture – only to be proved wrong. Why should they believe the Chinese now, especially when the studies they were publishing appeared to date back nearly ten years?

It was Dan Klayman, then head of medicinal chemistry in WRAIR's experimental therapeutics division, who decided to take a closer look at the Chinese study, and as he did his interest grew. Artemisinin was an endo-peroxide, a molecule consisting of two oxygen atoms, but in a form he had never seen before. On exposure to air endo-peroxides normally become unstable and fall apart, yet the Chinese were claiming that artemisinin could be crystallized into a drug that would persist in the body long enough to destroy the parasite.

China's refusal to share her techniques with the WHO was understandable given the presence of WRAIR representatives on the WHO chemotherapy and malaria steering group. Rightly or wrongly, the Chinese feared that if they handed over the formula for artemisinin WRAIR would patent it for the benefit of capitalist pharmaceutical firms. Under the circumstances Klayman had no choice but to gather his own samples of the plant. Thus it was that a new hunt was begun, not for a tree this time but for a weed.

Klayman recruited botanists from the Smithsonian Institute in Washington and begun scouring North America for *Artemisia annua*. Incredibly, they found it growing right under their noses at Harper's Ferry, just down the road from WRAIR headquarters. Klayman had Boy Scouts harvest the plant and then set about duplicating the

Chinese extraction process. It took him two years but in 1984 he cracked it, grabbing the May cover of the prestigious US journal *Science* with his announcement that artemisinin was a poorly water-soluble crystalline compound. The two oxygen atoms, he revealed, were like a bomb waiting to explode. All it took to set them off was iron, and where was iron found? Why, in the malaria pigment of course – the haem the parasite releases when it devours red blood cells. When artemisinin came into contact with the iron-rich haem the molecule fell apart, triggering the release of free radicals that were toxic to the parasite. Indeed, artemisinin was so explosive that Klayman speculated the parasite would have little time to recognize its structure and develop resistance.

Klayman's faith in artemisinin has since been justified many times over. Today artemisinin and other artemether-group drugs are the main line of defence against drug-resistant malaria all along the Thai–Myammar border. Unlike quinine, which can be toxic in the doses needed to clear severe falciparum, the artemether drugs are faster acting and have fewer side effects. The most rapid of all is artesunate, a water-soluble derivative of artemisinin originally isolated by the Chinese. Indeed, doctors at the Mae La refugee camp in north-west Thailand – the centre of some of the most potent drug-resistant malarias in south-east Asia – have found that artesunate clears falciparum parasites from the blood faster than any drug they have encountered. But although artesunate is manufactured in China and Vietnam, ironically only one Western pharmaceutical company has so far been willing to make it. The reasons are all too predictable. 'Because the Chinese isolated it first, artesunate is not patentable,' says Milhous. 'And without a patent pharmaceutical firms aren't willing to pick up the co-development costs.' Instead, WRAIR has concentrated on two other derivatives: artemotil and atelinic acid, both of which are patentable. Indeed, the Dutch company ARTECEF registered artemotil in Holland in March 2000 and WRAIR is hoping that Glaxo SmithKline will soon seek a similar registration for artelinic acid in the US. In addition, the WHO is seeking licences for its own artesunate suppository. The significance of the artemether-group drugs cannot be overstated. Aside from intravenous quinine, artemotil is the only treatment for severe falciparum malaria currently licensed for use in Europe. The pity is that it has taken so long – nearly twenty years – to become available.

According to Milhous there are two key lessons to be learned from the post-war history of malaria. The first, as he puts it, is that 'pharmaceutical companies simply aren't interested in developing drugs for people who cannot afford shoes.' In other words, there are so few profits in malaria that in order to have any hope of coming up with therapies for the drug-resistant strains of the future governments must take the lead in drug development. This is now beginning to happen. In 1999 WRAIR received a 'presidential uplift' of $3m on top of its present budget in recognition of the importance of its work on malaria, and extra money from NIH for the development of tafenoquine. Meanwhile, the WHO in partnership with the World Bank, the International Federation of Pharmaceutical Manufacturers, the UK Department for International Development, Holland and the Rockefeller Foundation has established a Medicines for Malaria Venture with the aim of raising at least $15m a year for new drug development in partnership with drug companies.

The second is that cutting corners by the money-saving trick of taking a partial, rather than a full course of drug treatment is simply no longer an option. Nor does it make sense to mortgage the farm on one drug – as occurred with chloroquine in the 1950s. The reason is that overuse is just as likely to lead to the emergence of drug-resistant strains as under-dosage. Indeed most scientists now accept that whatever drug they come up with its therapeutic life is bound to be limited. That is why WRAIR and others are increasingly advocating drug combinations. Thus when, in 1994, Professor Nick White of Bangkok's Mahidol University and his colleague François Nosten saw that mefloquine was no longer effective in half the cases of children infected with falciparum on the Thai–Myammar border they combined it with artemisinin and then artesunate. Their hope is that by combining the drugs malaria transmission will be greatly reduced and mefloquine's 'useful therapeutic life' – to borrow a phrase coined by White – will be greatly extended. But just in case he is wrong, White is now also conducting trials with artesunate in combination with Malarone, the new prophylactic developed by Glaxo Smith-Kline, in the hope that because Malarone is so new to the market there is still time to extend its therapeutic life before it encounters drug resistance.[7] In theory, drug combinations could slow the development of resistance in high malaria transmission areas 'by tenfold or more'. Says White: 'That means you need a new drug only every fifty years, not every ten.' The only problem is persuading hard-pressed African governments to accept the additional cost of funding two drugs where one would normally be sufficient to return a patient to health.

Where does all this leave the military? The answer is not much further advanced than at the beginning of the Second World War. Then the US and Britain had only quinine. Now they can deploy a whole range of anti-malarial drugs without fear of supplies suddenly falling into enemy hands. But the development of these drugs has not been driven so much by strategic necessity as by the evolution of the parasite. Moreover, no matter how effective the prophylactic there is still no guarantee soldiers will take it. As yet there is no resistance to mefloquine in Sierra Leone, for instance. But when Britain recently sent paratroopers to fight anti-government rebels there sixteen fell ill with malaria. The reason appears to be that the paratroopers discontinued the mefloquine rather than endure such unpleasant side effects as dizziness, sleeplessness and depression. Indeed, one soldier was reportedly driven to such distraction by nightmares and hallucinations associated with the prophylactic that he shot himself. Such problems are by no means confined to the British army. When the US deployed troops to Somalia during Operation Restore Hope, malaria was the number one cause of casualties. The US Air Force forbids pilots to take mefloquine because of the associated side effects and issues them instead with daily doses of doxycline. But as the US discovered during Operation Restore Hope a daily prophylaxis regime is difficult to enforce. Even under the most heavily enforced medical discipline in

Somalia, for instance, one marine unit suffered a staggering 10 per cent malaria attack rate in a single month.

There is one thing, however, that would guarantee that troops entering a war zone were fully protected against malaria and that is a vaccine. The problem is, malaria is a protozoan, not a virus, and so far no one has succeeded in developing a vaccine against any parasitical infection.

## Chapter Twelve

# THE VACCINE HUNTERS

There's no place on earth that's off the malaria map: Arctic circle, freezing mountaintop, burning desert, you name it, malaria's been there. We're not talking millions of cases here; more like hundreds of millions ... And even when it's properly diagnosed it's not like quinine is always going to get you home safe. With certain kinds of malaria you can mainline quinine all the livelong day and come nightfall you'll still be gathering freezer-burn in the mortuary.

Amitav Ghosh, *The Calcutta Chromosome*

IT IS EARLY EVENING in Cartagena and the XVth International Congress on Tropical Medicine and Malaria is about to get underway. Inside the modern, air-conditioned Convention Centre overlooking the harbour where in 1741 Admiral Vernon's fleet was repelled by the mosquito, nearly four hundred scientists from countries as diverse as Britain, the United States, Thailand and The Gambia have assembled to hear Colombian President Andreas Pastrana's opening address. It is the first tropical medicine congress to be convened in South America for nearly forty years and the fact that it is being held in a country racked by violence and political kidnappings is a testament to Pastrana's powers of persuasion. In ten days' time Bill Clinton will arrive in the beautiful and – as the conference brochure puts it – 'safe' city of Cartagena to unveil a $1.3 billion aid package aimed at eradicating Colombia's trade in cocaine. But for the moment the focus is on another global scourge — malaria — and why, despite the availability of more anti-malaria drugs than ever before, infant mortality from the disease in Africa has remained virtually unchanged in fifty years.

Pastrana runs through the familiar litany: 300—500 million cases a year and between 1.5 to 2.7 million deaths, half of them children in sub-Saharan Africa. 'Every thirty seconds somewhere in the world a child dies of malaria,' he says, before concluding his speech with a call for the establishment of a global fund to fight the disease.

The delegates applaud politely. Even though there are already many such global initiatives and they have heard the statistics many times before, that does not make the numbers any less shocking. In the last fifteen years, for instance, Aids has killed around 18 million people worldwide, whereas malaria has killed at least 23 million. Indeed, some parasitologists believe that malaria may have killed one out of every two human beings who ever lived on the planet. The only diseases that are bigger killers are dysentery and tuberculosis. But, of course, there is a vaccine for tuberculosis, albeit one that is increasingly ineffective in many parts of the tropics. As yet, however, there is no vaccine for malaria and thus little possibility of eradicating the disease. Nevertheless, a number of scientists believe they are very close. Indeed one man claims he is on the point of cracking the code governing the parasite's ability to evade the body's immune defences and is just waiting for the final pages of the code book. His name is Manuel Elkin Patarroyo and, remarkably, he is Colombian.

Patarroyo is making his way through the delegates emerging from the conference chamber now. A short man with unruly grey hair offset by a shiny bald spot, he is barely visible through the crowd thronging the steps. But you can tell it is him simply by the flash of press bulbs and the numbers of would-be Colombian beauty contestants trailing in his wake. Imagine Stephen Hawking, the wheelchair-bound English physicist, regularly featuring in the pages of *Hello!* or *Vogue* and you get some sense of the media frenzy that attends Patarroyo's every public appearance in Colombia. Dressed in an immaculate blue suit and red tie, he looks more like a banker than a scientist. According to national opinion polls, Patarroyo is the second most prominent Colombian this century, just behind his good friend, the celebrated novelist Gabriel García Marquez. Were he to run for the presidency tomorrow he would probably be elected.

What makes Patarroyo's celebrity so remarkable is that malaria is not usually considered a glamorous endeavour. Most of the break-throughs in malaria came at the end of the nineteenth century, as a result of Ross's painstaking dissection of mosquitoes and Italian researchers' close observation of blood slides. It was another hundred years before the revolution in molecular biology and biotechnology transformed our understanding of the malaria parasite and other infective organisms, and gave researchers new tools with which to probe its defences. But if you are seeking fame and publicity, far better to launch yourself at a cause that preoccupies the developed world, like the cure for cancer or Aids.

That Patarroyo has generated similar excitement with his search for a vaccine for malaria is a tribute to both his charisma and the controversy that surrounds his research institute in Bogotá. Located in a rundown district to the east of the city centre, Patarroyo's head-quarters are reached via a path overgrown with weeds that winds to the back of the grimy San Juan de Dios public hospital. One of the three buildings is little more than a shell with pigeons roosting in the eaves; on the others, the once grand porticoes are cracked and the plaster is peeling off. The moment you cross the threshold, however, it is a different story. Laboratory technicians deep in concen-tration scurry along the corridors, their pockets bulging with computer printouts. On one floor young women are carefully measuring white powders into a series of vials, while downstairs young men jot chemical equations on a blackboard. Meanwhile, in another part of the complex an electron microscopy machine is slowly scanning a key molecule of the *Plasmodium falciparum* parasite. In the three-dimensional image being generated on a nearby computer, it looks like something out of a science fiction film, a space-age insect with colour-coded legs.

Sitting in an office at the top of a marble staircase lined with contemporary Latin American art is the reason for all this frenetic activity: Patarroyo, or as his colleagues prefer to call him, el Jefe – 'the Chief'. For the past twenty-five years Patarroyo has devoted himself single-mindedly to the search for the cure for malaria. It is the Holy Grail of malaria research – the modern equivalent of the nineteenth-century hunt for cinchona – a one-shot vaccine that will provide complete protection against falciparum, and other human malaria parasites, for life. From Washington to Oxford and Paris to Sydney many other scientists are chasing the same goal. Whoever succeeds will almost certainly win the Nobel Prize. But according to Patarroyo his vaccine is the most advanced. 'I am already 80 per cent of the way there,' he says, handing me a sheaf of papers recording the trials of his synthetic chemical vaccine, SPf66. 'All I am waiting for are the remaining rules.'

Other scientists beg to differ. In Washington, for instance, the US Army and Navy both have their own advanced vaccine development programmes, making what Patarroyo claims is a one-horse race at least a three-horse race. And while Patarroyo's vaccine has reputedly performed well in South America, the results of independent trials in Africa and south-east Asia have been disappointing. But such is Patarroyo's celebrity in Colombia that few of his countrymen doubt him. Just as José Celestino Mutis put Colombia on the map with his botanical institute devoted to the taxonomy of cinchona, so Manuel Elkin Patarroyo's Institute of Immunology has brought Colombia to the attention of the international scientific community. The hundred and fifty scientists working out of his state-of-the-art laboratories have the support of both the Rockefeller Foundation and the WHO. As Howard Engers, the director of the WHO vaccination development programme, puts it: 'I am very impressed by his work. He is a very motivated hard-working person, and if he says he has succeeded we take him seriously.'

In order to understand what it would take for a vaccine against malaria to work you first have to understand how vaccines protect against bacteria and viruses. A virus's sole raison d'être is to colonize living cells. To prevent this happening vaccine-makers take attenuated or dead versions of the virus and use them to stimulate the immune system to produce antibodies. The same principle is also applied to bacteria. The idea is that if you can train the immune system to produce antibodies against an apparent threat – an attenuated version of a bacillus or a virus – then when the real thing comes along the immune response will be vastly accelerated and take it out before it has a chance to do any damage. The first and best example is the smallpox vaccine.

In 1796 Edward Jenner, an English country doctor, used cowpox – a disease related to smallpox that causes serious illness in cattle but not in humans – to inoculate workhouse children against its deadly human cousin. The result was that smallpox was eventually eradicated worldwide. However, Jenner had no concept of the viral nature of smallpox and only hit on inoculating with cowpox after seeing how milkmaids who were exposed to the bovine disease were protected. The real birth of immunology came with Louis Pasteur's observation in 1887 that you could prevent chickens from acquiring fowl cholera by inoculating them with a dying culture of the fowl cholera bacillus. By the 1960s Pasteur's insight had resulted in vaccines against a host of life-threatening bacterial and virulogical agents – from mumps to polio to yellow fever and measles.

Unfortunately, designing a vaccine against malaria is not as straightforward as designing a vaccine against a virus or a bacillus. A virus is simply a small strand of nucleic acid, either RNA or DNA, wrapped in a protein coat. Strictly speaking it is not alive but co-opts the machinery of living cells to produce copies of itself. A bacillus is more like the malaria parasite in the sense that both are single-celled organisms. However while a bacillus is always a bacillus (and a virus always a virus), the malaria protozoan comes in a myriad guises. It enters your bloodstream as a sporozoite, bursts from the liver as an asexual merozoite, then transforms itself into a gametocyte and jumps back into the mosquito to begin its life cycle again. This constant shape-shifting makes it extremely difficult for the immune system to recognize and mount a sustained attack. Normally antibodies would identify alien invaders in the bloodstream while killer T-cells would hunt down and destroy unwelcome cellular guests. But the sporozoites are only in the blood for half an hour – too short a time for our antibodies to destroy all of them – and by the time the T-cells are ready to remove them from the liver they have transformed themselves into merozoites and migrated to red blood cells where, once again, they are safe from attack.

Parasitologists believe that this extraordinary capacity to outwit and evade our immune system is proof of malaria's antiquity and its long association with man. Some biologists believe that falciparum, and other human malaria protozoa, evolved from a unicellular plant organism, like algae, as its DNA shows that a distant ancestor could manufacture chlorophyll, the substance that makes plants green and allows for photosynthesis. One theory is that it began as a parasite of a prehistoric plant-eating reptile that was later picked up by a mosquito; another is that it was a parasite of the mosquito first and subsequently became established in dinosaurs. Whatever, we know from the fact that anophelines transmit more than a hundred and seventy similar protozoa to a wide range of vertebrates from reptiles and birds to rodents and apes that the parasite has been around for at least thirty million years. More importantly, from our point of view, we also know that many of the surviving bird and monkey malarias are closely related to the plasmodia that infect us. *P. cynomolgi*, a malaria parasite carried only by the south-east Asian rhesus monkey, is very closely related to vivax malaria. And the DNA sequences of *P. reichenowi*, a malaria parasite of chimpanzees, are so close to falciparum they could almost be a forgery – as if someone had copied the gene strings as one would copy a sonata, hitting an occasional false note. Fortunately over evolutionary time man has evolved various strategies for living with malaria and it is these strategies that hold out hope that Patarroyo and other vaccine-makers may one day succeed in cracking the parasite's defences.

Take sickle-cell anaemia, an excruciating and usually fatal genet-ically transmitted blood disorder found only in black Africans and blacks of African descent. Victims of sickle-cell disease, who inherit sickle-cell genes from both parents, tend to die young, often before they have had the opportunity to bear children. Natural selection should therefore have led to the disappearance of sickle-cell genes, as those who develop the disease are less likely to reproduce than other members of the population. But this is not what happens. Instead, many African blacks still carry the sickle-cell 'trait'. The reason is people who get the gene from just one parent have partial protection against malaria: they can still be infected with falciparum but their sickle-cell gene stops them developing the full-blown version of the disease. The result is that in areas where malaria is endemic, infants with the trait have a greater chance of survival than those born without it, and thus have a greater chance of producing offspring who also carry the aberrant gene.[1]

Another reason for optimism is that if you survive malaria in infancy and continue to be exposed to it in early adulthood you will eventually develop partial immunity to the parasite. The reason is that repeated exposure to the disease keeps the immune system in a high state of alert so that there are always antibodies ready to attack the parasite immediately it invades. People with acquired immunity can still be infected with malaria and transmit it, but their symptoms are milder, with the result that the disease is rarely fatal. The only drawback is that the immune response is strain-specific. A Gambian teenager may be immune to the strains of falciparum in his village but if he travels to the village next door he may encounter a different strain and fall ill. These evolutionary differences between strains of the same parasite may represent the most formidable challenge of all facing Patarroyo and other immunologists.

In order to have any hope of training the body to fight malaria vaccine-makers must first decide which stage of the parasite's life cycle they wish to concentrate on. Thus you could develop a vaccine that stops the plasmodium infecting liver cells – the sporozoite stage – but has no effect on merozoites already in the blood. Or you could develop an asexual vaccine for the blood-stage parasites that would have no effect on the sexual gametocytes that actually transmit the disease. Finally, you could design a transmission-blocking vaccine that stimulates antibodies against gametocytes and stops mosquitoes being infected, but has no effect on either sporozoites or merozoites. Moreover, whichever stage you decide to concentrate on the vaccine has to be perfect. It's no use making a vaccine that kills most of the sporozoites as it takes only one parasite to reach the liver and begin manufacturing merozoites for your 'sporozoite-specific' vaccine to be useless.

For various reasons Patarroyo and other researchers decided to concentrate on the sporozoite stage. First, it was the most direct approach: a vaccine that stopped the sporozoites reaching the liver would kill infections at source and thus provide absolute protection both for non-immune travellers to malaria-endemic areas and for children most at risk of dying from the disease. Second, and more importantly, by the early 1970s scientists knew through experiments with radiation that it was possible to use attenuated sporozoites to confer complete protection.

In 1968 researchers at New York University found that if mosquitoes infected with malaria were dosed with X-rays the sporozoites in their salivary glands were inactivated: that is, they were still alive and capable of eliciting an immune response but they were no longer able to invade host cells. Having ascertained that the irradiated sporozoites conferred immunity in rodents and monkeys against their malarias, in 1971 US Army scientists began a series of experiments to see if they would work in people too. It took several trials but eventually WRAIR confirmed that if volunteers were bitten at least a thousand times by irradiated mosquitoes they were protected against malaria for up to six months, after which the immunity wore off. Unfortunately, the protection was strain-specific. Moreover, if you extracted the irradiated sporozoites from the mosquitoes and injected the dead parasites instead nothing happened. In other words, you had to use live mosquitoes. Short of building a massive insectary to deliver the vaccine this was obviously impractical. However, by now researchers had noticed that the key to the immune response was a series of proteins on the skin of the sporozoite. One, the circumsporozoite

(CS) protein, seemed to be particularly promising. If it could be cultured biologically, or better still synthesized chemically, you might be able to skip the mosquito altogether and manufacture sufficient quantities to make a vaccine viable.

By the early 1980s biotechnology had progressed to the point where you could extract any gene – be it from brewer's yeast or a nematode worm – and engineer a bacterial culture to 'express' it. In theory this meant you could grow the CS protein in a culture and then insert it into an inert virus – say smallpox or hepatitis – and see whether you got an immune response. Similarly, the new peptide-synthesizing machines meant that if you knew the sequence of amino acids along any section of the parasite's skin you could manufacture the same protein molecule chemically. When it was discovered that the key CS antigen consisted of a sequence of just four amino acids repeated over and over again this is exactly what Patarroyo and other researchers decided to do.

It is not so much Patarroyo's fame that has brought me to Bogotá as the intriguing parallels with José Celestino Mutis. Although Mutis is better known as a botanist and an early Colombian champion of the Newtonian and Copernican systems of physics, he was first and foremost a physician. Like Patarroyo, he was fascinated with disease. As well as experimenting with quinine to cure malaria, Mutis conducted the first South American trials on smallpox, inoculating patients in Cartagena with pus taken from the sores of smallpox victims in an attempt to provoke an immune response. More importantly, like Patarroyo, Mutis put Colombian science on the map. At his herbarium housing twenty thousand different New World plants he oversaw a team of thirty draughtsmen. Like the chemists and immunologists at Patarroyo's institute, they worked in shifts, sketching in painstaking and exquisite detail the different species of cinchona growing in the *montaña* of Colombia and Ecuador. It was Mutis's descriptions of cinchona that enabled Linnaeus to complete his classification and led him to described Mutis as '*nomen immortale*'. Had it not been for Mutis it would have taken very much longer for the world to discover the valuable new Colombian species of cinchona. And had it not been for Mutis, it is unlikely that Humboldt – the most eminent scientist of his day – would have felt compelled to visit Bogotá and linger as long as he did.

Today, it is not uncommon for eminent scientists and elder statesmen to make a similar pilgrimage to the San Juan Hospital. The walls of Patarroyo's office are cluttered with pictures of previous honoured guests: Nelson Mandela, the King and Queen of Spain, the President of Nigeria, and my own favourite, Princess Anne. Then there are the awards: the Robert Koch medal, the Edinburgh medal, the French Légion d'Honneur . . . the list goes on and on. As we sit talking, the fax machine vibrates into life and out pops another from the mayor of a town in southern Spain. 'They want to name a street and their new biotechnology institute after me,' says Patarroyo proudly. 'I must get two or three proposals like this a week.'

The institute is a world apart from Ataco, the small town in the Tolima region of Colombia where Patarroyo grew up. The eldest of eleven, his parents were middle-class business people who expected their children to follow in their footsteps. Instead, they ended up with five physicians, one nurse and a child psychologist. In Patarroyo's case the catalyst was an illustrated science book his parents gave him when he was eight. 'It was all about the discoveries of Pasteur, Koch and Ross,' he recalls. 'I was captivated. Some people want to be football stars. I decided then and there I wanted to be an immunologist.'

Patarroyo attended medical school in Bogotá but, by his own admission, he was a mediocre student. Then in the second year of his studies, during his internship at the San Juan Hospital, he met Ronald Mackenzie, the head of the Rockefeller Institute, and told him he was interested in pursuing a chemical approach to vaccines. In 1965 this was a radical idea. Ever since Pasteur, all vaccines had been cultured biologically. But what, wondered Patarroyo, if you could achieve the same effect by synthesizing key immunological antigens chemically? Then you would no longer have to worry about taking living material and attenuating it. Moreover, the resulting vaccine would be a lot cheaper to produce.

With this end in mind, in 1968 Patarroyo went to Yale University on a scholarship to study virology. Next he joined the immunology department of Rockefeller University. It was there that he came under the sway of Bruce Merrifield, the chemist whose pioneering work on synthetic peptides would lead to the award of the Nobel Prize in 1984. 'Merrifield was the single biggest influence,' says Patarroyo. 'He was the one who convinced me that the synthetic approach could work.' However, it was only when Patarroyo returned to Bogotá that he decided that the vaccine had to be malaria.

Patarroyo switches on a slide projector beside his desk and motions for me to wheel my chair across the room. 'Look, the biggest killer worldwide is tuberculosis,' he says, pointing to a diagram of a pie divided into 'disease slices'. 'Next is dysentery. But the third biggest is malaria.' He clicks to the next slide of an African baby with weeping eyes. 'Every year between one and a half and three million people, one third of them children in sub-Saharan Africa, die. The reason is that the principal drug, chloroquine, no longer works and resistance is growing to the alternatives. A vaccine is the only hope.'

In the mid-1970s Patarroyo convinced the San Juan Hospital to give him his own immunology wing funded by money from his private practice and began exploring ways of targeting the parasite. At this stage he was by no means the leader in the field. In 1979 the husband-and-wife team of Ruth and Victor Nussenzweig – the researchers at New York University who had conducted the first experiments with irradiated sporozoites in mice and monkeys – had identified the CS protein as the most likely target of a vaccine. A few years later they succeeded in synthesizing the protein in the lab and injecting it into mice. Not only did the mice produce antibodies against malaria but not a single sporozoite survived to colonize the rodents' liver cells. Excitement ran high. It looked as though the Nussenzweigs had solved the problem. However, the human trials in 1987 turned out to be a huge disappointment. Only one of three volunteers immunized by the Nussenzweigs remained free of malaria. In the case of the other two, the vaccine delayed the onset of the disease but failed to stop the emergence of merozoites. By now WRAIR and the National Institutes of Health (NIH) had also entered the stakes. Teaming up with one of the world's biggest pharmaceutical firms, SmithKline Beecham, they tried a different approach. Instead of synthesizing the CS protein they extracted the gene that encoded the protein from the parasite, grew it in bacteria and let the bacteria generate copies of it. They then injected the CS protein into six volunteers. Again, only one remained disease-free. The other five all developed malaria, albeit more slowly than they would have without the vaccine.

The failure set back the cause of malaria vaccine research in the US for years. The problem was that expectations had been pitched unrealistically high. In truth, the results were encouraging, but because the failure had been so public drug companies retreated to lick their wounds and the sources of research funding dried up. Patarroyo, however, was not hampered by such constraints. Just as Mutis answered only to the Viceroy of New Grenada, so Patarroyo answers only to the President of Colombia. As he told me: 'If I want something I simply call up Pastrana. Not even the Minister of Health can tell me what to do.'

In the eyes of the international scientific community, however, this strength is also Patarroyo's weakness. Unlike his rivals at more staid institutions in Washington and Oxford, Patarroyo is not subject to continual peer review. He can pursue a line of enquiry – possibly the wrong line of enquiry – for years without having to publish his findings and run the risk of being challenged. To his supporters this makes him like the gentlemen scientists of the nineteenth century. After all, would Darwin have arrived at his theory of natural selection if he had had to go cap in hand to the Medical Research Council for a travel grant to South America? But to his detractors, Patarroyo's methods are risky and wasteful. To them, his empirical approach to the vaccine – altering an amino acid here, an amino acid there – seems to have more in common with alchemy than science.

Nevertheless, in the early 1980s Patarroyo began churning out hundreds and then thousands of different amino acid sequences, turning down an offer of an assistant professorship at the Rockefeller Institute in New York in order to concentrate on his own research in Bogotá. In 1987, at around the same time that human trials were getting under way in the US, he reported that he had come up with his own synthetic vaccine, SPf66, that conferred 50 per cent protection in monkeys infected with falciparum. Then, in the first human trial, involving fifteen Colombian army volunteers, he reported that three out of five who received the vaccine were protected. Between 1988 and 1993 a series of major trials were conducted in Colombia, Venezuela, Ecuador and Brazil. The results were confusing. In some, the vaccine seemed to have an efficacy rate as high as 80 per cent; in others it was as low as 35 per cent, or else the results were statistically insignificant. Nevertheless, turning down lucrative offers from drug companies, in 1995 Patarroyo donated the rights to SPf66 to the World Health Organisation, boasting that the problem of malaria had been 'solved'.

Once again it was a false dawn. In randomized, double-blind trials sponsored by the WHO in The Gambia and Tanzania, SPf66 showed no protection in children under the age of five. Then, in a US Army sponsored trial in Thailand in 1996, twelve hundred Thai children given several inoculations of SPf66 were no more protected than those given a placebo. The verdict of the international scientific community was unanimous: SPf66 did not work.

To any other scientist such a setback would have been devastating. Patarroyo was roasted for his methodology and for the ethics of moving so quickly to human trials. His critics suggested that the reason he had obtained such promising results with his Colombian army volunteers was that he had 'challenged' the vaccine by injecting his study group with falciparum rather than by allowing them to be bitten with malaria-carrying mosquitoes. Moreover, critics said many of the Latin American trials had not been properly randomized, had inappropriate controls and neither his subjects nor the observers were blinded. Patarroyo quickly acknowledged that he had 'made mistakes' and had much to learn about epidemiology, but was adamant that he was on the right lines. Hitting out at the 'intellectual racism' of scientists in the North, Patarroyo argued that challenging the vaccine by intravenous injection was more accurate as it was impossible to tell in what quantities the parasite was harboured by mosquitoes. Believing that the vaccine's poor performance in Africa was due to his failure to take into account variations in local African strains of falciparum, he retreated to his peptide synthesizer in Bogotá determined to do better. Three years later, in 1999, he emerged from his self-imposed purdah to tell a British newspaper that he had developed an improved version of SPf66 and was ready to conduct new trials. Within two years, he confidently predicted, his vaccine would be available 'world-wide'.

Sitting in his office in Bogotá a year later Patarroyo remains acutely sensitive to criticism. He is still smarting from the conference in Cartagena where he claims members of the British media had been warned by other delegates not to take his claims about the vaccine 'seriously'. 'I don't mind being questioned by my peers. That's natural, I'm a scientist. But when people come at me with an agenda and don't tell me that's unfair.' As he says this I cannot help noticing a sketch on the wall depicting Patarroyo felling the malaria 'beast' with a hypodermic. The drawing bears the slogan 'David y Goliat' and the inscription, 'Para el doctor Patarroyo con mucho humor.' Humorous or not, don't such impressions play into the hands of his enemies?

Patarroyo admits that designing a vaccine has been very much more complicated than he, or anyone else, had imagined. 'But when we say there's a malaria vaccine, we are not saying, bingo, here is something we have just taken off the shelf. It has taken a hell of a lot of work to get this far.'

Patarroyo argues that the fundamental reason for SPf66's disappointing performance in Tanzania, The Gambia and Thailand are the variations in the African and south-east Asian strains of falciparum. It is these variations that he believes make all the difference between a vaccine that works in the laboratory and one that performs in the field. The obvious solution is to target the proteins on the surface of the parasite that do not vary – the so-called 'conserved' regions. These are the proteins that the parasite has to use to gain entry to the red blood cell. Unfortunately they are also the regions associated with the weakest antibody response.

'Imagine the parasite like a human hand and the conserved sequences like fingers,' explains Patarroyo, reaching for the door to his office. 'The parasite wants to unlock the door and find a way into the host cells. Our aim is to stop it; to keep the door locked. The problem is the parasite can open the door with these fingers' – Patarroyo grabs the door with his right hand – 'or with these fingers' – he grabs the handle with his left hand instead. 'My job is to train the immune system to recognize which hand the parasite is using so that its fingers no longer work.'

Since 1995 this is just what Patarroyo has been doing. He really believes that the conserved regions are governed by certain 'rules' that he is on the point of divining. If he can find just the right cocktail of antigens, Patarroyo believes he will have the equivalent of molecular gold: a vaccine that confers 100 per cent protection against any strain of the parasite anywhere in the world. At least, that is the theory.

It is 5.30 a.m. at Bogotá's El Dorado airport and Patarroyo is nowhere to be seen. He has told me to meet him bright and early at the Aero República ticket desk so that we can be sure of boarding a flight to Leticia in the Colombian Amazon. But the only other people on the concourse are a family of Amazonian Indians and an old man laden with boxes packed with rope, fabric and canned food – essential jungle supplies.

Leticia is where Patarroyo keeps the owl monkeys that are critical to his experiments with the vaccine. The monkeys are indigenous only to South America, from Panama to northern Argentina. More importantly, the owl monkey is one of only three primates that can be infected with falciparum. According to Patarroyo the owl monkey's immune system is nearly identical to our own, making it the 'perfect' animal model for testing his vaccine. If SPf66 clears falciparum from the blood of owl monkeys then – QED – it will clear the parasite in humans. Like Dr Moreau, Patarroyo even has his own island – Isla de Los Micos – dedicated to proving his thesis. The island is on the Amazon at the border of Colombia and Peru. But to get there first you have to fly to Leticia, an Amazonian trading town further down-river.

It has taken months of badgering by phone and fax to persuade Patarroyo. First he was preoccupied with the congress in Cartagena, then he had to attend a banquet in honour of Clinton, and in a week's time it is his daughter's wedding. The only reason he has agreed to fly with me today is that he has a new batch of vaccine to deliver and is anxious to get the results. But as the airport comes to life and the queue at the Aero República desk lengthens I am beginning to think he has had second thoughts. The flight to Leticia leaves at 7 a.m. and it is now 6.30 a.m. I am about to relinquish my place in the queue when I spot a man with a baseball cap pulled tightly around a shock of frizzy grey hair scoot across the concourse and duck behind the ticket desk. The man looks like Patarroyo but I cannot be sure. It is only when he removes his cap and the attendant, in a sudden flash of recognition, jumps to attention, that I recognize him too. 'We were up until ten thirty last night analysing new ideas,' says Patarroyo apologetically. 'The team wanted to know what the boss was cooking up.'

The young woman at the ticket desk hands us our boarding passes ahead of the old man with the boxes and we begin making our way toward the departure lounge. As we wander through the concourse I begin to understand Patarroyo's earlier furtiveness. On the way we are twice stopped by boys wanting his autograph and by mothers wanting him to bless their babies. He deals with each supplicant good-naturedly. His fame in Colombia is such that it crosses the political divide too. A few years ago, he tells me, he was taken hostage by the Fuerza Armadas Revolucionarias de Colombia (FARC) – the Marxist guerrillas who control the demilitarized zone in southern Colombia. But after just five hours they let him go. 'They wanted to tell me that malaria was a problem for their people too. They now send me faxes urging me to keep up the good work.'

Wherever Patarroyo goes his ledger book, containing the results of his vaccine trials, is never far from his side. Safely on board the plane, he opens it to show me. Each page is divided into neat rows and columns. The rows record the numbers of monkeys in each trial; the columns show the time it has taken for the vaccine to clear the parasites from their blood. The monkeys are given SPf66 in three doses over four weeks. Then on day thirty, Patarroyo 'challenges' their immune systems by injecting them with falciparum and waits to observe the effect on the parasites in their blood.

'See, in 1994 we gave the vaccine to fifty monkeys. But by day five after infection all showed signs of parasitaemia. As soon as they reach 6 per cent parasitaemia we stop the experiment, treat their malaria and release them. After all, we don't want them to die.'

Patarroyo turns to the next page, headed October 1994. 'I thought that maybe the problem was that the vaccine wasn't big enough so I added more peptides to make the molecule bigger, but that didn't work either.' He flips the page, running his finger along each row. 'See, every monkey comes down with malaria on day five, so I randomly changed the sequence of amino acids.' He turns to January 1995 and points to a row of zeros. 'Look, for the first time I began to see zero parasitaemia in a few monkeys. That was exciting. It meant we were on to something.'

All the monkeys with zero parasitaemia subsequently went on to develop full-blown malaria, but it was a significant development: the onset of the infection had been delayed. Working on a hunch that the key was the conserved protein regions, Patarroyo continued mixing up the amino-acid sequences in the hope of finding a 'cocktail' of antigens that would trigger a fully protective immunological response.

For two years he admits he was 'working in the dark'. Then in 1997 he started to see zero parasitaemia up to day ten in a number of monkeys, and in a few cases the monkeys never went on to develop an infection. Patarroyo was now convinced that —as he puts it — he had discovered 'half the rules'. But he still had a long way to go before he would be in a position to publish, let alone contemplate human trials. Instead, he continued playing with the amino-acid sequences. By 1999 he had synthesized some fourteen thousand peptides. Then, in June, he claims he got the breakthrough he had been waiting for. 'Look, row after row of zeros.' Patarroyo flips the page. 'In August it's the same, and in September.' By autumn 1999, Patarroyo says, only 20 per cent of the monkeys were developing infections. 'The vaccine was providing 80 per cent protection after three shots,' he says.

Since then Patarroyo has refined the vaccine further and now claims he is able to achieve the same results with just two shots. However, he will only be satisfied when he has a one-shot vaccine providing 100 per cent protection.

Gradually the Cordillera Central gives way to the Cordillera Oriental and then the mountains recede from view and we are flying over virgin jungle. Here and there the green canopy is broken by a snaking channel or the metallic glint of a lake, but after about an hour a haze envelops the forest and all I can see for miles in any direction are puffy white clouds. In the wet season Leticia is highly malarial but it is August and Patarroyo has assured me I do not need a prophylactic. What does he take for malaria? 'Nothing. I vaccinated myself in 1986 and haven't needed to worry since. It doesn't matter whether I am in Colombia or Tanzania, I never get ill.' Indeed, such is Patarroyo's confidence in SPf66 that he has vaccinated his whole family. So far, he insists, there have been no adverse side effects.

Two hours later the plane dips beneath the clouds and we begin the descent to Leticia. Patarroyo leans across the aisle and points out the starboard window at a mist-shrouded island far below. 'Isla de Los Micos,' he whispers.

After Bogotá the heat of the Amazon is oppressive. Raul Rodri-guez, the manager of Patarroyo's research station, is at the airport to meet us. A short, chubby man with gentle brown eyes, Rodriguez is dressed for the tropics in shorts and a tennis shirt, whereas we are still bundled up against the chill of El Dorado airport at seven in the morning. We quickly strip down to our shirtsleeves and I hop onto the back of Patarroyo's scooter for the five-minute drive into town. 'There are only eleven kilometres of road in Leticia,' explains

Patarroyo over the hum of the bike. 'This is the only way to get around.'

Patarroyo drops me at the Hotel Anaconda – a huge air-conditioned palace overlooking the town square. The manageress greets him warmly. Our arrival has already created quite a stir. As we stroll to a nearby restaurant for breakfast, Patarroyo pauses to shake hands with everyone from the corner cigarette seller to the manageress of the local bank. By the time we sit down for *caldas* and hot chocolate we have picked up a conga-line of shoeshine boys and are dripping perspiration. Fortunately, it is only a ten-minute walk to the research station.

On the way Rodriguez fills me in on the *Aotus*. The monkey, which is on the protected primate list, is the only truly nocturnal monkey in the world. 'That's why we call it the "owl",' says Rodriguez. 'We feed them eggs, papayas, bananas. You will see, they are very well cared for.'

In the wild, the monkeys sleep high up in trees, nestled in tangles of vines. The only way to catch them is to climb into the canopy and snag them with nets. It is a highly prized skill and one that is passed down from father to son. 'Here it costs me $40 to $50 for each monkey,' boasts Patarroyo. 'In America the same monkey would cost nearly $3,000.'

Patarroyo argues that this cheap and plentiful supply of primates gives him a huge advantage over his rivals. Whereas the US Army and Navy breed all their experimental monkeys in captivity, Patarroyo literally plucks his from the riverside. Moreover, because he argues the monkey and human immune systems are virtually identical he believes his results will automatically hold good for humans.

Patarroyo's critics disagree. They point out that his snatch and grab approach to animal testing means that he has no idea whether or not the monkeys in his experiments have already been exposed to malaria in the wild. Therefore, he has no way of knowing if some of the monkeys have heightened antibodies against falciparum – a factor that could influence the outcome of his trials. Moreover, there is evidence to suggest that some owl monkeys are not susceptible to falciparum infection at all. This means that SPf66 may not be protecting as many monkeys as Patarroyo thinks. Conversely, it is possible that a vaccine that has no protective effect in owl monkeys could be protective in people. But the most damning criticism of Patarroyo's monkey trials is that so far other experimenters have been unable to repeat his results. In 1990 researchers at the Centers for Disease Control in Atlanta inoculated monkeys with both their own version of SPf66 and a batch provided by Patarroyo. Neither of the groups was protected. Then in 1992 another Colombian researcher inoculated monkeys with the same batch of vaccine Patarroyo had used on the Colombian army volunteers. This time the monkeys did not even produce detectable antibodies.

Patarroyo is unmoved by such criticisms. He points out that owl monkeys live in small monogamous groups and that he deliberately selects his test subjects from different families so as to ensure as much diversity as possible. Moreover, he claims that the reason his vaccine did not perform well in human trials in Africa and Thailand is not due to differences in the monkey and human immune systems but because of differences in the African and south-east Asian strains of falciparum. Finally he claims that the latest batch of SPf66 is more potent than previous versions. 'We have manufactured a completely new molecule. One that has never before been seen in nature.'

We are now standing in front of a pretty walled compound. As Rodriguez opens the gate I feel as though I am about to step onto a set from *Planet of the Apes*. A sign above the entrance reads 'Experimental Primate Research Station'. The grounds are brimming with bougainvillaea, palms and ficus trees. To the left is a conference room; to the right, the laboratories and monkey barracks.

Rodriguez unlocks the door and shows me round. The monkeys are housed in small metal pens arranged one on top of the other in long, neat rows. They have just had breakfast and are smaller than I expected with greyish-brown coats, pale underbellies and long, delicate fingers. But their most distinctive feature is their large round eyes with white patches above the lids. The patches create the illusion that they are awake even when they are asleep – an important defence mechanism in the wild, presumably, but useless here.

Rodriguez opens the door to a cage and pulls one out. It emits a series of high-pitched screeches, but it quickly calms down once it realizes it cannot escape. Next door Patarroyo is already unpacking his vials of vaccine. The largest room contains two hundred and sixty monkeys, the one next door a hundred. But today Patarroyo plans to inject just fifty. Rodriguez takes the seat beside him. Breaking the seal on a vaccine bottle he sucks the fluid into a needle and, instructing his men to hold the monkeys outstretched on the table in front of him, begins injecting the vaccine into their soft undersides.

It takes an hour to vaccinate the fifty monkeys. As each one is brought through Patarroyo makes a careful note of its serial number in his ledger. Tomorrow Rodriguez will vaccinate a further two hundred. Then in twenty days' time all two hundred and fifty monkeys will be given a second dose of the vaccine, ready to be infected with falciparum ten days later. 'In forty days I will know the results,' says Patarroyo.

It is noon and Patarroyo's work for the day is almost over. He has only one more duty to perform: to return fifty monkeys from the last trial to the wild. While Rodriguez prepares the motorboat for the ride to monkey island, Patarroyo shows me round his private suite. His bedroom is simple but elegant: two low wooden beds, a writing desk and a large cupboard full of freshly pressed white shirts. 'This is where I count the blood cells when the results come back – ten thousand per monkey. It takes all day.'

Patarroyo changes into shorts and a loose-fitting shirt for the boat trip and tells me to help myself to a pair of deck shoes. Then he selects a baseball cap from the cupboard and we are ready to go.

The government gave Patarroyo the island in the late 1980s. In effect, Isla de Los Micos is a giant segregation compound, a way of ensuring that monkeys with vaccine-enhanced antibody levels do not become mixed up with the immunologically virgin monkeys Patarroyo needs for his trials. The only problem is the island is overcrowded.

Patarroyo has been vaccinating an average of fifty monkeys every three months for thirteen years. That makes two and a half thousand monkeys since 1987. 'We have asked the government for another island but they are not that easy to come by. We will just have to wait and see.'

It is now a perfect Amazonian afternoon and blisteringly hot. The jetty is only ten minutes from the research station but by the time we reach the boat we are soaked through. A large grey gunship lies moored in mid-river, marking the three-way border between Colombia, Peru and Brazil. Even in a baseball cap and shorts, however, Patarroyo is instantly recognizable and the customs guards wave us through with minimum fuss.

I notice that Rodriguez has loaded the monkeys into canvas sacks and dumped them on the floor of the boat. The temperature inside must be stifling. The bags bulge and leap about the deck as the monkeys wriggle for air and space. The island is sixty kilometres upriver. In the waterbus the journey takes an hour and a half but Rodriguez assures me that by launch it is just forty minutes. He cranks the motor and the nose of the boat leaps up into the water. Then another crank and we are off. He is right, the boat is very fast, and the breeze makes the heat less oppressive.

As the jungle skirts by it is hard to believe we are conducting an experiment that may transform the lives of children on the other side of the world. Music from a waterside cabana on the Peruvian side of the river mingles with the steady drone of the motor, lulling us into a trance. If the current batch of vaccine performs as well as Patarroyo expects he says he plans a human trial in Colombia later this year, followed by larger field-scale trials in Tanzania in 2001. 'We are very close,' he tells me, admiring the wake from the boat. 'I can feel it.' For a moment I think Patarroyo is talking about the island. Then I realize that he is talking about his vaccine. Despite all the disappointments and criticism his faith in SPf66 is unshaken.

The next thing I know we are skirting the island and Rodriguez is looking for a beach on which to land. Most of the banks are overgrown with giant lianas but eventually we find a clearing and Rodriguez parks the launch. A macaw sticks its beak from the jungle curious to see what the commotion is. The air is thick with mosquitoes and the croak of tree frogs. Gingerly, we form a chain and begin passing the sacks up the bank. The wriggling has grown more intense and it is an effort to keep my balance. As the sacks reach the shore, Rodriguez unties them and shakes free the contents. The monkeys shoot out with startling speed, scattering high into the treetops. Within minutes all the bags have been emptied and the job is done. Just one monkey seems reluctant to leave. He is lying on his side, breathing heavily. Rodriguez reaches out to touch him but he shoves his hand away like a petulant child. The monkey is hurt. 'Son los machos,' murmurs Rodriguez. 'The males are very territorial.'

We wait for the monkey to catch his breath, then prod him again. Gingerly, like a wounded trooper, he gets to his feet and limps slowly into the jungle, casting us accusing glances as he goes. 'Poor monkey,' I murmur. Patarroyo gives me a cold, clinical look. 'Think of the children dying of malaria every thirty seconds in Africa. That's whom you should reserve your sympathy for.'

The next morning Patarroyo boards the first flight out of Leticia. It will be forty days before the results of the trial are known and in the meantime he has appointments to keep in Bogotá. I am anxious to question him in more detail but we have run out of time. Throughout the trip he has been dropping constant hints that he has already found the magical mix of antigens and is just waiting for the right moment to publish. But now he is about to board the plane he is suddenly reticent. 'It's no use changing the molecule anywhere,' he says enigmatically. 'You have to know exactly where to make the change otherwise the vaccine doesn't work. That's the beauty of chemistry – it is so precise.'

Patarroyo is not the only scientist who believes he is close to a breakthrough. At the conference in Cartagena, Captain Stephen

Hoffman, a US Navy clinician and immunologist, also announced he had a new vaccine going to trial. Based at the US Navy Medical Research Center in Bethesda, Maryland – part of the same complex that houses WRAIR – Hoffman comes straight out of the same tradition of military doctoring that produced Walter Reed and William Gorgas. The difference is that whereas Reed and Gorgas fought malaria with petrol and quinine, Hoffman is deploying the most sophisticated weapon in the modern immunologist's arsenal – DNA.

A tropical medicine specialist with a passing resemblance to the actor Danny Kaye, Hoffman joined the navy in 1980 after stints in Bogotá, working with malnourished children, and the London School of Hygiene and Tropical Medicine – the school where Manson demonstrated the mosquito–man–mosquito transmission of malaria. His first posting was the US Navy medical research laboratory in Jakarta. It was supposed to be a three-year attachment. Twenty years later, Hoffman is still wearing the uniform.

It was in Indonesia that Hoffman found himself drawn to the study of malaria. He soon familiarized himself with the history: how the extraction of quinine in the early nineteenth century and the synthesis of chloroquine had led to the retreat of the disease only for it to rebound spectacularly after the Second World War. How despite the arsenal of therapeutics at the navy's disposal, the marines still lost more men to diseases, including malaria, than to enemy fire. And how a viable vaccine could eliminate the problem of prophylaxis indiscipline at a stroke. Then he looked at deaths from malaria in Africa. 'I studied the figures and realized that in the past fifty years no drug has been developed that has reduced the mortality rate from severe malaria in hospitals in the developing world one percentage point,' he says. Realizing that a vaccine that protected marines could also have incalculable benefits for African children, Hoffman decided to learn as much as he could about biotechnology and molecular immunology.

Hoffman joined the staff of the Navy Medical Research Center but found himself spending most of his time at WRAIR, where the efforts to develop a sporozoite vaccine were just beginning. It was an exciting time. Major Ripley Ballou, a WRAIR specialist in infectious diseases, had just teamed up with the NIH and SmithKline to conduct the first human trial of the CS vaccine using the latest gene-cloning technology. In the best traditions of army medicine, Ballou and Hoffman decided that the way to test the vaccine was on themselves. These were the first human trials that, along with the NYU experiment, were to go down as 'failures'.

In 1987 Hoffman, Ballou and four other volunteers took the vaccine and allowed themselves to be bitten repeatedly by infectious mosquitoes. After two weeks – the period it normally takes for the falciparum parasites developing in the liver to invade the blood – three of the volunteers fell ill. But not so Hoffman and Ballou, who believed they were protected. Hoffman flew to San Diego where he was scheduled to deliver a lecture while Ballou went for a run, after which he attended a party. No sooner had he arrived than he fell into a fever and had to leave. That evening his temperature soared to 104 degrees. There was no doubt about it, he had malaria and the next morning checked into hospital.

Meanwhile, in San Diego, Hoffman was enduring a more public torture. 'I was in the middle of my presentation when I developed the malaria rigour and the shaking chills. That was it.'

Although, as in the NYU trial, only one volunteer was fully protected against malaria, Hoffman and Ballou took encouragement from the fact that they had developed the disease far more slowly than they would have without the vaccine. 'We proved the principle that you could make these vaccines and you could induce protective immunity,' says Hoffman.

Undeterred, Hoffman and Ballou decided to see whether the antibody response could be boosted by repeated exposure to malaria in the field. Again the results were disappointing – the vaccine resulted in more antibodies but did not confer protection. Demoralized, Hoffman and Ballou retreated to their animal models. Like Patarroyo, Hoffman also conducts tests with owl monkeys. Some are kept at the joint army–navy building in Maryland; others at the navy's jungle research laboratory in Iquitos, in the Peruvian Amazon. The difference is that the monkeys are bred from birth in captivity so that their full medical history is known. However, because of the costs involved, most of the trials are conducted on mice infected with rodent malarias.

By the early 1990s these animal experiments were suggesting that antibodies were only one of the ways that irradiated sporozoites generated an immune response. The other was by stimulating killer T-cells to attack the parasites in the liver. The problem was that the recombinant and synthetic peptide vaccines so far developed were incapable of marshalling those T-cells into action. Then Hoffman heard about a new technology, DNA vaccines. Often known as gene vaccines, they consist of a gene from the pathogen, stitched into a circular stretch of bacterial DNA known as a plasmid. In theory all Hoffman had to do was select DNA from the parasite that encoded for key antigenic liver-stage proteins, splice them into plasmid and inject it directly into muscle tissue. The muscle cells would then transcribe the DNA into RNA and begin generating the same proteins the parasite produces when it is in the liver. When the parasite next came along the immune system would recognize its proteins as invaders and send in the marines – in this case, the killer T-cells. 'In essence DNA vaccines harness the machinery of the human cell and use it to stimulate the appropriate immune response for us,' explains Hoffman.

In 1995 Hoffman's navy research team began testing DNA malaria vaccines on animals for the first time. The results were encouraging. When they challenged mice with the most infectious strain of rodent malaria the mice showed no signs of disease. Next they moved to monkeys, with similarly impressive results. Then in 1997 they conducted the first safety trials on twenty human volunteers. Not only was the vaccine well 'tolerated' but the majority of volunteers had heightened T-cell responses. The next stage is to see if the vaccine actually confers protection when volunteers are challenged with malaria.

The advantage of DNA vaccines is that they are relatively easy to manufacture and can be tailored to be as complex as the parasite itself. In theory, if enough genes from the parasite are inserted into the vaccine the immune system will recognize the parasite at every stage of its life cycle, defeating its ability to change shape and evade the body's defences. So far, Hoffman's team has produced cocktails with genes from five, eight and fifteen different antigens. As yet, however, no one knows whether they will result in sufficiently large T-cell responses in humans.

Meanwhile, Walter Reed, in partnership with SmithKline, has been concentrating on boosting the antibody response of the CS protein using what Ballou calls 'molecular biology tricks'. In 1997 this effort resulted in RTS,S, the most promising vaccine yet. Like SPf66, the vaccine consists of synthesized sections of the CS protein. The difference is that the portions of the protein are fused with hepatitis B surface antigens and then mixed with adjuvants — chemicals known to boost the immune system. In 1997 Walter Reed reported that RTS,S had protected an unprecedented six out of seven volunteers in tests in Washington. Two years later SmithKline and the Medical Research Council held full-scale field trials in The Gambia. Recruiting three hundred and six men from six rural villages, the MRC administered the vaccine in three separate doses. After two months, almost two-thirds of the men were protected. Unfortunately, that rate fell to just 16 per cent after fifteen weeks. It was too short a time to be of practical use but for the first time a vaccine had provided some protection against malaria in the field. Not only that but the vaccine had worked in The Gambia — the place where many previous vaccines, including Patarroyo's, had met their Waterloo.

'The Gambia trial confirmed good and bad things about the vaccine,' says Ballou cautiously. 'Yes, it confers immunity on about half the people it is given to but it lasts only a couple of months. Nobody believes that we have a vaccine that is ready for licensing or that will meet sub-Saharan Africa's needs yet.'

Twenty or even ten years ago such humility in malaria vaccine research was unheard of. But as immunologists have begun to realize

the scale of the problem facing them it is increasingly the norm. This
is only partly due to the immunological challenges. In the laboratory
the parasite has been equally reluctant to give up its secrets. At the
Sanger Centre in Cambridge, where scientists have succeeded in
mapping the human genome, to date only two of the parasite's
fourteen chromosomes have been sequenced. The problem is its
genome is chock full of adenines and thymines, two of the four-
nucleotide bases that are the building blocks of DNA. In some places
these so-called 'A's and 'T's average 80 per cent and on chromosomes
2 and 3 nearly 100 per cent. The real sticking point for the sequencers,
however, has been a section known as the 'blob' – three chromosomes
that are so close in size they have to be treated as one. 'Falciparum
has been far more difficult than any other organism we've tackled,'
says Sharon Bowman, the molecular biologist in charge of Sanger's
falciparum-sequencing effort. 'Because of the concentration of 'A's
and 'T's it's very difficult for us to clone out the bits of the parasite
we need and then fit the pieces back together again.'

In theory, as more of these pieces of the parasite become available
it should become easier to identify proteins for drug development and
for splicing into a vaccine. However, many scientists are increasingly
coming round to the view that DNA vaccines alone are not the
answer. Instead, they are experimenting with what are known as
'prime-boost' techniques – priming with a DNA vaccine and boosting the immune system with a second vaccine, either a recombinant
protein or a recombinant virus. Hoffman, for instance, is now looking at boosting a DNA vaccine with RTS,S. Meanwhile, Adrian
Hill, Professor of Human Genetics at the Nuffield Department of
Medicine in Oxford, has begun field trials in The Gambia of a six-
part DNA vaccine inserted into an attenuated version of the vaccinia
virus – the virus that eliminated smallpox. One of several prime-
boost 'strategies' being studied by Hill, the vaccine has already performed well in trials involving forty volunteers conducted in Oxford
in 1999. Unlike Hoffman, Hill is not interested in the antibody
response but is focusing exclusively on boosting T-cells in the liver

stage of the infection. But he does not rule out combining his techniques with those of other researchers in future. 'At the moment the best vaccine is RTS,S. But at the end of the day we may find that we need to use several different approaches. My view is that malaria is so complex that for the moment everyone has to concentrate on what they are best at. We should not expect any one person to come up with the answer. Those days of vaccine discovery are over.'

One thing that would help is more money. The US currently spends $300m a year on HIV and Aids research. In contrast, it spends just $30m on malaria – of which only about $5m funds the military's work on the vaccine. In 1999 Bill Gates, the Microsoft computer billionaire, donated $50m for vaccine development via a non-profit organization established with his wife, Melinda, and his father, William. But while the money will accelerate research on vaccines already under way, it is a mere drop in the bucket set against the hundreds of millions of dollars poured by pharmaceutical companies each year into research into cures for more 'profitable' diseases.

However, money is not the only problem. In the 1970s the WHO succeeded in eradicating smallpox and came close to wiping out a host of other childhood diseases, like polio and measles, by mobilizing hundreds of health workers across the globe. Today, the level of organization that would be required for a global malaria vaccine campaign simply does not exist. 'We have to work in recognition that even if we had the best vaccine cheaply available, manufactured in large quantities, in our hand right now, we could not deliver it effectively to the children who are dying from malaria,' admits Dr Regina Rabinovich, the director of Gates's Malaria Vaccine Initiative.

In reality of course we are nowhere near that point. Unless, of course, Patarroyo is right and his critics are wrong.

'I like to think of vaccines in two stages,' says Hoffman. 'First we need a vaccine that provides temporary protection for non-immune travellers and military personnel entering malarial areas. Second, we need a vaccine that protects children, growing up in areas where they are continually exposed to malaria, from dying. It could be that we come up with a vaccine that does both. The point is it is a very complex puzzle. Whether we solve it this year, next year or in ten to fifteen years' time, is what remains to be seen.'

# EPILOGUE

## WARNING – MOZZIES 5 KM

IN THE TWO YEARS that it took to research and write this book, mosquitoes and malaria have rarely been out of the news. No sooner did I begin looking into the legend of the Condesa de Chinchón, for instance, than it was reported that two Boy Scouts in Long Island, New York, had come down with the disease. According to Suffolk County health officials, the scouts had almost certainly been inoculated by mosquitoes breeding near a marsh on Long Island not far from where their camp was located. If so, it was the first case of locally acquired as opposed to imported malaria Suffolk County had seen in ten years.

A few weeks later, in September 1999, New York's mayor Rudolph Giuliani ordered the entire city to be doused with insecticide following the deaths of three adults from another mosquito-borne disease. This time the prime suspect was not the *Anopheles* but the *Culex* mosquito. At first scientists believed they were looking at an outbreak of St Louis encephalitis, a rare avian virus normally confined to the southern United States. But within days investigators had established that the *Culex* were actually transmitting West Nile virus, an even rarer bird-to-human disease never before seen in North America.

The theme that linked these stories was global warming. Up until the end of the nineteenth century malaria was commonplace in the continental United States. From the Carolina swamplands all along the Mississippi to Illinois, and from Washington DC as far west as Iowa, newspaper caricaturists would poke fun at the 'gaunt, lantern-jawed' inhabitants with their 'careworn expression and languid mien'. With the advent of Federal dam and river projects, land clearance and the popularization of quinine by medical purveyors like Dr John Sappington, the disease – and the caricatures – gradually receded. But malaria was never completely eradicated in Florida and, as the recent New York outbreaks underline, it – or other exotic tropical diseases – could rebound at any time.

In Britain, because of its more temperate climate, malaria was always a more localized and seasonal occurrence. For the most part the disease was confined to the marshes and coasts of Kent, Essex, Norfolk and Somerset where it would flare up in summer and around harvest time before subsiding in winter. Nevertheless, by the early eighteenth century field hands migrating north with the harvests had introduced malaria to the Scottish borders and there were even reports of 'ague' in Aberdeen and Inverness.

As in North America, marsh reclamation reduced the anophelines' breeding areas, and the introduction of cinchona bark and later quinine reduced the pool of infectious parasites. But the key factor in Britain was probably the introduction of new root crops, like the turnip, which both increased the size and health of animal herds and encouraged farmers to winter cattle in stables away from human habitations. The result was that *Anopheles atroparvus*, the main vector of malaria in Britain, began feeding on cows and horses instead of people, dramatically reducing the incidence of infections. If the British climate were to warm by just a few degrees, however, those same anophelines might change their nesting habits. All it would take is for one or two feverish backpackers returning from Asia to be bitten by a mosquito and malaria could begin to take hold again in southern Britain – at least, that was the theory advanced by Britain's chief medical officer, Liam Donaldson, at a press conference in February 2001.

But global warming was not the only spectre that stalked this book. While researching the history of the British cinchona missions, I could not help but notice that drug resistance was spreading. From Venezuela to Colombia, Brazil, Thailand, Kenya and Tanzania, there were now strains of falciparum malaria that responded to neither chloroquine nor quinine. Moreover, the tensions between profit and philanthropy first highlighted by Markham's bureaucratic battles with the India Office a hundred and fifty years ago had not gone away. Indeed, if anything, they were even more pressing.

Up until the end of the nineteenth century there was only one cure for malaria: quinine. The only question was how to bring it within reach of the masses. Today, no single drug is 100 per cent effective against all strains of the disease and developing a promising new anti-malarial is an expensive proposition – at least $150 million spread over three years. Because of the rate at which resistance is spreading, some health economists argue that we should be investing at least $500 million a year on new malaria drugs. Instead, we are only spending about $84 million. That translates into $42 per fatal case, significantly less than we spend on either cancer or Aids. Despite the fact that the G8 countries are now devoting substantial resources to malaria control – $750 million under the WHO's 'Roll Back Malaria' programme over the next ten years – it is still not enough. Sooner or later, argue leading malaria experts, we will face a major 'health calamity'.

When it comes, it is in Africa that the impact will be most acute. The WHO estimates that at present some three thousand people die of malaria in sub-Saharan Africa a day for want of rapid and effective treatment. That is the equivalent of a small stadium full of people every week, or about 1.1 million a year – the majority of them children under the age of five. Thanks to global warming and the collapse of public health systems, however, those numbers are about to get a lot worse. In the mountains of western Kenya, for instance, malaria-carrying mosquitoes have been found breeding at eighteen hundred metres for the first time in living memory, leading to an explosion of untreated cases. Doctors in Kisii, one of the worst affected areas, blame abnormal rainfall patterns and the high cost of new anti-malaria drugs.

Then there are the more frequent natural disasters, like the floods in Mozambique in March 2000, in which whole families were left stranded in trees, their bodies swarming with mosquitoes and other disease-carrying insects, as they waited for the arrival of helicopters that could airlift them to safety. Those floods resulted in a four-fold increase in malaria in Mozambique. Similarly high rainfall in the northern highlands of Burundi in November 2000 resulted in a quarter of a million new cases and threatened even greater levels of infection in 2001. In the worst-case scenario, we are talking about five hundred million infections worldwide. That's half a billion new fever cases every year.

But morbidity is not the only measure of malaria's impact; it is also a huge drag on economic productivity. According to a recent study by Harvard University health economist Dr Jeffrey Sachs, if the WHO had succeeded in its aim of eradicating the disease thirty-five years ago Africa's gross domestic product would be about $100 billion greater than it is now. In the words of the WHO's director, Dr Gro Harlem Brundtland, malaria is an 'economic handicap' that not only hurts the living standards of Africans today but is 'preventing the improvement of living standards for future generations.'

One of the places where the issues of drug resistance, global warming, and the role of philanthropy in twenty-first-century malaria control increasingly come together is at the London School of Hygiene and Tropical Medicine (LSHTM). Founded in 1899, the school has long been at the forefront of research into malaria and other tropical diseases. It was here that in 1900 Sir Patrick Manson arranged for his son, Patrick Thorburn Manson, and a laboratory assistant to be bitten by a malaria-infected *Anopheles* forwarded from the Santo Spirito Hospital in Rome, thus proving that the disease was transmitted from mosquito to man. And it was here that researchers first began warning in the early 1980s of the risk of a resurgence in tropical diseases due to global warming and increasing drug resistance.

In recognition of the school's importance as a world centre for malaria research and training, Bill and Melinda Gates recently donated $40 million to fund its work on new chemotherapy treatments, insecticides and vaccines, and to strengthen its existing links with scientists and health ministries in malaria-endemic regions. One possibility is to use the latest satellite mapping technology to pick out areas of unusually high rainfall in Africa as a way of predicting sudden outbreaks of the disease. Another is a project with Imperial College to produce the world's first genetically modified mosquito (the idea is to engineer a mosquito that is resistant to malaria that could invade wild mosquito populations). But, interestingly, the solution that offers one of the best chances of reducing morbidity and mortality in Africa is also one of the least complex: the mosquito net.

Long before the discovery that mosquitoes were the vectors of malaria, the mosquito net was an essential part of the explorer's kit. Livingstone, for instance, slept under a 'mosquito curtain' through-out his travels in Africa and was so thankful for the rest it brought him that he later remarked that its inventor 'deserve[d] a statue in Westminster Abbey'. In the summer of 1900, two researchers from the LSHTM proved that a mosquito screen provided perfect protec-tion from malaria when they spent four months shut up in a wooden hut on the Roman Campagna.[1] The result is that today the WHO is just as wedded to the invention as Livingstone, seeing the provision of bed nets as a key component of Roll Back Malaria – a programme that aims to cut mortality from malaria in Africa in half by 2010.

One of the campaign's leading supporters is Chris Curtis, LSHTM's Professor of Entomology. A short, dark-haired man with a permanently bemused expression, Curtis can usually be found showing graduate students around the school's vaults under Gower Street. There Curtis breeds some of the deadliest mosquitoes in the world: *Anopheles gambiae* from Africa, *A. stephensi* from Asia, and *A. albimanus* – the species that decimated French canal workers in Panama. The only clue that you are about to enter an insectary is a mock yellow triangle on the door which reads, 'WARNING – MOZZIES 5KM'. That and the humid 26-degree centigrade atmosphere.

According to Curtis, the office workers tramping to work along Gower Street have absolutely nothing to fear from the killers lurking beneath their feet. 'None of the mosquitoes carry malaria,' he says. Instead Curtis, who is a leading authority on mosquito resistance to insecticides, is breeding the anophelines to find more efficient ways of killing them. One of the best methods of all, he believes, are bednets dipped in pyrethroids – a naturally occurring insecticide derived from the pyrethrum plant that, like cinchona, is found at higher altitudes in Ecuador, Kenya and Tanzania.

Studies show that bed nets treated with pyrethroids can reduce infant mortality from malaria by as much as half in malaria endemic areas. If every child in Africa were provided with his or her own bednet, Curtis calculates, half a million lives would be saved each year.

There is just one problem. A bednet treated with a synthetic pyrethroid like permethrin costs $4 (£2.50) a child. Even if you halve that through subsidies, it is still more than most Africans living in poor, rural areas of Tanzania, Kenya, Nigeria and the Congo can afford. Then there is the question of how to provide the chemicals to re-treat the bednets once the permethrin wears off.

The answer, according to Curtis, is to follow the example of governments like Vietnam who provide both the nets and the re-treatments free of charge. But although studies show that the more people who have nets the greater the protection from malaria for the community as a whole, few African nations can afford such largesse. The result is a compromise. Under the Roll Back Malaria programme, governments are being urged to create more private–public partner-ships to reduce the cost of nets while increasing subsidies to the poor. The WHO's aim is that every African child should have his or her own bednet within ten years. But Curtis worries that because bed nets are seen as a form of 'personal protection' African governments will try to shuffle off responsibility to the very people who are most in need of help – subsistence farmers. 'It's a vicious circle,' says Curtis. 'I hope the WHO's programme succeeds but my suspicion is that it will take a lot more donor money.'

There is no starker illustration of the imbalance between rich and poor than the wealth of anti-mosquito merchandise on display at camping stores in Europe and North America. At Black's in London, for instance, the shelves groan with mosquito nets, sprays, coils and ever more sophisticated electronic devices for diverting anophelines from the 'unsalted' blood of affluent Western tourists. That such protections are available for less than the cost of the air tax from Heathrow to Nairobi only makes it the more baffling that every year some two thousand people return to Britain infected with the parasites that spread malaria.

The point is that with the exception of parts of Thailand, Cambodia, Brazil and other regions where drug resistance is growing, malaria is by and large an avoidable disease. All it takes is a few simple precautions. Before setting off for Venezuela to retrace Spruce's route along the Orinoco and Casiquiare in January 2000, for instance, I asked my GP for a course of mefloquine – a prophylactic that is still highly effective against most South American strains of the disease. I also amassed an impressive collection of sprays and creams and invested in a jungle-green permethrin-soaked net. The net, unfortunately, turned out to be quite useless – a Venezuelan entomologist laughed when she saw it, saying it was the sort of thing she used to 'trap mosquitoes'. But the mefloquine protected me until I found a replacement, and swamped in Deet and my shop-bought repellents I found the mosquitoes were more of a nuisance than anything else.

If I wanted proof of the consequences of ignoring such simple precautions, however, I did not have to look very far. At Tamatama, a Protestant mission post near Esmeralda – the village where Spruce was driven to distraction by 'plagues' of mosquitoes in 1853 – I discovered that scores of people had been hospitalized with falciparum malaria in the first week of January alone. As the missionaries admitted, they had no one to blame but themselves. Although malaria is widespread in the region – particularly among the Yanomami and other Indian communities living on the river – there had never been an outbreak at Tamatama before. In consequence no one bothered with prophylactics. 'Our sleeping quarters are screened in and the grounds are sprayed regularly so we assumed it wasn't necessary,' explained the mission nurse, Brenda Barkman.

However, just behind the compound lies a lagoon – the ideal breeding ground for anophelines. When in the second week of December missionaries began arriving at Tamatama from all over the Orinoco to celebrate the last Christmas of the twentieth century it was in the lagoon that many of their Indian charges chose to camp. Although no one can be sure, it was probably here that the malaria became established and began to spread to the rest of the post.

The decisive moment came on Christmas Eve when the Indians, the missionaries and their children – some hundred people in all – gathered for dinner in the refectory. Unlike the barracks, there were no screens on the refectory. As it was a special occasion the festivities lasted well into the night.

The first case of falciparum malaria occurred five days later. By the end of the first week of the New Year some seventy people had the disease. Barkman prescribed chloroquine and primaquine, then mefloquine. But nothing worked.

It was only when she administered repeated courses of quinine that she at last saw the parasite loads begin to fall. It took five weeks for all her patients to recover. Afterwards, Barkman ordered the refectory to be screened in and banned night-time volleyball – up until then a fixture of the missionaries' California-sur-jungle lifestyle. As far as I know, the curfew is still in force.

The missionaries were not the only casualties I encountered during the journey upriver. Two days after our stop at Tamatama, my Venezuelan guide, Hugo, also began to complain of headaches and fever. By the time we reached San Carlos on the Río Negro he was sweating profusely. This time the diagnosis was vivax malaria.

Although Hugo had slept under a mosquito net, like the missionaries he had also failed to take a prophylactic.

Hugo's malaria eventually responded to chloroquine and proguanil. But it is only a matter of time before strains that are resistant to chloroquine, mefloquine and quinine invade the Orinoco too. The question is, what drugs will we look to then and who will provide them? One answer is the WRAIR in Washington, another is the WHO's Medicines for Malaria Venture. But as laudable as these organizations and initiatives are, ultimately they will count for little unless they also win the backing of pharmaceutical companies.

It is not all doom and gloom, however. The free market has been harnessed in the cause of philanthropy before, and for concrete proof you need wander only a few blocks north of the LSHTM to the junction of Gower Street and Euston Road. There, overlooking the traffic-clogged artery opposite Euston Station, are the offices of the Wellcome Trust – the largest medical research charity in the world. Each year the Trust donates nearly £550 million to medical research, of which about 4 per cent is spent on malaria. That the source of this money is the Wellcome Foundation – a business organization built on the profits of the pharmaceutical company Wellcome plc (now known as GlaxoSmithKline) – is a tribute to the acumen and vision of one man.

Henry Solomon Wellcome was born in Garden City, Minnesota, in 1853. The son of a Methodist preacher, he is best remembered today for coining the term 'tabloid' to describe the marketing, with his partner Silas Burroughs, of the world's first compressed medicines in 1880. The pills – which included such essentials as 'tabloid' quinine sulphate – were an instant hit and it was not long before everyone, from kings to presidents to explorers, was extolling their virtues. Tabloid quinine found its way into King Edward VII's automobile, the saddlebags of Theodore Roosevelt and the supply pack of the African explorer Henry Morton Stanley. The result was that London-

based Burroughs-Wellcome became one of the most profitable pharmaceutical concerns of all time.

But Wellcome was not merely a brilliant businessman and
publicist, he was also — like Sir Clements Markham — a humanitarian
with a strong philanthropic streak. During a trip down the Nile in
1901 he had seen at first hand how malaria, smallpox and famine had
blighted the lives of the Sudanese following Kitchener's brutal
suppression of the 1898 uprisings. As Wellcome later told a Con-
gressional committee, that experience convinced him that 'in times
of distress, the whole world is akin'. Two years later he founded
the Wellcome Tropical Research Laboratories in Khartoum and
instructed Andrew Balfour to supervise the draining and clearance of
the *Anopheles* breeding grounds. The result was that within a few
years mortality from malaria in and around Khartoum had been cut
by 90 per cent.

But for the roots of Wellcome's fascination with malaria we have
to go back much further, to his experiences as a travelling salesman in
South America. It was this that gave birth to his lifelong empathy for
the sufferings of indigenous peoples and the catalyst, as for so many
travellers before and since, was the legend of the Condesa de
Chinchón.

After graduating from the Philadelphia College of Pharmacy in
1874, Wellcome went to work for a small company in New York.
Then, in 1876, he was offered a trial with McKesson & Robbins, at
the time one of America's largest pharmaceutical firms. His job was
to promote the company's new gelatin-coated pills to doctors and
druggists. The pay was just $16 a week, but as well as taking him all
over North America the job offered him the opportunity to travel to
South America and investigate local Indian remedies.

Concerned about the growing shortage of cinchona bark, in 1877
Wellcome's superiors decided he should visit Ecuador and report on
the condition of the bark forests. Thus it was that in June Wellcome
and a companion landed at Guayaquil and caught a steam launch
up a branch of the Guayaquil River to Pueblo Nueva. Wellcome
had long been fascinated with the story of quinine's origins and was

anxious to question the Lojans about the legend of the Condesa's cure. But first he had to climb through the cloudforests and cross over the freezing sierra.

In effect Wellcome retraced Spruce's route in reverse, trekking around the summit of Chimborazo from west to east. It was there, just below the narrow-gauge railway that cuts across the sierra in the shadow of the volcano, that he saw his first cinchona tree. As he subsequently recalled in an article on his travels, he was picking his way down a slippery mud slope when, 'suddenly our guide shouted "cascarilla" and we were gladdened by the sight of several fair-sized trees of *cinchona succirubra.*'

Like Humboldt and Spruce, Wellcome was mesmerized by the bright green and red foliage and the way the leaves seemed to 'glisten' in the harsh Andean light. Unfortunately, when he reached Loja he found that hillsides had been stripped of mature trees and that the 'outlook for bark supplies was exceedingly discouraging'. Nevertheless, he used his time profitably, questioning the local inhabitants about the origins of the cure.

Wellcome was suspicious about the absence in the Spanish chronicles of any reference to the Indians' medicinal use of cinchona bark and pointed out that 'it was the policy of the conquistadors to appropriate to themselves all creditable things.' Speculating that the use of cinchona was probably confined to local tribes living near the bark forests, he concluded: 'It is a general belief among the natives that cinchona bark was well known and highly regarded as a remedy by their ancestors long before the Spaniards, under the daring Pizarro, invaded their coast.'

Interestingly, however, Wellcome's most lasting memory of Ecuador was not of the cinchona tree but of the fevers and sufferings of the Indians. 'The malaria,' he wrote, '. . . is simply fearful, and owing to the great exposure and want of nutritious food the Indians yield very quickly to its influence.' As if that were not bad enough, the gorges were strewn with the skeletons of Indians who, overloaded with cinchona bark, had lost their footing struggling to carry the valuable febrifuge out of the forests. 'It is only by extreme poverty,' he noted, 'or obligation as peons, that they are induced to enter the bark forests to encounter the dangers for the meagre pittance of ten to twenty-five cents per day.'

Later on, in his travels in Africa, Wellcome also experienced the scourge of other insect-transmitted diseases – notably leishmaniasis, sleeping sickness and yellow fever. But malaria always remained a central concern. He twice succumbed to the disease and following a visit to Panama in 1910 on behalf of the US War Department he became a passionate supporter of Gorgas's sanitation campaign against mosquitoes.

It is little wonder then that on his death in 1936 Wellcome stipulated that his shares in Burroughs-Wellcome be used to fund medical research aimed at 'the discovery, invention and improvement of medicinal agents ... and the control or extermination of insects and other pests which afflict human beings and animal and plant life in tropical and other regions.'

Today that bequest is worth approximately £15 billion.

For all his interest in medical research and medical history, however, Wellcome died convinced that Sebastiano Bado's story of the Condesa's cure was true. It was only after his death that, ironically, a researcher at the Wellcome medical museum unearthed the Conde's diary and other documents in Seville, showing that the Condesa de Chinchón was almost certainly never treated for malaria in South America.

Fortunately, however, her legacy lives on – not just in the quinine still used to treat severe cases of falciparum malaria, but in medical research into new anti-malarials funded in part by Henry Wellcome's slick marketing of her cure.

# End Note

In 1866 Sir Clements Markham also decided to investigate Bado's story. Boarding an omnibus in Madrid, he travelled to Chinchón and questioned local villagers about the legend's provenance. To his gratification, he found that the story of how the Condesa had distributed the bark on her husband's estates had passed into local folklore.

Markham later called for the Linnean botanical nomenclature to be overturned and for the correct spelling – 'chinchona' – to be reinstated in its place. But it never was. Instead, at the 1886 International Botanical Congress in London delegates voted to retain Linnaeus' spelling on the grounds of 'priority'.

Interestingly, Peru never blamed Markham for the theft of the cinchona tree. Instead in 1921 the embassy presented the Royal Geographical Society with a bust of Markham in thanks for the support he had given Peru during its war with Chile. In his speech, Peru's chargé d'affaires praised Markham's role in the cinchona missions, saying they had rendered 'a great service to humanity'.

In 1971 botanists from all over the world gathered at Coneysthorpe, in the shadow of Castle Howard, to unveil a plaque in honour of Spruce at the cottage where he spent the last seventeen years of his life. The inscription reads: 'Richard Spruce of Ganthorpe, Welburn and Coneysthorpe: Distinguished botanist, fearless explorer, humble man.'

In 1986, ACF Chemiefarma, a Dutch company that was then the leading manufacturer of quinine in the world, erected a new tombstone to Charles Ledger at Rookwood Methodist Cemetery in Sydney. It reads: 'Here rests Charles Ledger. He gave quinine to the world.'

As yet, there is no monument to Manuel Incra Mamani.

*Timeline*

| *Related Event* | SPRUCE |
| --- | --- |
| | *August 1817*<br>Born Ganthorpe |
| *1820*<br>Pelletier and Caventou isolate<br>quinine from cinchona bark | |
| *1829*<br>Discovery of Wardian case —<br>problem of plant transportation<br>solved | |
| | *1849*<br>Leaves for Brazil on the *Britannia*<br>accompanied by Henry Wallace |

| LEDGER/MAMANI | MARKHAM |
|---|---|
| | |
| *March 1818*<br>Born Bermondsey | |
| | |
| | *July 1830*<br>Born Stillingfleet |
| *1836*<br>Leaves Southampton for Peru on<br>the *Swallow* | |
| | *August 1851*<br>Leaves for Peru, via Halifax,<br>Boston and New York |

| Related Event | SPRUCE |
|---|---|

*April 1853*
Dutch-botanist Justus Charles
Hasskarl arrives on the Peruvian-
Bolivian border disguised as a
German businessman

*May 1853*
Livingstone takes quinine to cure
himself of malaria at Luanda

*Christmas Day 1853*
Arrives at Esmeralda on the
Orinoco

| LEDGER/MAMANI | MARKHAM |
|---|---|

*November 1851*
While exploring a possible route
for the export of alpaca, stumble on
fifty huge trees of *calisaya roja* — the
'red bark' of Bolivia

|  | *May 1852*
Sees first cinchona tree while
following an old Inca trail in
a valley east of Cusco |

*December 1852*
Leaves for Australia to explore
possibility of exporting alpaca to
New South Wales

*July 1853*
Returns to South America.
Reunited with flock

| *Related Event* | SPRUCE |
|---|---|
| *May 1854*<br>In an article in a Venezuelan journal, Dr Louis Daniel Beauperthuy suggests mosquitoes may be the cause of malaria | *May 1854*<br>Leaves San Carlos for San Fernando de Atabapo |
| *June 1854*<br>Dr William Balfour Baikie employs quinine prophylaxis to navigate Niger River, resulting in zero fatalities | |
| | *July 1854*<br>Suffers malaria fever attack at Maipures |

LEDGER/MAMANI                    MARKHAM

*November 1855*
Reunited with alpaca in Bolivia
and begins driving herd south to
Salta in Argentina

*May 1857*
Herd arrives at Laguna Blanca
in Chilean Andes

*May 1858*
After treacherous journey over
cordillera, herd reaches coast
of Chile

*November 1858*
Leaves for Australia with Alpaca

| *Related Event* | SPRUCE |
|---|---|
| | *April 1859*<br>Commissioned by India Office to collect *cascarilla roja* from Ecuador |
| | |
| | *April 1860*<br>'The Break Down': suffers sudden mysterious paralysis at Ambato |
| | *June 1860*<br>Crosses Chimborazo by mule; then descends western cordillera on foot |
| | *July-August 1860*<br>Collects seeds and plants of *Cinchona succirubra* at Limon |
| | *October 1860*<br>Despatches collection to Kew Gardens |

| LEDGER/MAMANI | MARKHAM |
| --- | --- |
| | *April 1859*<br>Commissioned by India Office to lead cinchona missions |
| | *January 1860*<br>Arrives at Lima |
| | *March 1860*<br>Reaches Arequipa |
| | *April 1860*<br>Reaches Sandia |
| | *May 1860*<br>Collects calisayas on banks of Tambopata River |
| | *June 1860*<br>Loads plants onto steamer at Islay and dispatches them to Britain via Panama |
| | *July–August 1860*<br>John Weir arrives at Southampton with 270 calisayas. Immediately despatches them to India via Egypt |

*Related Event*                            SPRUCE

*April 1861*
Spruce's collection reaches Indian
plantations – 463 healthy plants

*May 1864*
Returns to Britain

*1872*
*Cinchona succirubra* establishes itself
as favoured species in India

*1877*
Granted £100 annual pension from
India Office

| LEDGER/MAMANI | MARKHAM |
|---|---|
| | *December 1860*<br>On arrival at government plantations in Mysore all Markham's calisayas are dead |
| | |
| | |
| *May 1865*<br>Mamani delivers 40lb of cinchona seeds to Ledger in Tacna | |
| *July 1865*<br>British reject Mamani's seeds. Instead, George Ledger sells 1lb bag to Dutch for just £20 | |
| | |
| *1877*<br>Mamani dies in Coroico after being beaten by chief of police. Bark from his trees fetch twice their reserve price at auction in Amsterdam | |

| *Related Event* | SPRUCE |
|---|---|
| **1880**<br>Alphonse Laveran discovers malaria parasite in blood of a French soldier in Algiers | |
| **1886**<br>International Botanical Congress in London rejects Markham's plea for 'Chinchona' to be instated as botanical nomenclature for tree | |
| **1890**<br>Price of quinine begins to fall | |
| | *December 1893*<br>Dies at home in Coneysthorpe |
| **20 August 1897**<br>'Mosquito Day' – the British army surgeon Ronald Ross connects malaria parasite to the mosquito | |
| **1902**<br>Ross wins Nobel Prize | |

| LEDGER/MAMANI | MARKHAM |
|---|---|

---

*1880*
Half a million trees of *Calisaya*
*ledgeriana* thriving in Java

---

*1881*
Calisayas renamed *Cinchona*
*ledgeriana*

---

---

---

*May 1897*
Awarded £100 annual pension by
Dutch

---

---

---

*Related Event*                      SPRUCE

---

*1913*
European quinine manufacturers
and Dutch planters reach accord to
regulate supply of quinine

---

*August–Septemebr 1916*
Allied troops decimated by malaria
at Solonika

---

*1918*
Kina Bureau agrees Second
Quinine Convention

---

*1920*
Quinine prices reach record levels

---

| LEDGER/MAMANI | MARKHAM |
|---|---|

*May 1905*
Dies a pauper in Sydney

 

                             *January 1916*
                             Dies in a fire while reading by
                             candlelight at home in London

# Notes

One THE FEVER

1. The consequences are also potentially far graver as the sand flies transmit leishmaniasis, a parasitic skin disease.

2. Or as one British sailing directory put it as late as 1883, 'poisonous exhalations from the land'. The canard was only finally laid to rest in 1897 when the British army surgeon Sir Ronald Ross succeeded in showing that malaria was caused by a parasite harboured in the mosquito's salivary gland and injected into its human host each time the insect took a blood meal.

3. Neither Spruce nor Wallace record any further details of the encounters. In the edited account of his fever in his *A Narrative of Travels on the Amazon and Rio Negro* (London; New York: Ward, Lock, 1890) Wallace does not say whether he had the quinine with him, writing simply: 'The ague, however, now left me, and in another week, as I could walk with a stick down to the river-side, I went to Sao Gabriel, to see Mr Spruce, who had arrived there, *and kindly been to see me a short time before* [my italics].' However, the passage leaves open the possibility that Spruce was the provider.

4. The exact date of Wallace's revelation is not known. It is thought that the theory came to him in the Spice Islands in either February or March 1858, but the precise date is lost because Wallace's diary is vague (possibly because he was confused by fever). As soon as he had recovered, however, he sent a 4,000-word synopsis to Darwin, who received the letter on 18 June 1858. Wallace's ideas were so similar to his own as yet unpublished *On the Origin of Species* that two weeks later Darwin hastily submitted their ideas in a joint paper to the Linnean Society in London.

5. Humboldt was also the first to note the way in which the different species

of biting flies on the Orinoco stagger their attacks. 'What appeared to us very remarkable, and is a fact well known to the missionaries, is that at different hours of the day you are stung by different species. Every time the scene changes and ... other insects "mount guard," you have a few minutes, often a quarter of an hour, of repose. The insects that disappear have not their places instantly supplied by their successors.' (Humboldt and Bonpland, p. 276.)

6. It is a pity the mosquitoes undermined Spruce's determination to climb the Cerro Duida. When the mountain was finally explored by two Americans in 1928 it yielded no fewer than 700 different plants, of which over 200 were new to science.

7. The road itself is a bleak reminder of the fevers that plague this region. Built in 1924 by the Venezuelan dictator Juan Vicente Gómez, hundreds of workers died from malaria during its construction and it is said their souls still haunt the carriageway.

8. To escape the mosquitoes and press his botanical specimens in peace, Humboldt's travelling companion, Aimé Bonpland, was forced to crawl into a *hornito*, a smoke-filled oven without doors or windows. Humboldt writes that 'the absence of the mosquitoes is purchased dearly enough by the excessive heat of the stagnated air, and the smoke of the torch of copal, which lights the oven during your stay in it.' (Humboldt and Bonpland, p. 281.) In fact, Bonpland probably already had malaria. Humboldt writes that he had been feeling lethargic ever since coming down to Maypures from San Fernando and by the time they reached Angostura (Ciudad Bolívar) a few weeks later he was seriously ill. After taking quinine and Angostura bitters, however, he recovered.

9. Before the identification of malaria with specific plasmodia, the disease was defined by the interval between attacks: thus *vivax* was known as 'benign tertian' because of the relative mildness of the paroxysms and the fact that the fever occurred every second day with the remission coming on the third day; *malariae* was known as 'quartan' because the attacks occurred every fourth day; while *falciparum* was known as 'malignant tertian' or 'pernicious fever' because of the severity of the attacks, lasting anywhere from twenty-four to thirty-six hours with only about twelve hours of intermission.

10. The hammock can still be seen in a display case at Castle Howard.

*Two* THE CURE

1. Linnaeus named the genus *Cinchona* in his *Genera Plantarum* of 1742. One theory is that in so doing he relied on Sebastiano Bado, the Italian physician who first popularized the legend of the Condesa's cure in his 1663 book and who used the spelling 'cinchon', the Spanish 'ch' sound being 'ci' in Italian. However, although 'cinchona' is now the accepted botanical nomenclature, confusion still reigns over the correct pronunciation with English-speaking botanists saying 'sin-kona' or 'sin-chona' and Spanish speakers saying 'cheen-chona'.

2. The best barks were reserved for the exclusive use of the royal pharmacy at Madrid, hence the appellation 'Crown' barks, while other less valuable barks were sold at auction for export overseas. Crown barks originally sold at Panama for five and six dollars, and at Seville for twelve dollars the pound, but they were later adulterated with less valuable barks and the price fell to one dollar the pound.

3. Writing in 1663 Gaspar Caldera de Heredia, a Portuguese trader based in Seville, claimed that cinchona was first used by Indian miners in Ecuador for the relief of cold. In order to reach the rock face the miners had to wade through freezing water and alleviated their '*rigor et frigor*' by taking pulverized cinchona bark. Observing this, the Jesuits requested samples of the bark and applying logic decided to test whether it was also beneficial in the cold and shivering of intermittent fevers.

4. In another, even more fanciful version of the legend, which first achieved popularity in 1817 as a play entitled *Zuma ou la Découverte du Quinquina* by Mme de Genlis, a governess in the Duke of Orleans' household, it is the Condesa's beautiful Indian servant girl, Zuma, who imparts the secret to her mistress. The most salient feature of this version is Zuma's reluctance at first to share the bark's miraculous healing powers with the hated conquistadors. Indeed she has been sworn not to, the Indians taking great pleasure in watching their Spanish oppressors die from fevers to which they alone have the cure. It is only when Zuma is consumed by the same fever and her husband smuggles some of the precious bark into the palace at Lima to treat her that she takes pity on the Condesa and cures her too. Ironically, in Mme de Genlis's play the court physicians suspect Zuma of poisoning her mistress and condemn her to be burnt at the stake. Luckily, the Condesa recovers in

the nick of time, pardons Zuma and the Caciques come forward to reveal the virtues of the bark to the Spaniards.

5. In yet another version of the legend it was not the Corregidor of Loja but the Viceroy's physician, Dr Juan de Vega, who suggested the Condesa take the cure and who, on her recovery and return to Spain in 1640, brought a quantity of the bark with him, selling it at Seville, a then very malarious area of Spain, for an English sovereign an ounce (about £75 an ounce in today's money). In fact, as scholars have since shown, de Vega never left Peru but continued to practise medicine in Lima until at least 1650.

6. The problem with this argument is that if the cure was known to the Incas why don't we find similar reverence for cinchona as for the coca leaf? The earliest finds suggest that coca was used on the coast of Peru by 2000 BC. Remains of coca leaves have been found at Indian sites dating back to AD 600, and lime pots and ceramic figurines depicting people chewing leaves have been found at virtually every major site from every era of pre-Colombian civilization. We also know that for the Inca the coca leaf was a living manifestation of the divine. Coca fuelled the construction of the Incas' monumental stone cities, kept its armies on the march and enabled the imperial runners, the *chasquis*, to relay messages six and a half thousand kilometres in a week. Perhaps the lack of reverence for the bitter-tasting cinchona bark simply reflects the fact that the Inca were a highland people and that prior to the Spanish conquest malaria was not a problem.

7. See John Thurloe, *A Collection of State Papers of John Thurloe, Esq.*, ed. Th. Birch, 7 vols (London: Woodward and Davis, 1742, 4:18).

8. For a detailed account of Cromwell's symptoms and an analysis of his post-mortem see L. J. Bruce-Chwatt, 'Oliver Cromwell's Medical History', *Transactions and Studies of the Royal College of Physicians of Philadelphia*, 5. ser, v. 4, 1982.

9. The key foreign ingredient of course was quinine bark but what was the other? One intriguing possibility is that Talbor added the leaves of sweet wormwood, *Artemisia annua*, a powerful antimalarial recently 'rediscovered' in China where it is known as *quinghaosu*. For a fascinating discussion of Talbor's remedy for malaria, see Mary Dobson, 'Bitter-sweet solutions for malaria: exploring natural remedies from the past', *Parassitologia* 40: 69–81, 1998. According to Dobson, Talbor may have used wormwood to offset the bitterness of the cinchona.

10. Unfortunately Sydenham rather spoils the effect of this endorsement in the next sentence when, in what is clearly a swipe at Talbor, he continues: 'which the physicians of London not being pleased to take notice of in my book, or not believing me, have given an opportunity to a fellow that was but an apothecary's man, to go away with all the practice on Agues, by which he has gotten an estate in two months, and brought great reproach on the faculty.'

11. It is also said that Torti was the first to refer to intermittent fevers as *mal'aria*, from the Italian for 'bad air'. But the term never appears in his writings and appears to have already been in use in Italy more a century before his birth. (See Saul Jarcho: Quinine's Predecessors.)

## *Three* The Curse

1. His nickname 'Old Grog' came from his habit of wearing a grosgrain cape in foul weather. But it was as a result of his introduction of rum diluted with four parts water that the term 'grog' passed into the English language as a cognate for rum. In an effort to curb drunkenness at sea, Vernon replaced the standard issue of neat rum with the diluted mixture, and made the issue take place twice a day rather than once. He thus hoped to avoid the accidents that occurred when men drank half a pint of neat rum in one go.

2. To ensure that the men would not take advantage of the directive and get drunk, the Admiralty stipulated that the medicated chests be kept under lock and key below deck, as was the practice with other spirits, and brought up only when a ship entered malarious waters or sailors went ashore.

3. Indeed, it was the first time Linnaeus had seen the flowers of the cinchona tree and he wrote immediately to Mutis to thank him. 'I received in due time, eight days ago, your letter dated 24th day of September of 1764, and was greatly moved and overjoyed by it, as it contained a beautiful drawing of the quina bark, together with leaves and flowers, which flowers, never seen by me until now, really have given me an idea of a very rare genus, and very different from that which I acquired through the figure of Monsieur Condamine. I am very grateful for everything.' (Jaramillo-Arango, *Basic Facts in the History of Cinchona*, p. 302.)

4. In fact, as subsequent analysis has confirmed, red bark contains four alkaloids in near equal amounts: quinine, quinidine, cinchonine and cinchon-

idine, while yellow bark contains much quinine and a little cinchonine. Grey bark contains cinchonine and tannin.

5. These are the presence of curly hairs bordering the laciniae of the corolla, the characteristic upwards dehiscence of the capsule and the little pits at the axils of the veins on the undersides of the leaves.

## Four THE VISION

1. See Weddell: *Historie Naturelle des Quinquinas.*

2. This appears to be the explanation for the mysterious death of Hasskarl's plants. In 1865 Ledger overheard Henriquez, the Indian who had assisted the Dutchman, boasting how he had mixed arsenic with the earth in the Wardian cases and in the pots that Hasskarl used for watering his cinchonas. 'Lucky for Hasskarl,' writes Ledger, 'that they did not poison him, as they could have done.'

## Five THE PHILANTHROPIST

1. Ruiz and Pavon named it *Cinchona uritusinga* after the mountain near Loja in which it was most abundant. In fact, it was identical to the variety sketched by La Condamine in the forests of nearby Cajunuma and named *C. officinalis* by Linnaeus. Markham later proposed that *uritusinga* should be known as *condaminea* to avoid confusion. However, his suggestion was not adopted.

2. 'It is a curious coincidence that at the very time when Dr Royle was writing this report I was actually exploring some of the chinchona forests of Peru,' Markham later recalled in his popular account of the cinchona missions, published in 1880. 'But the object of my travels was of an antiquarian and ethnological character, and I was in ignorance of the desire of the Indian government to procure supplies of those plants, which I then only admired for their beauty.' (*Peruvian Bark*, p. 88.)

3. Livingstone's experiments with quinine resulted in his formulation of the famous 'Livingstone' or 'Zambezi Rousers', consisting of eight grains (520 mg) each of resin of julap and calomel mixed with four grains each of quinine and

rhubarb. The pill's name was inspired by his remark that 'two ordinary sized pills would be a rousing dose for a woman.'

4. Despite being administered quinine 354 soldiers were admitted to Varna general hospital suffering intermittent fevers between June and August 1854 and more than 100 died. But considering that as many as 30,000 soldiers had been camped in the malarious Danube delta since January, the casualty figures were low, particularly when compared to deaths from other diseases like cholera and typhus.

5. Before setting sail from England in 1849 Spruce had seen a huge quantity of bark from these very forests lying unsold in a warehouse in Liverpool. The bark had been exported to England by a young Peruvian businessman, Don Luis Lopez, in the belief that it was identical to the *Cascarilla roja* of Huánuco and that he was about to make his fortune. But when the bark arrived at Liverpool after an epic journey down the Amazon and across the Atlantic, it turned out that it was a false quina, *Condaminea corymbosa*, with no febrifugal powers whatsoever. 'There had not been wanting people on the spot who warned Don Luis of his mistake; but he was too opinionated to listen to them, and persevered to his disastrous overthrow,' Spruce wrote to Bentham.

## *Six* THE QUEST

1. See *Peruvian Bark*, pp. 266–7.

2. Every time you purchase goods in Peru you are honouring this legacy, for the national coat of arms, complete with cinchona tree, appears on the reverse side of the Peruvian *sol* (silver dollar).

3. Don B. Vicuna Mackenna in a review of *Cuzco and Lima* published 4 February 1860 in the *Commercio de Lima*.

4. The doctors treated the stricture with enemas and opiates, but the years of misdiagnosis had taken their toll and for the remainder of his life Spruce was unable to sit up at a microscope without the risk of internal bleeding and could only write by reclining in a chair with his papers spread on his lap.

## *Seven* SPRUCE'S RIDGE

1. The boy's fever subsequently fell and he was taken to Guanujo. Spruce never learnt what became of him but writes that 'marsh fevers are generally cured, as if by magic, by simply removing the patient to the cool rarefied atmosphere of the Andes.' (*Report on the expedition to procure seeds and plants of the cinchona succirubra . . .*, p. 75.)

2. Markham later wrote: 'If I had received any proposal from him I should, without hesitation, have taken upon myself the responsibility of engaging Mr Ledger's services, and he would then certainly have received some, though probably inadequate, remuneration.' (*Peruvian Bark*, p. 214.)

3. Ledger later wrote that although he could ill afford to help Markham he 'could not resist the temptation of obtaining what was so much wanted'.

## *Eight* THE SHADOW IN THE FOREST

1. The Royal Pharmaceutical Society notation identifies it as a picture of Santiago but Gabrielle Gramiccia, who researched Ledger's life extensively, believed it to be a picture of Manuel. Either way the picture is a graphic illustration of the confusion surrounding Mamani's life and identity. See Gramiccia.

## *Nine* A TALE OF TWO SEEDS

1. Nine years later, in 1873, Nightingale presented an almost identical paper, entitled *Life or death in India*, to the National Association for the Promotion of Social Science in Norwich.

2. McIvor calculated that Money's pouch of *Cinchona ledgeriana* contained some 20,000 seeds. If he had followed the same procedures as Van Gorkum, in theory he could have raised four million plants. In the end, however, only 60,000 seedlings were planted and only a small proportion of these were forwarded to Sikkim.

3. One hundred years later the Pasteur Institute would broadly vindicate the

results. In in vitro studies in 1987 against *Plasmodium falciparum* using the most up to date techniques, the Institute found that, depending on the strain tested, quinidine and cinchonine were between five and ten times more active than quinine, and that a combination of all the alkaloids was between two to ten times more effective against strains that showed marked resistance to quinine.

4. 'A thin flexible surgical instrument made of waxed linen, india-rubber, metal, etc., for introduction into the passages of the body, for the purpose of exploration, dilatation, or medication.' (*OED*)

## *Ten* THE GREAT WHITE HOPE

1. Why Laveran observed exflagellation when everyone else had missed it is not clear. He was not the first to examine live blood from a malaria patient but he may have been the first to wait fifteen minutes before doing so. This is just long enough to permit the male gametocytes to transform themselves into gametes, a process that usually takes place inside the stomach wall of the mosquito.

2. The reason is that the mature gametocytes do not ingest haemoglobin and there is thus no toxic waste process for quinine to interfere with.

3. For these reasons quinine is considered a suppressive as opposed to a 'causal' prophylactic.

4. It was not a new idea. From the earliest days of the British Raj, British officers stationed in India had been dissolving quinine in carbonated water. And inspired by their example, Schweppes had begun manufacturing Indian tonic water in 1870. Other quinine-flavoured drinks soon followed, including bitter lemon, and in France Dubonnet. The practice eventually led to the invention of gin and tonic – one of the most popular drinks of all time, although of course the amount of quinine in the tonic water today is minimal.

5. A unit was the standard measure for pricing bark and was equivalent to five grams of quinine (1 per cent of quinine per one half kilo of bark). In 1920s prices, one Dutch cent was equivalent to 0.46 US cents.

## *Eleven* THE MALARIA FIGHTERS

1. The problem was that there was still far too much bark being produced. To reduce the supply and help maintain an economically viable price, in 1929 the Association of Bark Producers in Java began a campaign to persuade planters to retire from the business. Their plantations were then uprooted.

2. 125,000 lb and 1,500,000 lb. See Hehir, p. 291: 'It is clear that the world could not at present meet this, the Indian demand, and also that the demand will never be realised while present world prices continue.'

3. Notwithstanding this agreement, the Netherlands Indies government issued a series of ordinances six years later, further restricting bark exports.

4. Unfortunately while Atabrine was a success against falciparum malaria, it merely suppressed the vivax form of the disease. Hence, when troops were put on malaria-free islands to recover and Atabrine was stopped, they all relapsed.

5. Recently, however, DDT has been making a comeback. In December 2000 the United Nations approved limited use of DDT to control mosquitoes despite calls for a worldwide ban on the pesticide by Greenpeace and the World Wildlife Fund. The UN's decision followed intense lobbying by South Africa and the Malaria Foundation International who argue that spraying houses with DDT is still one of the most effective and affordable methods of malaria control.

6. From a military point of view a key advantage of chloroquine, and later the 'CP' tablet, was that it only had to be taken once a week, meaning that it could be administered as easily in combat as in garrison. One of the reasons for the 'failure' of quinine and Atabrine is that the pills had to be taken daily – a discipline that was hard to enforce in the field.

7. Novartis is marketing yet another artemisinin derivative, artemether, in combination with lumefantrine, while the WHO and the UK Department of International Development, in partnership with Glaxo SmithKline, are conducting trials in Africa with a chlorproguanil–dapson combination called Lapdap.

*Twelve* THE VACCINE HUNTERS

1. Biologists have found similar correlations between malaria and the incidence among Polynesian islanders and people of southern Mediterranean descent of thalassaemia, another inherited recessive blood trait that results in a failure to manufacture haemaglobin. However, while thalassaemia provides some protec- tion against malaria, biologists are divided over whether its prevalence is due to selection pressure exerted by malaria.

EPILOGUE

1. Dr G. Carmichael Low, Dr L. Sambon and the artist Signor A. Terzi erected the hut at Castel Fusano, near Ostia, a notoriously malarial area. They lived there from July to October 1900, venturing outside during the day but making sure they were always back inside the hut before sunset. Their only view of the night sky was through a small wire-screen gauze. They took no quinine and when at the end of four months they were found to be free of malaria the experiment was declared a success.

# Bibliography

## Note on Sources

The primary source for Spruce was his two-volume *Notes of a Botanist on the Amazon and the Andes*, edited by Alfred Russel Wallace (London: Macmillan, 1908). However, in some places Wallace omits important passages or else skirts over key details of Spruce's travels and in order to fill these in I also consulted his original journals and letters at Kew Gardens. Similarly, for Spruce's journey over Chimborazo I made extensive use of his *Report on the Expedition to Procure Seeds and Plants of the Cinchona Succirubra, or Red Bark Tree* to the Under-Secretary of State for India, 3 January 1862. For an overview of Spruce's life and contribution to botany I also referred to M. R. D. Seaward and S. M. D. Fitzgerald, eds, *Richard Spruce (1817–1893): Botanist and Explorer* (Royal Botanic Gardens, Kew, 1986).

For Ledger's life and travels I referred to Gabriele Gramiccia's *The Life of Charles Ledger 1818–1905: alpacas and quinine* (Basingstoke: Macmillan, 1988) and Ledger's voluminous correspondence with John Eliot Howard at the Royal Pharmaceutical Society of Great Britain. I also found Norman Taylor's *Cinchona in Java: the story of quinine* (New York: Greenberg, 1945) useful for the subsequent history of his *Cinchona ledgeriana* seeds.

Markham published two books on the cinchona missions, *Travels in Peru and India while superintending the collection of chinchona plants and seeds in South America and their introduction into India* (London: John Murray, 1862) and *Peruvian Bark: a popular account of the introduction of chinchona cultivation into British India 1860–1880* (London: John Murray, 1880). In addition, he arranged for all correspondence on the introduction of the cinchona plant into India to be entered in the parliamentary record. These records are contained in the 'Blue Books' published by Her Majesty's Stationery Office and covering the period 1852 to

1870. As in all Markham's works on cinchona the titles adopt his preferred 'ch' spelling. For the narrative of his expedition to Tambopata in Peru and an insight into his motives and fears I also consulted his *Private Journals* and *Chinchona Notebooks I and II* (1859–60) at the Royal Geographical Society, London. For an overview of Markham's 'other' career as a geographer and patron of polar exploration I referred to Albert H. Markham's *The Life of Sir Clements Markham* (London: John Murray, 1917).

Humboldt's description of the cinchona tree and his reflections on the origin of the cure are contained in his paper, *An account of the cinchona forests of South America drawn up during five years residence and travels on the South American continent*, translated by Alymer Bourke Lambert (London: Longman, 1821).

La Condamine's description of the cinchona tree, *Sur l'arbre du quinquina*, was published in the *Mémoires de l'Academie Royale des Sciences de Paris*, 1738, pp. 226–43 (Amsterdam: P. de Coup, ca 1745). For his subsequent voyage with the seeds to Brazil, see his paper, *Relation abrégée d'un voyage fait dans l'intérieur de l'Amérique Méridionale … en descendant la Rivière des Amazones*, read before the Academy on 28 April 1745 (Paris: Veuve Pissot, 1745).

I found de Jussieu's description of the cinchona tree in *Description de l'arbre à quinquina: mémoire inédit de Joseph de Jussieu* (Paris: Société du traitement des Quinquinas, 1936).

Many scholars have tried to unravel the provenance of the story of the Condesa's cure and the etymology of the word 'quinaquina'. These questions are unlikely ever to be finally resolved but I found the best forensic analyses were A. W. Haggis's *Fundamental errors in the early history of cinchona* (*Bull. Hist. Med.*, 1942, 10, pp. 586–92) and Jaime Jaramillo-Arango's *A critical review of the basic facts in the history of cinchona* (Academic Press for the Linnean Society of London, 1949, pp. 272–311). For a more recent analysis, see Fernando Ortiz Crespo's *Fragoso, Monardes and pre-Chinchonian knowledge of Cinchona* (*Archives of Natural History*, 1995, 22 (2), pp. 169–81). The information on the Kina Bureau and quinine pricing between the wars was taken from the United States Department of Commerce's Trade Information Bulletin, *Quinine Production and Marketing* (No. 273, October 1924).

FURTHER READING

*Botanical Exploration*

COATS, Alice M.: *The Quest for Plants: a history of botanical explorers* (London: Studio Vista, 1969)

CUTRIGHT, P. R.: *The Great Naturalists Explore South America* (New York: Macmillan, 1940)

DAVIS, Wade: *One River: explorations and discoveries in the Amazon Rain Forest* (New York: Simon & Schuster, 1996)

FURNEAUX, Robin: *The Amazon: the story of a great river* (London: Hamish Hamilton, 1964)

HAGEN, Victor Wolfgang von: *South America Called Them: explorations of the great naturalists* (London: the Scientific Book Club, 1949)

HUMBOLDT, Alexander von and Bonpland, Aimé: *Personal Narrative of Travels to the Equinoctial Regions of America, During the Years 1799–1804* (London: Henry G. Bohn, vols 1 and 2 1852, vol. 3 1853)

MUSGRAVE, T; Gardner, C.; Musgrave, W.: *The Plant Hunters: two hundred years of adventure and discovery around the world* (London: Orion, 1998)


*Cinchona and Quinine*

ACOSTA SOLIS, Misael: *La Cinchona, planta nacional del Ecuador* (Quito: Impr. del Ministerio del Tesoro, 1950)

ANDERSSON, Lennart: 'A Revision of the Genus Cinchona (Rubiaceae–Cinchoneae)', *Memoirs of the New York Botanical Garden*, Vol. 80, 30 Jan 1998

BADO, Sebastiano: *Anastasis Corticis Peruviae, Seu Chinae Chinae Defensio* (Genoa: P. J. Calenzani, 1663)

DE VRIJ, Dr J. E. (trans. Clements Markham): *On the cultivation of quinine in Java and British India* (London: Eyre and Spottiswoode, 1865)

DURAN-REYNALS, Marie Louise de Ayala: *The Fever Bark Tree: The Pageant of Quinine* (New York: Doubleday, 1946)

HOBHOUSE, Henry: *Seeds of Change: six plants that transformed mankind* (London: Macmillan, 1999)

HODGE, W. H.: 'Wartime Cinchona Procurement in Latin America', *Economic Botany*, Vol. 2, July–September 1948

HOWARD, John Eliot: *Illustrations of the Nueva quinologia of Pavon* (London: L. Reeve, 1862)

—— *The Quinology of the East Indian Plantations* (London: L. Reeve, 2 vols, 1869–76)

JARCHO, Saul: *Quinine's predecessor: Francesco Torti and the early history of cinchona* (Baltimore: John Hopkins University Press, c. 1993)

LAMBERT, Aylmer Bourke: *An illustration of the genus Cinchona: comprising descriptions of all the official Peruvian barks, including several new species* (London: J. Searle, 1821)

MARKHAM, Clements R: *A memoir of the Lady Ana de Osorio: countess of Chinchon and vice-queen of Peru, 1629–39, with a plea for the correct spelling of the chinchona genus* (London: Troubner, 1874)

MUTIS, José Celestino: *Expedición Botánica* (Colombia: El Ancora Editores, 1983)

RAINEY, Froelich: 'Quinine hunters in Ecuador', *National Geographic* magazine, March 1946

RUIZ, Hippolito (trans. Bruce Dahlgren): *Travels of Ruiz, Pavon and Dombey in Peru and Chile, 1777–1788* (Chicago: Field Museum of Natural History, 1940)

TAYLOR, Norman: *Quinine: the story of Cinchona* (New York: Cinchona Products Institute, 1943)

VAN GORKOM, Karel Wessel (trans. B. D. Jackson): *A Handbook of Cinchona Culture* (London: Trübner, 1883)

VARIOUS AUTHORS: *Three Centuries of Cinchona: proceedings of the celebration of the three hundredth anniversary of the first recognized use of cinchona held at the Missouri botanical garden, St Louis, October 31–November 1, 1930* (St Louis: Missouri Botanical Garden, 1931)

WEDDELL, Hugh Algernon: *Histoire Naturelle des Quinquinas* (Paris: V. Masson, 1849)

——: *Voyage dans le nord de Bolivie et dans les voisins de Perou* (Paris: P. Bertrand, 1853)

Malaria: Science, History and the Military

BARTLETT, Elisha: *The history, diagnosis, and treatment of the fevers of the United States* (Philadelphia: Lea and Blanchard, 1847)

BAYNE-JONES, Stanhope: *The evolution of preventive medicine in the United States*

*Army, 1607–1939* (Washington: Office of the Surgeon General, Dept. of the Army, 1968)

BLANCO, Richard L.: *Wellington's surgeon general: Sir James McGrigor* (Durham, N.C.: Duke University Press, 1974)

BOYCE, Sir Rupert W.: *Mosquito or Man? The conquest of the tropical world* (London: John Murray, 1909)

BRUCE-CHWATT, Leonard Jan: *Essential Malariology* (William Heinemann Medical Books, London, 1st ed. 1980; 2nd ed. 1985)

— and de Zulueta, Julian: *The Rise and Fall of Malaria in Europe: a historico-epidemiological study* (Oxford and New York: Oxford University Press, 1980)

CANTLIE, Neil: *A history of the Army Medical Department* (Edinburgh: Churchill Livingstone, 2 vols, 1974)

CELLI, Angelo (trans. John J. Eyre): *Malaria according to the new researches* (London: Longmans, Green and Co., 1900)

CUTHBERT, Christy: *Mosquitoes and Malaria: a summary of knowledge on the subject up to date* (London: Sampson Low, Marston & Co., 1900)

DESOWITZ, Robert S.: *The Malaria Capers: tales of parasites and people* (New York: Norton, 1991)

DOBSON, Mary: '"Marsh Fever" – the geography of malaria in England' (*Journal of Historical Geography*, 1980, pp. 357–89)

DRAKE, Daniel: *Malaria in the interior valley of North America* (Urbana: University of Illinois Press, 1964)

FALLS, Cyril & Becke, A. F.: *History of the Great War* (London: HMSO, Vol. 1 1933; Vol. 2 1935)

HARRISON, Gordon: *Mosquitoes, Malaria and Man: a history of the hostilities since 1880* (London: John Murray, 1978)

HARRISON, Mark: 'Medicine and the Culture of Command: the case of Malaria Control in the British Army during the two World Wars' (*Medical History*, 1996, 40, pp. 437–52)

HEHIR, Sir Patrick: *Malaria in India* (London: Oxford University Press, 1927)

JARAMILLO-ARANGO, Jaime: *The Conquest of Malaria* (London: Heinemann, 1950)

JOY, Robert J. T.: 'Malaria in American troops in the south and southwest Pacific in World War II', *Medical History*, 1999, 43, pp. 192–207.

LEMAITRE, Eduardo: *A Brief History of Cartagena* (Colombia: Editorial Colina, 1994)

LLOYD C. & COULTER, J. L. S.: *Medicine and the Navy*, Vol. 3: *1745–1815* (London: Livingston, 1961)

MACPHERSON, W. G. & Mitchell, T. J: *History of the Great War, Medical Services General History*, Vol. 4 (London: HMSO, 1924)

NYE, Edwin and Gibson, Mary: *Ronald Ross: malariologist and polymath* (London: Macmillan, 1997)

RUSSELL, Paul F.: *Man's Mastery of Malaria* (London and New York: Oxford University Press, 1955)

——: *Practical Malariology* (London: Oxford University Press, 2nd ed., 1963)

SHEPHERD, John: *The Crimean Doctors: A history of the British medical services in the Crimean War*, Vols 1 and 2 (Liverpool University Press, 1991)

SPURGEON, Neel: *Vietnam Studies, medical support of the U.S. Army in Vietnam 1965–70* (Washington: Department of the Army, 1973)

*Disease: Migration, Conquest and African Exploration*

ACKERKNECHT, Erwin H.: *History and Geography of the Most Important Diseases* (New York: Hufner Publishing Co., 1965)

BAIKIE, William Balfour: *Narrative of an Exploring Voyage up the Rivers Kwo'ra and Bi'nue (commonly known as the Niger and Tsa'dda) in 1854* (London: John Murray, 1856)

CAMERON, Ian: *The Impossible Dream: the building of the Panama Canal* (London: Hodder and Stoughton, 1971)

CARLSON, Dennis G.: *Africa Fever: a study of British science, technology and politics in West Africa, 1784–1864* (Canton, MA: Science History Publications USA, 1984)

CARTWRIGHT, Frederick F. & Biddiss, Michael: *Disease and History* (Guildford, Surrey: Sutton, 2000)

CHILDS, St Julien Ravenel: *Malaria and Colonization in the Carolina Low Country 1526–1696* (Baltimore: John Hopkins Press, 1940)

CURTIN, Philip D.: *Disease and Empire: the health of European troops in the Conquest of Africa* (Cambridge University Press, 1998)

DIAMOND, Jared: *Guns, Germs and Steel* (London: Vintage, 1998)

GELFAND, Michael: *Livingstone the Doctor, his life and travels* (Oxford: Basil Blackwell, 1957)

HEMMING, John: *The Conquest of the Incas* (London: Macmillan, 1970)

KLEIN, Herbert S.: *African slavery in Latin America and the Caribbean* (New York, London: Oxford University Press, 1986)

McCULLOGH, David: *The Path Between the Seas: the creation of the Panama Canal (1870–1914)* (New York: Simon and Schuster, 1977)

RANSFORD, Oliver: *David Livingstone: the dark interior* (London: John Murray, 1978)

# Index